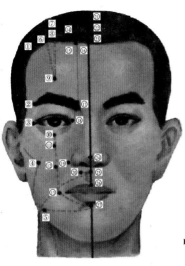

① Tóuwéi (S 8)　　　② Sīzhúkōng (TE 18)
③ Tóngzǐliáo (G 1)　④ Quánliáo (SI 18)
⑤ Dàyíng (S 5)　　　⑥ Běnshén (G 13)
⑦ Mùchuāng (G 16)　⑧ Tóulínqì (G 15)
⑨ Yángbái (G 14)　　⑩ Chéngqì (S 1)
⑪ Sìbái (S 2)　　　　⑫ Jùliáo (S 3)
⑬ Dìcāng (S 4)　　　⑭ Wǔchù (B 5)
⑮ Qūchā (B 4)　　　⑯ Méichōng (B 3)
⑰ Cuánzhú (B 2)　　⑱ Jīngmíng (B 1)
⑲ Yíngxiāng (LI 20)　⑳ Kǒuhéliáo (LI 19)
㉑ Xìnhuì (GV 22)　　㉒ Shàngxīng (GV 23)
㉓ Shéntíng (GV 24)　㉔ Sùliáo (GV 25)
㉕ Shuǐgōu (GV 26)　　㉖ Duìduān (GV 27)
㉗ Chéngjiāng (CV 24)

**Diagram of the Distribution of the Points of the
Fourteen Meridians (The Frontal View of the Head)**

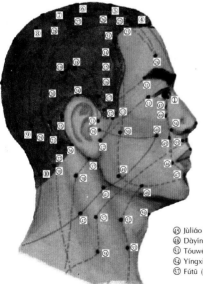

① Jīngmíng (B 1)　　② Cuánzhú (B 2)
③ Méichōng (B 3)　　④ Qūchā (B 4)
⑤ Wǔchù (B 5)　　　⑥ Chéngguāng (B 6)
⑦ Tōngtiān (B 7)　　⑧ Luòquè (B 8)
⑨ Yùzhěn (B 9)　　　⑩ Tiānzhù (B 10)
⑪ Tóngzǐliáo (G 1)　⑫ Tīnghuì (G 2)
⑬ Shàngguān (G 3)　⑭ Hànyàn (G 4)
⑮ Xuánlú (G 5)　　　⑯ Xuánlí (G 6)
⑰ Qūbìn (G 7)　　　⑱ Shuàigǔ (G 8)
⑲ Tiānchōng (G 9)　⑳ Fúbái (G 10)
㉑ Tóuqiàoyīn (G 11)　㉒ Wángǔ (G 12)
㉓ Běnshén (G 13)　　㉔ Yángbái (G 14)
㉕ Tóulínqì (G 15)　　㉖ Mùchuāng (G 16)
㉗ Zhèngyíng (G 17)　㉘ Chénglíng (G 18)
㉙ Nǎokōng (G 19)　　㉚ Fēngchí (G 20)
㉛ Sīzhúkōng (TE 23)　㉜ Ěrhéliáo (TE 22)
㉝ Ěrmén (TE 21)　　㉞ Jiǎosūn (TE 20)
㉟ Lúxī (TE 19)　　　㊱ Chìmài (TE 18)
㊲ Yìfēng (TE 17)　　㊳ Tiānyǒu (TE 16)
㊴ Tīnggōng (SI 19)　㊵ Quánliáo (SI 18)
㊶ Tiānróng (SI 17)　㊷ Tiānchuāng (SI 16)
㊸ Chéngqì (S 1)　　㊹ Sìbái (S 2)

㊺ Jùliáo (S 3)　　㊻ Dìcāng (S 4)　　㊼ Chéngjiāng (CV 24)
㊽ Dàyíng (S 5)　　㊾ Jiáchē (S 6)　　㊿ Xiàguān (S 7)
�51 Tóuwéi (S 8)　　�52 Rényíng (S 9)　　�53 Shuǐtū (S 10)
�54 Yíngxiāng (LI 20)�55 héliáo (LI 19)�56 Shuǐgōu (GV 26)
�57 Fútū (LI 18)　　�58 Tiāndǐng (LI 17)�59 Liánquán (CV 23)

**Diagram of the Distribution of the Points of the
Fourteen Meridians (The Lateral View of the Head)**

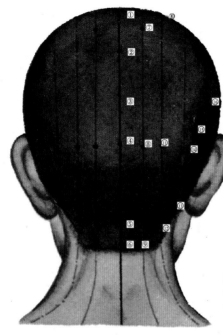

① Bǎihì (GV 20)

② Hòudǐng (GV 19)

③ Qiángjiān (GV 18)

④ Nǎohù (GV 17)

⑤ Fēngfǔ (GV 16)

⑥ Yǎmén (GV 15)

⑦ Luòquè (B 8)

⑧ Yùzhěn (B 9)

⑨ Tiānzhù (B 10)

⑩ Chénglíng (G 18)

⑪ Nǎokōng (G 19)

⑫ Fēngchí (G 20)

⑬ Wángǔ (G 12)

⑭ Tóuqiàoyīn (G 11)

⑮ Fúbái (G 10)

⑯ Tiānchōng (G 9)

Diagram of the Distribution of the Points of the Fourteen Meridians (The Posterior View of the Head)

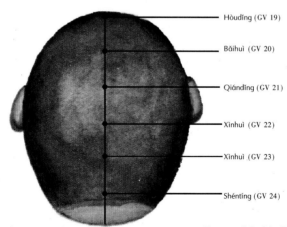

Hòudǐng (GV 19)

Bǎihuì (GV 20)

Qiándǐng (GV 21)

Xìnhuì (GV 22)

Xìnhuì (GV 23)

Shéntíng (GV 24)

Diagram of the Distribution of the Points of the Fourteen Meridians (The Parietal Region)

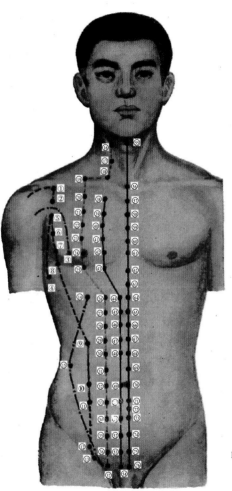

① Yúnmén (L 2)
③ Tiānchí (P 1)
⑤ Zhōuróng (Sp 20)
⑦ Tiānxī (Sp 18)
⑨ Fù'āi (Sp 16)
⑪ Fùjié (Sp 14)
⑬ Chōngmén (Sp 12)
⑮ Zhāngmén (Liv 13)
⑰ Shuǐtū (S 10)
⑲ Quēpén (S 12)
㉑ Kùfáng (S 14)
㉓ Yīngchuāng (S 16)
㉕ Rǔgēn (S 18)
㉗ Chéngmǎn (S 20)
㉙ Guānmén (S 22)
㉛ Huáròumén (S 24)
㉝ Wàilíng (S 26)
㉟ Shuǐdào (S 28)
㊲ Qìchōng (S 30)
㊴ Yùzhōng (K 26)
㊶ Língxū (K 24)
㊸ Bùláng (K 22)
㊺ Fùtōnggǔ (K 20)
㊼ Shígān (K 18)
㊾ Huāngshū (K 16)
㊿ Sīmǎn (K 14)
㊾ Dàhè (K 12)
⑤ Liánquán (CV 23)
⑤ Xuánjī (CV 21)
⑤ Zǐgōng (CV 19)
⑥ Tánzhōng (CV 17)
⑥ Jiūwěi (CV 15)
⑥ Shàngwǎn (CV 13)
⑥ Jiànlǐ (CV 11)
⑥ Shuǐfēn (CV 9)
⑦ Yīnjiāo (CV 7)
⑦ Shímén (CV 5)
⑦ Zhōngjí (CV 3)

② Zhōngfǔ (L 1)
④ Dàbāo (Sp 21)
⑥ Xiōngxiāng (Sp 19)
⑧ Shídòu (Sp 17)
⑩ Dàhéng (Sp 15)
⑫ Fǔhè (Sp 13)
⑭ Qīmén (Liv 14)
⑯ Rényíng (S 9)
⑱ Qìshè (S 11)
⑳ Qìhù (S 13)
㉒ Wūyì (S 15)
㉔ Rǔzhōng (S 17)
㉖ Bùróng (S 19)
㉘ Liángmén (S 21)
㉚ Tàiyǐ (S 23)
㉜ Tiānshū (S 25)
㉞ Dàjù (S 27)
㊱ Gūilái (S 29)
㊳ Shūfǔ (K 27)
㊵ Shéncáng (K 25)
㊷ Shénfēng (K 23)
㊹ Yōumén (K 21)
㊻ Yīndū (K 19)
㊽ Shāngqū (K 17)
㊿ Zhōngzhù (K 15)
⑤ Qìxué (K 13)
⑤ Héng gǔ (K 11)
⑤ Tiāntū (CV 22)
⑤ Huágài (CV 20)
⑥ Yùtáng (CV 18)
⑥ Zhōng tíng (CV 16)
⑥ Jùqué (CV 14)
⑥ Zhōng wǎn (CV 12)
⑥ Xiàwǎn (CV 10)
⑦ Shénquè (CV 8)
⑦ Qìhǎi (CV 6)
⑦ Guānyuán (CV 4)
⑦ Qūgǔ (CV 2)

**Diagram of the Distribution of the Points of the
Fourteen Meridians (The Chest and the Abdomen)**

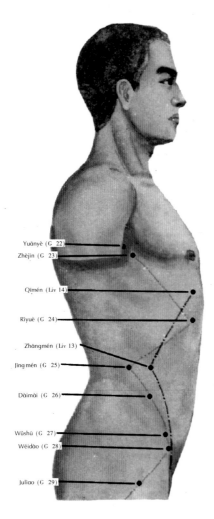

Yuānyè (G 22)
Zhèjīn (G 23)

Qīmén (Liv 14)

Rìyuè (G 24)

Zhāngmén (Liv 13)
Jīngmén (G 25)

Dàimài (G 26)

Wǔshū (G 27)
Wéidào (G 28)

Jūliáo (G 29)

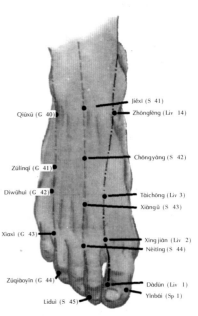

Qiūxū (G 40)

Jiěxī (S 41)
Zhōngfēng (Liv 14)

Chōngyáng (S 42)

Zúlínqí (G 41)

Dìwǔhuì (G 42)

Tàichōng (Liv 3)
Xiàngǔ (S 43)

Xiáxī (G 43)

Xíngjiān (Liv 2)
Nèitíng (S 44)

Zúqiàoyīn (G 44)

Dàdūn (Liv 1)
Yǐnbái (Sp 1)

Lìduì (S 45)

**Diagram of the Distribution of the Points of
the Fourteen Meridians (the Lateral View of
the Chest and the Abdomen)**

**Diagram of the Distribution of the Points of
the Fourteen Meridians (the Instep)**

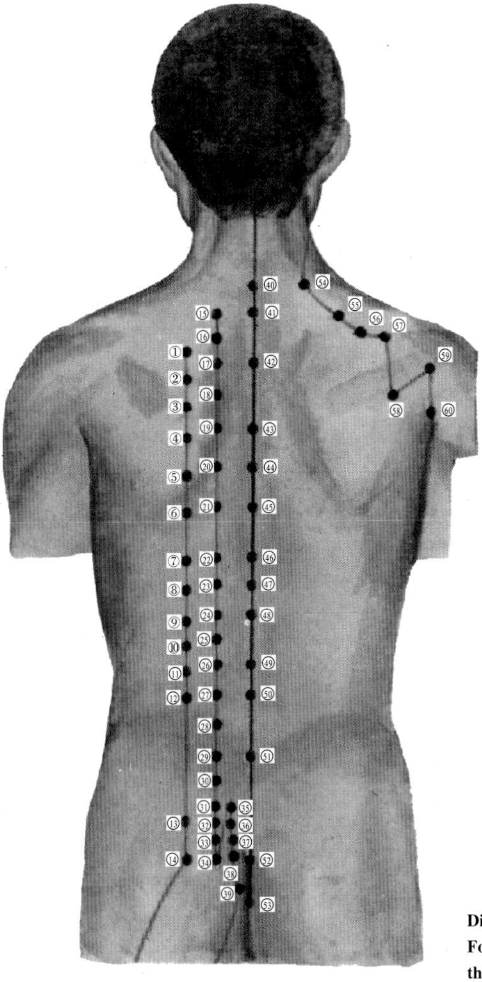

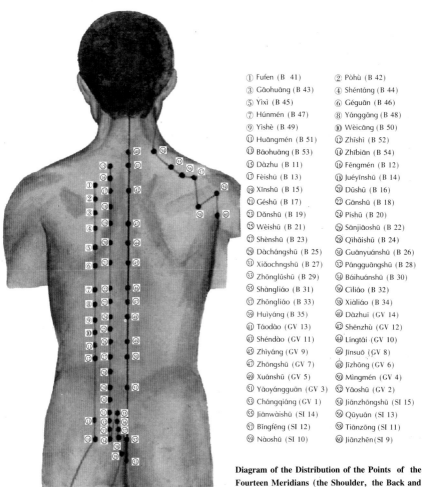

① Fufen (B 41) ② Pòhù (B 42)
③ Gāohuāng (B 43) ④ Shéntáng (B 44)
⑤ Yìxì (B 45) ⑥ Géguān (B 46)
⑦ Húnmén (B 47) ⑧ Yánggāng (B 48)
⑨ Yìshè (B 49) ⑩ Wèicāng (B 50)
⑪ Huāngmén (B 51) ⑫ Zhīshì (B 52)
⑬ Bāohuāng (B 53) ⑭ Zhībiān (B 54)
⑮ Dàzhu (B 11) ⑯ Fēngmén (B 12)
⑰ Fèishū (B 13) ⑱ Juéyīnshū (B 14)
⑲ Xīnshū (B 15) ⑳ Dūshū (B 16)
㉑ Géshū (B 17) ㉒ Gānshū (B 18)
㉓ Dǎnshū (B 19) ㉔ Píshū (B 20)
㉕ Wèishū (B 21) ㉖ Sānjiāoshū (B 22)
㉗ Shènshū (B 23) ㉘ Qìhǎishū (B 24)
㉙ Dàchángshū (B 25) ㉚ Guānyuánshū (B 26)
㉛ Xiǎochngshū (B 27) ㉜ Pángguāngshū (B 28)
㉝ Zhōnglǔshū (B 29) ㉞ Báihuánshū (B 30)
㉟ Shàngliáo (B 31) ㊱ Cìliáo (B 32)
㊲ Zhōngliáo (B 33) ㊳ Xiàliáo (B 34)
㊴ Huìyáng (B 35) ㊵ Dàzhuī (GV 14)
㊶ Táodào (GV 13) ㊷ Shēnzhù (GV 12)
㊸ Shéndào (GV 11) ㊹ Língtái (GV 10)
㊺ Zhìyáng (GV 9) ㊻ Jīnsuō (GV 8)
㊼ Zhōngshū (GV 7) ㊽ Jīzhōng (GV 6)
㊾ Xuánshū (GV 5) ㊿ Mìngmén (GV 4)
(51) Yāoyángguān (GV 3) (52) Yāoshū (GV 2)
(53) Chángqiáng (GV 1) (54) Jiānzhōngshū (SI 15)
(55) Jiānwàishū (SI 14) (56) Qūyuán (SI 13)
(57) Bǐngfēng (SI 12) (58) Tiānzōng (SI 11)
(59) Nàoshū (SI 10) (60) Jiānzhēn (SI 9)

Diagram of the Distribution of the Points of the Fourteen Meridians (the Shoulder, the Back and the Buttocks)

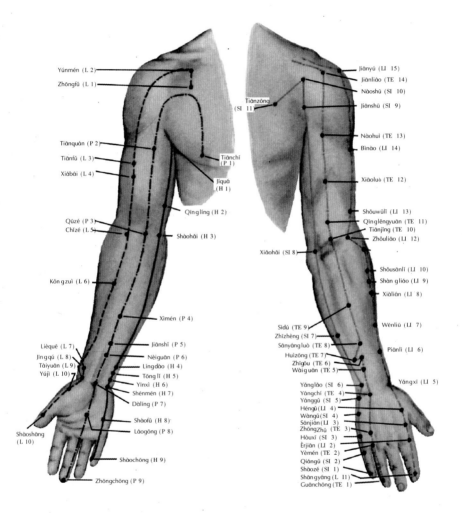

Yúnmén (L 2)
Zhōngfǔ (L 1)
Tiānzōng (SI 11)
Jiānyú (LI 15)
Jiānliáo (TE 14)
Nàoshū (SI 10)
Jiānshū (SI 9)

Tiānquán (P 2)
Tiānfǔ (L 3)
Xiábái (L 4)
Tiānchí (P 1)
Jíquá (H 1)

Nàohuì (TE 13)
Bìnào (LI 14)

Xiāoluò (TE 12)

Qīnglíng (H 2)

Qūzé (P 3)
Chǐzé (L 5)
Shàohǎi (H 3)

Shǒuwǔlǐ (LI 13)
Qīnglěngyuān (TE 11)
Tiānjǐng (TE 10)
Zhǒuliáo (LI 12)

Xiǎohǎi (SI 8)

Kǒngzuì (L 6)

Shǒusānlǐ (LI 10)
Shàngliáo (LI 9)
Xiàlián (LI 8)

Xīmén (P 4)

Sìdú (TE 9)
Zhīzhèng (SI 7)
Sānyángluò (TE 8)
Huìzōng (TE 7)
Zhīgōu (TE 6)
Wàiguān (TE 5)

Wēnliù (LI 7)

Lièquē (L 7)
Jīngqú (L 8)
Tàiyuān (L 9)
Yújì (L 10)
Jiānshǐ (P 5)
Nèiguān (P 6)
Língdào (H 4)
Tōnglǐ (H 5)
Yīnxì (H 6)
Shénmén (H 7)
Dàlíng (P 7)

Piānlì (LI 6)

Yángxī (LI 5)

Yǎnglǎo (SI 6)
Yángchí (TE 4)
Yánggǔ (SI 5)
Héngǔ (LI 4)
Wàngǔ (SI 4)
Sānjiān (LI 3)
ZhōngZhǔ (TE 3)
Hòuxī (SI 3)
Èrjiān (LI 2)
Yèmén (TE 2)
Qiángǔ (SI 2)
Shàozé (SI 1)
Shàngyáng (L 11)
Guānchōng (TE 1)

Shàofǔ (H 8)
Láogōng (P 8)

Shàoshāng (L 10)

Shàochōng (H 9)

Zhōngchōng (P 9)

Diagram of the Distribution of the Points of the Fourteen Meridians (the Medial View of the Upper Limbs)

Diagram of the Distribution of the Points of the Fourteen Meridians (the Medial View of the Upper Limbs)

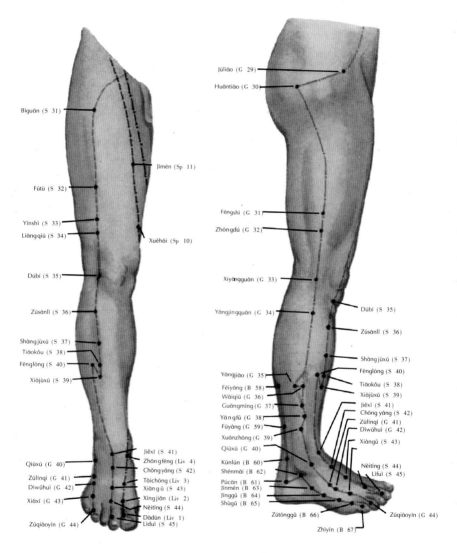

Diagram of the Distribution of the points of the Fourteen Meridians (the Anterior View of the Lower Limbs)

Diagram of the Distribution of the points of the Fourteen Meridians (the Anterior View of the Lower Limbs)

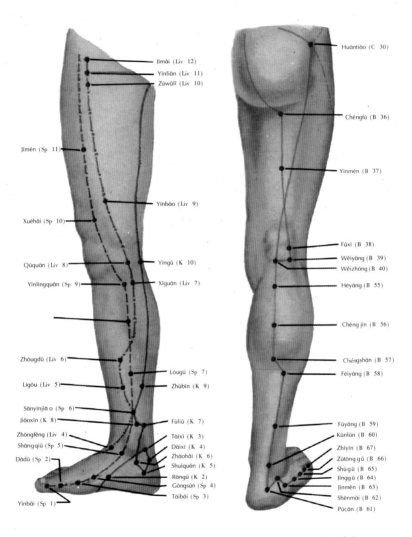

Jǐmài (Liv 12)
Yīnlián (Liv 11)
Zúwǔlǐ (Liv 10)

Huántiào (C 30)

Chéngfú (B 36)

Jīmén (Sp 11)

Yīnmén (B 37)

Yīnbāo (Liv 9)

Xuéhǎi (Sp 10)

Qūquán (Liv 8)

Yīngǔ (K 10)

Fúxì (B 38)
Wěiyáng (B 39)
Wěizhōng (B 40)

Yīnlíngquán (Sp 9)

Xīguān (Liv 7)

Héyáng (B 55)

Chéngjīn (B 56)

Zhōngdū (Liv 6)

Lòugǔ (Sp 7)

Chéngshān (B 57)

 Lǐgōu (Liv 5)

Zhùbīn (K 9)

Fēiyáng (B 58)

Sānyīnjiāo (Sp 6)
Jiāoxìn (K 8)

Fùliū (K 7)

Fùyáng (B 59)

Zhōngfēng (Liv 4)
Shāngqiū (Sp 5)

Tàixī (K 3)
Dàxī (K 4)

Kūnlún (B 60)
Zhìyīn (B 67)
Zútōnggǔ (B 66)

Dàdū (Sp 2)

Zhàohǎi (K 6)
Shuǐquán (K 5)
Rángǔ (K 2)
Gōngsūn (Sp 4)
Tàibái (Sp 3)

Shùgǔ (B 65)
Jīnggǔ (B 64)
Jīnmén (B 63)
Shēnmài (B 62)

Yǐnbái (Sp 1)

Púcān (B 61)

Diagram of the Distribution of the points of the Fourteen Meridians (the Medial View of the Lower Limbs)

Diagram of the Distribution of the points of the Fourteen Meridians (the Medial View of the Lower Limbs)

A PRACTICAL ENGLISH DICTIONARY OF ACUPUNCTURE-MOXIBUSTION
针灸学辞典

Shuai Xuezhong

Cheng Zhiming

湖南科学技术出版社

HUNAN SCIENCE & TECHNOLOGY PRESS

First Edition   1997

ISBN 7—5357—2046—3/R · 385

Published by

Hunan Science &. Technology Press

Printed by

Hunan Xinhua 2nd Printing Factory

Distributed by

China International Book Trading Corporation

35 Chegongzhuang Xilu, Beijing 100044, China

P. O. Box 399, Beijing, China

Printed in the People's Republic of China

CONTENTS

CONTENTS

目　录

PREFACE

As early as the 6th century Chinese acupuncture-moxibustion had handed to the Asian countries near China, and then to the Europe in the 17th century. Since the 1950's Chinese acupuncture-moxibustion has moved towards the whole world along with the gradual enlargement of the international contact. It has been propagated over 130 countries in the five continents. In the course of this propagation, it is no doubt that the translation, particularly English translation, has played an important role in bridging acupuncture and the whole world. This is because English language is most widely used in the world. Medical workers in the most countries can touch Chinese acupuncture science just by directly or indirectly regarding English as the medium. In the present world, acupuncture works translated or compiled or written in English are enumerous. Some other acupuncture works are translated from English edition. The above-mentioned works have assuredly promoted the propagation of Chinese acupuncture over the whole world. However, frankly speaking, their contents do not exceed the rudimentary knowledge of acupuncture. As compared with the rich and profound contents of acupuncture specialty, they are far from being special. This makes foreign medical workers understand that academy of Chinese acupuncture is just so so and they need not to study it deeply. The reason to cause this state are many. The most radical one is the barrier of language, and quite a few acupuncture terms lack of proper English translation and explanation.

In recent years, the Chinese-English dictionaries of traditional Chinese medicine have been continually published. Although they include acupuncture terms, these terms are quite limited that they can not meet the need of acupuncture specialty. Hence, it is actually an urgent task to translate or compile an acupuncture dictionary.

It is nothing easy to translate an acupuncture dictionary into English or compile it in English. This is because the translators or compilers can hardly find out the corresponding English words and expressions. They have to search for them widely and repeatedly deliberate them. This requires the translators to master not only English but also acupuncture. Prof. Shuai is the one of them. He is an eminent English specialist for traditional Chinese medicine in China and has been frequently in charge of English translation for international acupuncture conferences. Being responsible for English teaching and research in the acupuncture department for dozens of years, he has a deeper understanding of acupuncture academy. Ten years ago, he was once in charge of compilation and translation of Chinese-English Terminology of Traditional Chinese Medicine, which has been warmly welcome by the readers. Nowadays, he is once again in charge of compiling and translating A Practical English Dictionary of Acupuncture. It contains over 3,000 entries, each of which is more minutely explained in English. It is very suitable for the medical practitioners' need in study on Chinese acupuncture. As for the translators of English for Chinese acupuncture it is also a must. I believe that it will certainly promote the popularization of acupuncture over the world and make the essence of Chinese acupuncture understood by the people the world over. For this reason I wrote the Preface with great pleasure.

Wang Xuetai
at China Academy of Traditional
Chinese Medicine,
on April 1, 1996

序

　　中国针灸早在公元 6 世纪就传到邻近的亚洲国家，17 世纪又传到欧洲。自从 20 世纪 50 年代以来，随着国际之间的交往日益扩大，针灸走向了全世界，至今已经传到 130 多个国家，遍及五大洲。在这个传播过程中，毫无疑问翻译工作起着非常重要的桥梁作用。尤其是英文翻译起的作用最大，因为在全世界，英文的使用面最广。大多数国家的医务人员，正是直接或间接地以英文为媒介，才接触到中国针灸学术的。

　　现在世界上，以英文翻译或编著的针灸书籍很多，还有一些是从英文转译为其他语种的针灸书籍。这些书籍的确促进了中国针灸向全世界的传播。然而毋庸讳言，这些书籍的内容并未超出针灸的基础知识，与针灸专业的丰富而精深的内涵相比，尚相去甚远。致使国外医界人士误以为中国针灸学术不过如此，用不着深入钻研。造成这种状况的原因非一，而最根本的原因还是语言文字的障碍，许多针灸学的名词术语还缺少恰当的英文翻译与解释。

　　近几年，我国陆续出版了几种中英对照的中医辞书。这些辞书虽然也包括针灸学的名词术语，可是收词量有限，不可能满足针灸专业的需要。因此，用英文翻译或编写一部针灸辞书，实乃当务之急。

　　翻译或编写英文针灸辞书很不容易，许多名词术语由于难以找到相应的英文词句，不得不广泛搜寻，反复推敲。这就要求从事翻译的人，不但要有深厚的英文功底，而且还要掌握针灸学术。帅学忠教授正是具备这些条件。他是全国知名的中医外语专家，多次在国际针灸学术大会上担任英语翻译主持人。由于他长期在针灸系主持英语教学，所以对针灸学术有较深的理解。十余年前，他曾主持编译过一本《英汉双解常用中医名词术语》，深受读者欢迎。现在，帅君又主持编译了一部《针灸学辞典》，收词三千余条，对每条词句都用英文写出较详细的释义，很适合国外医界人士钻研中国针灸的需要。对于从事中医针灸的翻译工作而言，也是一部必不可少的工具书。我相信这部词典问世以后，必将促进针灸向全世界的传播，使华夏的针灸真髓为世人所理解，故而欣然作序。

王雪苔
1996 年 4 月 1 日
于中国中医研究院

FOREWORD

Acupuncture science is an integral component of traditional Chinese medicine. For several thousand years, Chinese nation has accumulated extremely theoretical knowledge and clinical experiences in prevention and treatment of diseases in this field. Acupuncture works and literatures are enumerable and their terms are so many. The author can only collect some practical ones. So, this dictionary is just a middle-sized one (only over 3, 000 terms that are practically used were collected). Quite a few names of acupuncture experts and those of acupuncture books have not yet been collected. In recent years, varieties of acupuncture dictionaries in Chinese language have been published at home. They are mainly for the domestic readers. Hence, so many foreign readers (because of their ignorance of Chinese language) can not read them. In order to meet their urgent need, we wrote this book in English on the basis of a large reference literatures of Chinese medicine including Chinese acupuncture from the readers' practical need. We sincerely hope that it will be liked and treated as a must in your learning, research, and clinical practice. For foreign readers' convenience, we adopted the index for English entries and that for Chinese *pinyin* entries (the index for the strokes of the Chinese characters are omitted).

Up to now, English nomenclature of acupuncture terms have not been standardized except the names of the fourteen meridians and their points, which have been standardized by WHO. What we have tried for may lay a foundation for English nomenclature of interna- tional standardization of acupuncture terms. We still hope that it will promote the realization of the internal standardization of the acupuncture terms and contribute to the cause of popularization of Chinese acupuncture the world over.

Here, I would like to express my sincere thanks to my favourate students, Miss Jiang Xiaofang, Mr. Nie Feng, Miss He Lijuan, Mr. Zhang Jiping, and Miss Yang Qianyun for their helping us in compiling the indexes.

I'll be very grateful for the readers at home and abroad if they bring out their suggestions and criticism after reading the book.

Shuai Xuezhong
at Hunan College of Traditional
Chinese Medicine, Changsha, China
on October 13, 1995

A

Abdomen 腹 [fù] An ear point at the slightly medial side between Lumbar Vertebra and Sacral Vertebra.

abdominal midline 腹正中线 [fù zhèng zhōng xiàn] The line of locating the meridian points, at the area where CV passes through. Distributed over the line are Jiuwei (CV 15), Juque (CV 14), Shangwan (CV 13), Zhongwan (CV 12), Jianli (CV 11), Xiawan (CV 10), Shuifen (CV 9), Shenque (CV 8), Yinjiao (CV 7), Qihai (CV 6), Shimen (CV 5), Guanyuan (CV 4), Zhongji (CV 3), Ququ (CV 2).

abdominal pain 腹痛 [fù tòng] Generally referring to pain in the abdomen, the extremely common symptom in clinic. It may be accompanied with various visceral disorders.

abnormalities of micturition 淋证 [lín zhèng] It is mainly manifested by frequency of urination, urgency of urination, painful micturition or incontinence of urination. It may be classified into five types, such as dysuria caused by calculus, dysuria caused by dysfunction of the bladder, chyluria, chronic dysuria, and hematuria with pain, and includes such distress as infection, calculus and tuberculosis of the urinary system, chyluria and prostatitis, etc.

abrupt pulse 促脉 [cù mài] The pulse is rapid and irregular. It often indicates excessive yang heat, heart disease, etc.

absorbing cup 吸筒 [xī tǒng] The bamboo cup used for cupping. It can be steamed and boiled.

accumulation of dampness and heat in the bladder 膀胱湿热 [páng guāng shī rè] The pathologic manifestations due to accumulation and stagnation of the pathogenic damp and heat in the bladder. The main symptoms are frequency and urgency of urination, painful urination with scanty fullness and distension of the hypochondrium, yellowish glossy coating of tongue, rapid pulse, etc.

accessary manipulation 辅助手法 [fǔ zhù shǒu fǎ] Contrary to the basic manipulations. Some cooperative manipulations are used during the operation for a certain point and aiding in inserting and withdrawing the needle and regulating needling sensation. E. g. , fingernail pressing, searching and pinching, springing, and scratching the handle of the needle, kneading and closing the needling hole, etc.

acquiring *qi* 得气 [dé qì] It means that sunken and tense sensations are felt by the doctor beneath the inserted needle during acupuncture. That is, the patient feels sour, numb, distending and heavy while the doctor feels sunken and tense beneath the needle.

acromion of scapula 髃骨 [yù gǔ] Referring to the acromion of the scapular bone.

Acupuncture Classic of Midnight-noon Ebb-flow 子午流注针经 [zǐ wǔ liú zhù zhēn jīng] A special book written by He Ruoyi in Jin Dynasty (1115—1234), noted by Yan Mingguang, three volumes, a book specially dealing with theory of midnight-noon ebb-flow, checked and approved by Dou Guifang in Yuan Dynasty (1271—1368), one of "Four Acupuncture Books". Its chief contents were collected in the acupuncture books written in latter generations.

acupuncture and moxibustion in hottest summer 伏针、伏灸 [fú zhēn, fú jiǔ] Referring to administering acupuncture and moxibustion in the middle summer because it is very hot in the middle summer and yang *qi* ascends and evaporates, during which acupuncture and moxibustion have the favourable effect for chronic diseases, cough and asthma easily attack in autumn and winter.

acupuncture technique of midnight-noon ebb-flow 子午流注针法 [zǐ wǔ liú zhù zhēn fǎ] 1. A kind of point-combined method according to time. It consists of the five-*shu* points matching the five elements and Heavenly Stems and Earthly Branches matching the viscera and the time interval. 2. The name of the book written by Cheng Danan and others.

acupuncture stone 针石 [zhēn shí] "If the trouble is at the muscle, it can be treated by the stone needle." (Plain Questions) "If one's defensive *qi* is retained and full, it can be reduced by needling. If suppurative blood is stangant, it can be broken by the stone needle. Stone means the stone needle, that is the *bian* (sharp) stone." (Wang Bin's Notes)

acupuncture doctor 针师 [zhēn shī] Referring to the doctors who were in charge of acupuncture techniques. There was the acupuncture position, in the Impirical Health Institute in ancient China.

acupuncture science 针灸学 [zhēn jiǔ xué] 1. One of the subjects of Chinese medicine, including the two main parts, basic theories and clinical practices. The 1st one mainly contains the meridians, *shu* points, etc.; The 2nd, puncturing techniques, moxibustion techniques, and their treatment, etc. The outstanding advance has been achieved in research on its mechanism, acupuncture anesthesia and acupuncture methods. 2. A name of the book compiled by Acupuncture Teaching-Research Section of Jiangshu Provincial School of Traditional Chinese Medicine, published by Jiangshu People's Press. It contains six chapters, the meridians, *shu* points, needling techniques, moxibustion techniques, treatments and reference data. It is characterised by the description and identification of the meridians, analysis of the indications of *shu* points enumerating of acupuncture and moxibustion methods, collection of clinical cases

and records. 3. A name of the book compiled chiefly by Nanjing College of Traditional Chinese Medicine, the trial textbook of national medical and pharmaceutical colleges, published by People's Health Press in 1961, and revised in 1964,1975,1979,1980 and published by Shanghai Science & Technology Press. It contains three chapters, respectively describes the origin of acupuncture science, meridians and points, needling and moxibustion methods and treatment of diseases, of which some research achievements and new therapies in recent years have been cited.

Acupuncture Prescriptions 针方 [zhēn fāng] A book written by Zhen Quan in Tang Dynasty (618—907), one volume, lost.

acupuncture assistant 针助教 [zhēn zhù jiào] The position of the staff in the Imperical Health Institute in ancient China.

acupuncture-moxibustion 针灸 [zhēn jiǔ] A collective term for acupuncture techniques and moxibustion techniques. The former is a therapeutic method of applying the special needling tool that acts on the meridians and points; The latter is a therapeutic method by using mugwort as the main material to scorch the meridians and points. It is generally called acupuncture-moxibustion treatment.

acupuncture point 穴位 [xué wèi] 1. The *shu* point, also referring to the area where the *shu* point is located. For details, see *shu* point; 2. *Xue*, an abbreviation for *shu xue*. It refers to the small location on the body through which the viscera and meridians are connected.

acupuncture sensation 针感 [zhēn gǎn] Also termed *zhenci ganying*. Referring to the local or larger scale of sensations, such as soreness, distension, heaviness and numbness, etc., produced by the patient due to acupuncture, and the sunken and tense reactions beneath the tip of the needle that are felt by the doctor's hand (i.e., a kind of being slightly absorbed by the needle).

Needling sensations appear due to the anatomical characteristics of different locations. E. g. , at the location of the thick muscle, sore and distending sensations and sunken and tense sensations may usually appear; At the location of dull sensation, distending and heavy sensations may usually appear; At the location of the ends of the four extremities and sensitive location, painful sensation may usually appear.

Acupuncture Classic 针经 [zhēn jīng] A name of the book. 1. An ancient term for Miraculous Pivot; 2. A book written by Fu Wong in Eastern Han Dynasty (25—220 A. D.), lost.

acupuncture reinforcing-reducing manipulations 针刺补泻法 [zhēn cì bǔ xiè fǎ] A name of classified acupuncture manipulation. In clinic the acupuncture method is divided into reinforcing and reducing manipulations for the purpose of reinforcing *xu* (deficency) and reducing *shi* (excess). Since Internal Classic appeared it has been described in acupuncture books in the succeeding dynasties. E. g. , "slight twirling" and "pressing after withdrawing the needle" were classified into reinforcing manipulation, "finger-pinching and twirling" and "widening the hole of the point by shaking the needle" were classified into reducing manipulation; In Plain Questions, inserting the needle in association with taking out air and withdrawing the needle in association with taking air in were classified into reinforcing manipulation, inserting the needle in association with taking air in and withdrawing the needle in association with taking air out were classified into reducing manipulation. In Difficult Classic "after acquiring *qi* insert the needle and retain it" is called reinforcing manipulation. Later it was brought out that "slowly thrusting the needle and swiftly inserting the needle" is reinforcing manipulation while " swiftly thrusting the needle and slowly inserting the needle " is reducing manipulation; "left-twirling" (clockwise twirling) is reinforcing manipulation while " right-twirling . " (counter-clockwise) is reducing manipulation. Varieties of reinforcing and reducing manipulations are mainly differentiated by the speed (quick or slow) of inserting and withdrawing the needle, the power (light or heavy) of thrusting and inserting the needle, the amplitude of an direction of rotating the needle. Some are ruled in combination with the direction of puncture (along or against flow of *qi*), frequency of administering puncture (the number of nine or six), and the strength of the stimulation volume is also related to reinforcing and reducing manipulations. In ABC of Medicine "It is advisable to insert the needle slightly and superficially in the case of reinforcing manipulation and heavily and deeply in the case of reducing manipulation. " Hence slight stimulation is adopted for deficiency syndrome while strong stimulation is adopted for the excess syndrome. Yet, there was also the record that the stimulation volume of reinforcing manipulation is somewhat strong but that of reducing manipulation is weak in ancient times. E. g. , "Heaviness is reinforcing while slight weakening is reducing. " (Supplements to Gold Prescriptions Worth a Thousand Gold). In clinic the proper reinforcing and reducing manipulation should be selected according to the condition.

acupuncture prohibited points 禁针穴 [jìn zhēn xué] Referring to the points where acupuncture is prohibited. According to Systematic Classic of Acupuncture, they are Shenting (GV 24), Shangguan (GB 3), Luxi (TE 19), Renying (ST 90), Yunmen (LU 2), Qichong (ST 30), Futu (ST 32), Sanyangluo (TE 8), Fuliu (KI 7), Chengjin (BL 56), Rangu (KI 2), Ruzhong (ST 17), Jiuwei (CV 15), women's Shimen (CV 5), Shouwuli (LI 13), and Quepen (ST 12). Since most of them near important organs and arteries, they are prohibited to be punctured or punctured too deeply. Besides Ruzhong (ST 17) and Qichong (ST 30), others can be used according to the condition in clinic.

acupuncture point injected therapy 穴位注射法 [xué wèi zhù shè fǎ] A therapeutic method to inject drug fluid into the point. In general, glucose injection of low-consistancy water for injection of drug fluid suitable for muscular injection are selected. Inject them slowly into the point with a syringe with a comparatively small and long syringe needle,   (e. g., No. 5 syringe needle). Do not injure the nerve stem, inject drug fluid wrongly into the vessel, etc. The volume of injection is decided by different kinds of drug fluid and the selected point approx. 0. 1—0. 5 cc for the point at the four limbs, approx. 2—15 cc for the point at the waist and hip where the muscles are thick. If the point injection is done with a small amount of injection, the dosage is approx. 1/10—1/2 of the routine dosage, while applying this therapy, one must be familiar to the action of drug fluid. As to certain drugs the hypertensive test should be first done (e. g., procaine hydrochlorise, etc.) It is not advisable to apply oily injection or the drug with extremely stimulative action.

acupuncture manipulations 针刺手法 [zhēn cì shǒu fǎ] It generally refers to the operating method on treatment of acupuncture. To insert and withdraw the needle and apply reinforcing and reducing manipulations can not depart from the fingers. In modern times the main and single method is called the basic manipulation while that combined by certain simple method is called the synthetical method, that playing an accessary role in the course of acupuncture is called the accessary method. And that specially differentiating reinforcing and reducing manipulations is called reinforcing-reducing manipulation.

acupuncture fainting 晕针 [yūn zhēn] Fainting phenomenon caused by acupuncture. The symptoms are dizziness, blurred vision, palpitation, nausea, pale complexion, profuse cold sweat, yarning, lowering of blood pressure, sunken and hidden pulse, etc. When these phenomena are seen the inserted needle must be quickly withdrawn and let the patient lie down and have a rest. It generally occurs in a sultry ill-ventilated room and in the patient who is weak in constitution, very tired and very nervous (such as accepting acupuncture treatment for the first time) or under the circumstance of too heavy manipulation, prolonged sitting and prolonged standing.

acupuncture prohibition 刺禁 [cì jìn] Including the areas (the important internal organs, big vessel and cerebral cortex medulla) and the opportune moment,   (e. g., over hunger, over full, over fatigue, violent change of emotion, etc.).

acupuncture-moxibustion techniques 刺灸法 [cì jiǔ fǎ] A general term for varieties of techniques of acupuncture and moxibustion, an important part of acupuncture-moxibustion science.

acupuncture anesthesia 针刺麻醉 [zhēn cì má zuì] Briefly termed "*zhen ma*". A method to make the patient be able to accept the surgical operation in the state of mental consciousness by puncturing the point to produce the analgesic and regulating actions.   It is a research achievement that developed on the basis of acupuncture treatment of disease by Chinese medical practitioners.   It needs not complicated appratuses and instruments, simple, convenient and safe in operation. During the operation, less or none anesthetics is used, the accidental anesthesia and the side-effect of anesthesia would not occur in the patient. The patient keeps conscious, and besides painful sensation becomes dull, other sensations and motor functions keep normal. The pain due to the operation is comparatively mild. In general, the reactions such as nausea, vomiting would not appear, and the patient can take food earlier and more earlier. Moreover, as acupuncture has the action of mobilizing and strenthening the antibacterial factor in the body, it can shorten the recovery course after the operation. In clinic it suits the operations such as thyroidectomy, maxillary antrum operation, glaucoma, craniocerebral (anteroposterior cranial fossa) operation, anterior laryngectomy, pulmonary lobectomy, removal of the major part of stomach, splenectomy, cesarean section, abdominal urethral ligation, prostatectomy, meniscectomy of the lateral knee, etc. It is generally thought that the effect is favourable when it is used for the operations on the head, neck and chest. Its application benefits the safety of the patient during the operation and after the operation, who is hypersensitive to anesthesitics or is hypofunctional in the heart, lungs, liver and kidneys, or is severely ill or is old and asthenic, or suffers from shock. The stimulating methods used for acupuncture anesthesia are administering puncture with the manipulation, electroacupuncture point injection, etc. Sometimes a small amount of accessary drugs are adopted (e.g., the sedative, analgetics, local anesthetic drug or that being able to influence the transmitter of the central nerve). Yet, at present there are still the problems such as incomplete analgesia, inadequate relaxation of the muscle at the operated area, imcomplete control of traction, reflection of the viscera, which are to be further improved.

acute convulsion 急惊风 [jí jīng fēng] The infantile convulsion with sudden onset. Its chief manifestations are: sudden onset, coma, rolling upwards of the eyes, lockjaws, rigidity of the neck, convulsion of limbs, occasional high fever, frothy salivation, rattling sound due to phlegm in the throat, etc.

Adam's Apple 结喉 [jié hóu] The prominence situated in the anterior medial aspect of the neck, corresponding to the thyroid cartillage.

administering acupuncture 行针 [xíng zhēn] 1. Referring to administering and applying acupuncture therapy; 2. Referring to the manipulation after acupuncture, also called *yunzhen.*

Adrenal Gland 肾上腺 [shèn shàng xiàn] An ear point located 1/2 below the lateral side of the tragus.

adverse acupuncture 逆针灸 [nì zhēn jiǔ] Referring to administering acupuncture on the health person.

adverse moxibustion 逆灸 [nì jiǔ] A term of moxibustion techniques. Referring to administering moxibustion without disease for reinforcing the human body's anti-disease ability.

against and depriving 迎而夺之 [yíng ér duó zhī] A term for needling technique, opposite to 'along and strengthening.' It is the principle of reducing manipulation with the needle against the direction of *qi* flow. It implies that in reducing manipulation the tip of the needle should be against the flow of meridian *qi*, so as to deprive its excess.

all the vessels meet in the lungs 肺朝百脉 [fèi cáo bǎi mài] In the course of circulation and respiration, the blood from all over the body flows to the lungs via the vessels to exchange gases. This explains the close relationship between the lungs and vessels.

along the meridian *qi* **and tonifying** 随而济之 [suí ér jì zhī] A term of needling, contrary to 'against and depriving'. The principle of reinforcing along or against the direction of the tip of the needle. In reinforcing manipulation, the tip of the needle should be along the flow of meridian *qi* so as to tonify it.

amenorrhea 经闭 [jīng bì] 1. Menstruation has not been seen by the woman at the age of 18; 2. Menstruation ceases for more than three monthes accompanied by illnesses excluding such causes as pregnancy and breast feeding.

ancestral sinew 宗筋 ［zōng jīn］ Referring to the large tendon in the centre of the abdomen and at the lateral umbilicus. Its lower part gathers at the genital organ.

ancestral meridian 宗脉 ［zōng mài］ The meridian gathering to the ocular and auricular regions.

ankle 踝骨 ［huái gǔ］ Referring to the medial and lateral ankle at the lower ends of tibia and fibula, also referring to the higher part of the styploid process of ulna and that of radius.

Ankle joint 踝关节 ［huái guān jié］ An ear point below Toe and Heel to form a triangle.

anterior angle of ear 耳前角 ［ěr qián jiǎo］ Also called *qujiao*. Referring to the protruding part above the hair on the temples.

anterior yin 前阴 ［qián yīn］ Referring to external genitalia. It is collectively called two yin together with posterior yin （anus）.

anterior referred points 募穴 ［mù xué］ Referring to the specific points at the chest and abdomen concerning the viscera. Since they are near the viscera, they are where *qi* in the viscera gathers. When a viscus is in disorder, abnormal reflections such as tenderness or hypersenitivity, etc., may appear at the anterior referred points concerned. They can be used for diagnosis and treatment. E. g., for epigastric pain Zhongwan （CV 12） can be selected, for abnormal micturition Zhongji （CV 3） can be selected. They can also be used in cooperation with back *shu* points, called *shu-mu* combined points. The twelve meridians have one anterior referred point each （Fig 1）. Their names are as follows:

Bilateral Anterior Referred Points	Middle Anterior Referred Points
Lungs—Zhongfu （LU 1）	Pericardium—Danzhong （CV 17）
Liver—Qimen （LR 14）	Heart—Juque （CV 14）
Gallbladder—Riyue （GB 24）	Stomach—Zhongwan （CV 12）
Spleen—Zhangmen （LR 13）	Triple Energizer—Shimen （CV 5）
Kidneys—Jingmen （GB 25）	Small Intestine—Guanyuan （CV 4）
Large Intestine—Tianshu （ST 25）	Bladder—Zhongji （CV 3）

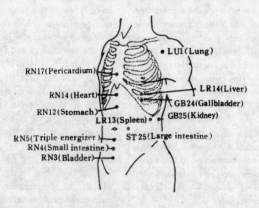

Fig 1

arteries of the twelve meridians 十二经动脉 [shí èr jīng dòng mài] The arteries along the courses of the twelve meridians, of which the pulse can be easily felt. They are those arteries located superficially. The points at the arteries of the various meridians are as follow: Lung Meridian of Hand-*taiyin*: Zhongfu (LU 1), Yumen (LU 2), Tianfu (LU 3), Xiabai (LU 4), Chize (LU 5) and Jingqi (LU 8); Heart Meridian of Hand-*jueyin*: Laogong (PC 8); Large Intestine Meridian of Hand-*yangming*: Hegu (LI 4), Yangxi (LI 5) and Wuli (LI 13); Small Intestine Meridian of Hand-*taiyang*: Tianchuang (SI 16); Triple Energizer Meridian of Hand-*shaoyang*: Heliao (SJ 22), Renying (ST 9), Qichong (ST 30) and Chongyang (ST 42); Bladder Meridian of Foot-*taiyang*: Weizhong (BL 40); Gallbladder Meridian of Foot -*taiyang*: Weizhong (BL 40); Gallbladder Meridian of Foot-*shaoyang*: Tinghui (GB 2) and Shangguan (GB 30); Spleen Meridian of Foot-*taiyin*: Jimen (SP 11) and Chongmen (SP 12); Kiddney Meridian of Foot-*shaoyin*: Taixi (KI 3) and Yinggu (KI 10); Liver Meridian of Foot-*jueyin*: Taichong (LR 3), Xingjian (LR 2), Wuli and Yinlian (LR 11).

anteroposterior point-combined method 前后配穴法 [qián hòu pèi xué fǎ] One of point-combined methods. 'Anterior' refers to the head and face while the 'posterior' to the occiput, nape, waist and back. The cooperation of the points at the anteroposterior regions is usually applied for treating disorders of the five-sense organs, internal organs. E. g. , for ocular trouble Jingming (BL 1) and Fengchi (GB 20) are selected; For stiff tongue Lianquan (CV 23) and Yamen (GV 15) are selected; For stomachache Zhongwan (CV 12) and Weishu (BL 21) are selected. Coupled puncture and *shu-mu* point-combined method can also be classified into this category.

anti-pathogenic *qi* 正气 [zhèng qì] A collective term for various kinds of functional active and body resistance against diseases.

Anus 肛门 [gāng mén] An ear point at the middle of Lower Segment of Rectum and Urethra.

Anxie 安邪 [ān xié] An alternate term for Pucan (BL 61).

aperture point 孔穴 [kǒng xué] A common term for the *shu* point. 'Kong' means the aperture or interspace, referring that the acupuncture point is used in the hollow place of the muscle and joint.

apoplexy 中风 [zhòng fēng] 1. Diseases such as cerebral vascular accident, etc. It is also called *zuzhong*; 2. A disease or symptom complex due to external affection by pathogenic wind. It is maifested as fever, headache, perspiration, slow and floating pulse, etc.

appearance of deficiency in extreme excess 大实有羸状 [dà shí yǒu léi zhuàng] At the critical stage of the excess syndrome, the pseudodeficiency symptoms appear.

Appendix 阑尾 [lán wěi] An ear point between Large Intestine and Small Intestine.

Appendix point 阑尾点 [lán wěi diǎn] An ear point. One located slightly above Finger, another superior to Shoulder, still another inferior to Clavicle. All of them are in the scaphoid fossa.

arisaema tuber 天南星 [tiān nán xīng] One of drugs for dressing. It is poisonous in nature. So, "it can reduce the swelling and resolve the mass and is used for treating deviated mouth and erosive tongue. " (Outline of Materia Medica)

acropecia areata 斑秃 [bān tū] A skin disease that in a short period of time the hair falls off, forming circular patches of smooth, glossy bald scalp of various sizes.

arrangement of fingers 布指 [bù zhǐ] The arrangement of the physician's index, middle and ring fingers for pulse diagnosis.

arrival of *qi* **at the affected area** 气至病所 [qì zhì bìng suǒ] Referring that needling induction tends to arrive at the affected area.

If the patient suffering from febrile disease feelsthat the needling sensation arrives at the affected area, twirl the needle to make it run downward to the affected area. In case the disease is distal, it must first make *qi* run directly to the affected area.

arrow-head needle 镵针 [chán zhēn] One of the ancient nine needles, called the arrow-head needle in latter generations. Mainly used for superficial puncture to cause little bleeding. Indication: Febrile symptoms of the head and body. It has developed into the cutaneous needle in contemprary times.

arrow-head stone 镵石 [chán shí] An ancient needling instrument made of stone.

Ascites point 腹水点 [fù shuǐ diǎn] An ear point in the middle of Kidney, Pancreas-Galladder and Small Intestine.

assembled *qi* 宗气 [zōng qì] It is formed by a combination of respiratory gases and the essence from water and grain.

asthma 哮喘 [xiào chuǎn] A disease with a combination of wheeping and dyspnea.

Asthma point 喘点 [chuǎn diǎn] An ear point approx. 0.2 m lateral to Uterus.

Ashi point 阿是穴 [ā shì xué] Referring to selecting the point by pressing the tender point. The painful or diseased area that is pressed or pinched and the patient feels comfortable or painful can be taken as the point for acupuncture. "Oh" is a cry due to painful sensation. It is same in meaning with "Where there is a pain there is a point", and the painful spot is taken as a *shu* point and "Tianying Point"called in latter generations.

atractylodes rhizome 苍术 [cāng shù] One of the interposing things used for moxibustion. The dried rhizome of Atractylodes lancea (Thumb) DC or Atractylodes chinensis Kodz. It can be used to treat sudden deafness.

auklandia root paste 木香饼 [mù xiāng bǐng] One of drug pastes used for moxibustion.

auscultation and olfaction 闻诊 [wén zhěn] One of the four diagnostics by listening and smelling to ascertain the clinical status.

aversion of the liver to wind 肝恶风 [gān wù fēng] The liver dislikes and fears pathogenic wind since pathologic changes of the liver are often manifested with unsteady and abrupt symptoms like wind, such as convulsions, spasm, pruritus, numbness, dizziness, apoplexy, etc.

B

Bachong 八冲 [bā chōng] Also term for Bafeng. They are located at the interspaces of the five toes on the dorsal foot, at the dorsal planter boundary of the edge of the toe webs, 4 on each foot, 8 in total. Indications: Headache, toothache, snakebite, redness and welling of the dorsal foot, numbness of the toe, etc. Puncture: 1.5—3 cm obliquely upward or to cause little bleeding with a triangular needle. (Fig 2)

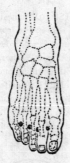

Fig 2

back-*shu* points 背俞穴 [bèi shú xué] *"Shu"* denotes that *qi* in the viscera transports and flows into certain points on the back. All of them are located at the 1st lateral line of the back, pertaining to Bladder Meridian of Foot-*taiyang*, and their positions are almost to the same with the those of the viscera from the upper arrangement to the lower. The abnormal reactions such as tenderness or hypersensitivity often appear at the corresponding back-*shu* points in disorders of various viscera, so that the diagnosis and treatment can be carried on. E. g., for cough, asthmatic breath, select Feishu (BL 13), for cardialgia, and palpitation with fright, select Xinshu (BL 15). 1. The *shu* points of the five storing viscera can also be

used for treating the diseases and symptoms concerning the five storing viscer e. g., since the liver is related to the eye, ocular trouble can be treated by selecting Ganshu (BL 18). Since the kidneys are related to the ear, ocular trouble can be treated by selecting Shenshu (BL 23). They can also be applied in cooperation with the anterior referred points, called combination of back-*shu* and anterior referred points (Fig 3). The names of the back *shu* points of the viscera are as follows. 2. Generally referring to various merisian points at the back, including various points at the midline of the back (GV), the 1st lateral line, the 2nd lateral line. 3. Referring to Dazhu (BL 19) and Fengmen (BL 12).

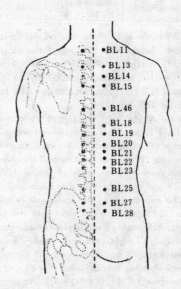

Fig 3

Bafeng (EX-LE 10) 八风 [bā fēng] An extra point, i. e., Bachong, located in the depres-

Viscera	Back-*shu*	Sequence of Vertebra
Lungs	Feishu (BL 13)	3th
Pericardium	Jueyinshu (BL 14)	4th
Heart	Xinshu (BL 15)	5th
Liver	Ganshu (BL 18)	9th
Gallbladder	Danshu (BL 19)	10th
Spleen	Pishu (BL 20)	11th
Stomch	Weishu (BL 11)	12th
Triple Energizer	Sanjiaoshu (SP 6)	13th
Kidneys	Shenshu (BL 23)	14th
Large Intestine	Dachangshu (BL 25)	16th
Small Intestine	Xiaochangshu(BL 27)	18th
Urinary Bladder	Pangguangshu (BL 28)	19th

sion at the ends of the toes on the dorsal foot. Indications: Swelling of the dorsal foot, numbness of foot. Puncture: 0. 9 cm obliquely. Moxibustion can be done on it.

Baguan 八关 [bā guān] An alternate term for Baxie (EX-UE 9).

Bahua 八华 [bā huá] An extra point, located at the back. Form an equilateral triangle with 1/4 of the distance between the two nipples (26 cm) as the length of the side, put the top of one angle on Dazhui (GV 14) and make the base side horizontally. The two angles of the lower side is the point. Measure twice, eight ones will be got. Indications: Weakness and emaciation, arthralgia, night sweat and cough. Moxibustion: 3—7 moxa cones or 5—15 minutes with warming moxibustion. (Fig 4)

Baicongwo 百虫窝 [bái cóng wō] 1. An alternate term for Xuehai (SP 10). 2. An extra point, also termed Xuexi. Located at the medial side of the thigh, 3 cm directly

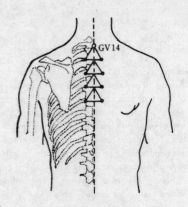

Fig 4

above Xuehai (SP 10). Indications: Eczema, itching skin, sore at the lower part of the body. Puncture: 3—4. 5 cm perpendicularly. Moxibustion: 3—7 moxa cones or 5—15 minutes with warming moxibustion.

Bailao 百劳 [bái láo] 1. An alternate term for Dazhu (GV 14); 2. Selecting the point at the painful spot; 3. The extra point located 3 cm bilateral and 6 cm lateral to Dazhui (GV 4). (Fig 5)

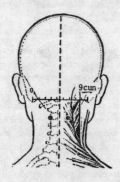

Fig 5

Baliao 八髎 [bā liáo] The four pairs of points, Shangliao, Ciliao, Zhongliao and Xialiao, 8 in total bilaterally.

bao 胞 [bāo] 1. Referring to uterus, also called *baogong*; 2. Same with *pao*, referring to the urinary bladder.

Baohuang 包肓 [bāo huāng] I. e., Baohuang (BL 53).

Baohuang (BL 53) 胞肓 [bāo huāng] A point of Bladder Meridian of Foot-*taiyang*. Location 9 cm lateral to the midline of the sacral region, at the level with the posterior foramen of the sacrum. Regional anatomy: At the greatest gluteal muscle. The middle gluteal muscle and the least gluteal cutaneous nerve are distributed. The superior gluteal nerve is in the deeper. Indications: Borborygmus, abdominal distension, pain in the lumbar spine, abnormal defecation and micturition, swelling in the pubic region. Puncture: 3—4.5 cm perpendicularly. Moxibustion: 3—7 moxa cones or 5—15 minutes with warming moxibustion.

Baomen 胞门 [bāo mén] 1. An alternate term for Qixue (KI 13); 2. The name of the extra point, see Baomen-Zihu.

Baomen-Zihu 胞门、子户 [bāo mén zǐ hù] An extra point. Same with Shuidao (ST 28) in location. Indications: Sterility, abdominal pain, dystocia, profuse leukorrhea, abdominal masses. Puncture: 3—4.5 cm perpendicularly (It is prohibited for women). Moxibustion: 3—5 moxa cones or 5—15 minutes with warming moxibustion. (Fig 6)

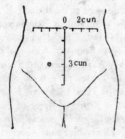

Fig 6

Baihuanshu (BL 30) 白环俞 [bái huán shū] A point of Bladder Meridian of Foot-*taiyang*, also termed Yuhuanshu. Location: 4 cm lateral to the sacral midline, at the level with the 4th posterior sacral foramen. Regional anatomy: In the greatest gluteal muscle. There is the inferior gluteal artery and vein. The medial artery and vein in the pubic region are in the deeper. The inferior clunical nerve, the lateral branch of the posterior branches of the 3rd and 4th sacral nerve, and the inferior clunical nerve are distributed. Indications: Leukorrhea, hernia, spermatorrhea, irregular menstruation, pains in the waist and legs. Puncture: 3—4.5 cm perpendicularly. Moxibustion: 3—7 moxa cones or 5—15 minutes with warming moxibustion.

Baihui (GV 20) 百会 [bái huì] A GV point, the confluence of GV and foot-*taiyang* meridian, also termed Sanyangwuhui, Tianman, Dianshang, Niwangong. Location: At the midpoint of the line connecting the tips of the two ears, 15 cm to the anterior hairline, on the midline of the head. Regional anatomy: In the falea aponeurotica, there is the left and right superficial temporal artery and vein as well as the anastomotic branch of the left and right occipital artery and vein. The branch of the greater occipital nerve is distributed. Indications: Headache, vertigo, palpitation with fright, amnesia, mania, tinnitus, stuffy nose, aphasia due to apoplexy, prolapse of anus, polapse of uterine, hemorrhoids, diarrhea, epilepsy, hysteria. Puncture: 1—2 cm harizontally. Moxibustion: 4—5 moxa cones or 5—10 minutes with warming moxibustion. (Fig 7)

basic manipulations 基本手法 [jī běn shǒu fǎ] Contrary to the accessay manipulations and synthetical manipulations, referring to some major and single manipulations, including rotating, lifting and thrusting, inserting and withdrawing. Many compound manipulations are based on them.

Baxie (EX-UE 9) 八邪 [bā xié] An extra point, also termed Baguan, located between the two fingers on the dorsal hand at the dorso-palmar boundary. There is the pal-

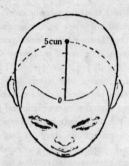

Fig 7

mar interosseous muscle, the dorsal nerve and artery of palm and the common nerve of the digital-palmar side. Each hand has four, eight in total. Indications: Congestion and swelling of the dorsal hand, toothache, malaria, snakebite. Puncture: 1 cm perpendicularly or prick to cause little bleeding. (Fig 8)

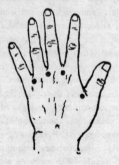

Fig 8

Bazhuixia 八椎下 [bā zhuī xià] An extra point, located on the posterior midline in the depression below the spinal process of the 8th thoracic vertebra. Indication: Malaria. Puncture: 1.5—3 cm obliquely. Moxibustion: 3—5 moxa cones or 5—10 minutes with warming moxibustion.

Beijiazhongjian 背胛中间 [bèi jiǎ zhōng jiān] An extra point, located at the inferior fossa of the scapular bone, i. e., in the cen-

tre of the scapula. Indication: Mania. Puncture: 1—1.5 cm perpendicularly. Moxibustion: 3—5 moxa cones or 5—10 minutes with warming moxibustion.

Beijie 背解 [bèi jiě] An alternate term for Yaoshu (GV 2).

Beinao 背臑 [bèi nào] I. e., Binao (GV 2).

Benshen 本神 [běn shén] A meridian point of Gallbladder Meridian of Foot-*shaoyang*, the confluence of foot-*shaoyang* meridians and Conception Vessel of Yang. Location: 1 dm lateral to Shenting (CV 24), 1.5 cm in the hairline of the midline of the forehead. Indications: Headache, vertigo, stiffness of the neck and nape, pains in the chest and hypochondrium, apoplexy - and unconsciousness, epilepsy, infantile convulsion. Puncture: 1—2 cm horizontally. Moxibustion: 1—3 moxa cones or 3—5 minutes with warming moxibustion.

Beiyangguan 背阳关 [bèi yáng guān] I. e., Yaoyangguan (GV 3).

Benchi 本池 [běn chí] An alternate term for Lianquan (CV 23).

benjie 本节 [běn jié] The round protuberance of the metacarpophalangeal joint or metatarsophalangeal joint. Its anterior part is called the anterior basic segement while its posterior part, the posterior segement.

bi 髀 [bì] 1. Another name of the thigth; 2. the upper half of the thigh.

Bian Que's Miraculous Acupuncture Classic 扁鹊神应针灸玉龙经 [biǎn què shén yìng zhēn jiǔ yù lóng jīng] A medical book written by Wang Guorui in Yuan Dynasty (1271—1360). The book contains Jade Dragon of One Hundred and Twenty Points in Rhythm, Notes to Bianyor Fu. Tianxing Eleven Points in Rhythm, Indications of Sixty-six Points, Secrects of *Panshijin Zhici*, Acupuncture-Moxibustion in Rhythm, and Essentials of Miscellaneous Moxibustion Techniques. It is full of experiences for clinical treatment. It was completed in 1329.

Biandu 便毒 [biàn dú] An extra point, located

at the flexor aspect of the forearm, 12 cm above the transverse crease of wrist, between the long palmar muscle and the radial flexor muscle of wrist. Indication: Enlargement of the inguinal lymph nodes. Puncture: 1.5—3 cm perpendicularly. Moxibustion: 3—5 moxa cones or 5—10 minutes with warming moxibustion.

Biangu 扁骨 [biǎn gǔ] An alternate term for Jianyu (LI 15).

bian **method** 砭法 [biǎn fǎ] A method to press the body surface with a sharp stone or a flat stone or a small piece of porcellain.

Bian Que 扁鹊 [biǎn què] I. e., Qin Yueren, a medical expert during the Warring States Periods. (772—221 B. C.). All ancient famous physicians are called 'Bianque'.

bian **stone** 砭石 [biǎn shí] A medical tool made of stone in ancient China, made of a cone-shaped or edged stone. Used for puncturing the body surface for treating diseases and pain or draining pus and lettintg bleeding.

biao **and** *ben* **of twelve meridians** 十二经标本 [shí èr jīng biāo běn] The locations of the twelve meridians. The six meridians of the hand and foot have their *ben* and *biao* locations. '*Ben*' refers to the location where *qi* of the meridians originates and '*biao*' of the three meridians of hand and foot is located at the head and face, while that of *ben* of the six meridians of hand and foot at the back-*shu* points. *Ben* of the six meridians of hand and foot is generally located below the elbows and knees. Şimilar to *gen* (root) and *jie* (branch). Their connection is comparatively wider. I. e., *gen* refers to the well-like points at the ends of the limbs while *ben* is distal or proximal; *Jie* is at the head, face, chest and abdomen while *biao* reaches at the back-*shu* point, and exceeds the scale of the meridian it pertains to.

biao-ben **of hand-*shaoyang*** 手少阳标本 [shǒu shào yáng biāo běn] One of *biao-ben* of twelve meridians. '*Ben*' of hand-*shaoyang* is located 3 cm between the small finger and ring finger, approx. at Zhongzhu (TE 23) and Yangchi (TE 4) while '*biao*' of hand-shaoyang at the upper corner of the posterior ear and below the outer canthus, approx. at Jiaosun (TE 23) and Tongziliao (GB 1).

Twelve Meridians	Ben	Biao
Foot-*taiyang*	1.5 dm above the heel	
Foot-*shaoyang*	between Qiaoyin	anterior to Chuanglong (ear)
Foot-*yangming*	at Lidui (ST 45)	at Renying (ST 9), cheek along *hansan*
Foot-*taiyin*	1.2 dm anterosuperior to Zhongfu (LU 1)	at back-shu and tongue proper
Foot-*shaoyin*	9 cm above the inferior ankle	at back-shu and sublingual vessel
Foot-*jueyin*	1.5 dm above Xinjian (LR 2)	at back-shu
Hand-*taiyang*	Posterior to the lateral ankle	3 cm above Mingmen (eye)
Hand-*shaoyang*	6 cm above the interspace between the small and ring fingers	at the superior corner of the posterior ear and inferior to the external canthus
Hand-*yangming*	in the elbow bone up to Bieyang	inferior to the cheek
Hand-*taiyin*	at *cunkou* section	in the medial axillary artery
Hand-*shaoyin*	at the end of processous styloid ulnae	
Hand-*jueyin*	in the interspace (6 cm) between two tendons	9 cm below the axilla

biao-ben of hand-*taiyang* 手太阳标本 [shǒu tài yáng biāo běn] One of *biao-ben* of the twelve merdians. "Ben" of hand-*taiyang* meidian is located "in the posterior of the lateral ankle", approx. at Yanglao (SI 6); "*Biao*" is located 3 cm above Mingmen (GV 4)", approx. at Zanzhu (BL 2).

biao-ben of hand-*jueyin* 手厥阴标本 [shǒu jué yīn biāo běn] One of *biao-ben* of the twelve meridians, approx. at Neiguan (PC 6) and Tianchi (PC 1).

biao-ben of foot-*shaoyin* 足少阴标本 [zú shào yīn biāo běn] One of *biao-ben* of the twelve meridians, Approximately at Sanyinjiao (BL 22) or Rangu (KI 2), Lianguan (CV 23).

biao-ben of hand-*shaoyin* 手少阴标本 [shǒu shào yīn biāo běn] One of *biao-ben* of the twelve meridians, approx. at Shenmen (HT 7) and Xinshu (BL 15).

biao-ben of foot-*taiyang* 足太阳标本 [zú tài yáng biāo běn] One of *biao-ben* of the twelve meridians. "*Biao* of foot-*taiyang* is located 5 cm above the heel." "Ben is located between the two eyes."

biao-ben of hand-*taiyin* 手太阴标本 [shǒu tài yīn biāo běn] One of *biao-ben* of the twelve meridians. '*Ben*' of hand-*taiyin* meridian is located at the *cunkou* setion; '*Biao*' is located at the artery in the axilla. Approx. at Taiyuan (EX-HN 5) and Zhonggu.

biao-ben of hand-*yangming* 手阳明标本 [shǒu yáng míng biāo běn] One of the *biao-ben* of the twelve meridians. "*Ben*" of hand-*yangming* meridian is located, approx., at Quchi (LI 11); "*Biao*" is located, approx., Renying (ST 9). '*Biao*' of foot-*jueyin* is at the back *shu* point, approx., at Zhongfeng (LR 4) and Ganshu (BL 18).

biao-ben of foot-*yangming* 足阳明标本 [zú yáng míng biāo běn] One of *biao-ben* of the twelve meridians. '*Ben*' of foot-*yangming* is located at Lidui (ST 450); '*Biao*' of foot-*yangming* is at Renying (ST 9).

biao-ben of foot-*taiyin* 足太阴标本 [zú tài yīn biāo běn] One of *biao-ben* of the twelve meridians. '*Ben*' of foot-*taiyin* is located 12 cm anterosuperior to Zhongfeng (LR 4); '*Biao*' of foot-*taiyin* is located between Backshu and Sheben, approx. at Sanyinjiao (SP 6), Pishu (BL 20) and Lianquan (CV 23).

biao-ben of foot-*shaoyang* 足少阳标本 [zú shào yáng biāo běn] One of *biao-ben* of the twelve meridians. '*Ben*' of foot-*shaoyang* is located between Qiaoyin; '*Biao*' of foot-*shaoyang* is located in front of Chuanglong (in front of the ear, approx., at Tinghui.)

biao-ben of foot-*jueyin* 足厥阴标本 [zú jué yīn biāo běn] One of *biao-ben* of the twelve meridians. '*Ben*' of foot-*jueyin* is 5 cm above Xingjian (LR 2).

biao-ben of six meridians 六经标本 [liù jīng biāo běn] See *biao-ben* of twelve meridians.

Bichuan 鼻穿 [bí chuān] I. e., Shangyingxiang (EX-HN 8).

Bichong 鼻冲 [bí chōng] An alternate term for Qucha (BL 4).

Bieyang 别阳 [bié yáng] 1. Binao (LI 14) that Large Intestine Meridian of Foot-yangming connects with; 2. Another name of Yangchi (TE 4) and of Yingjiao (GB 35).

big collateral of spleen 脾之大络 [pí zhī dà luò] One of the fifteen collateral meridians. The name of its point is Dabao (SP 21). It splites 9 cm below Yuanyue (GB 22) and disappears at the chest and hypochondrium. (Fig 9)

bigu 蔽骨 [bì gǔ] Referring to the xiphoid process of stern.

biguan 髀关 [bì guān] 1. The anteroposterior portion of the thigh; 2. The name of the point Biguan (ST 31).

big yin collateral meridian 大阴络 [dà yīn luò] I. e., the *taiyin* collateral meridian.

big yin meridian 大阴脉 [dà yīn mài] The meridian during the early period. Referring to foot-*taiyin* meridian.

big collateral meridian of stomach 胃之大络 [wèi zhī dà luò] See Xuli.

big elbow tip 大肘尖 [dà zhǒu jiān] Referring to olecranon.

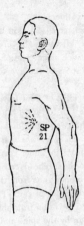

Fig 9

big hollow 大谷 [dà gǔ] Referring to the big hollow appearing between the muscles.

Biguan (ST 31) 髀关 [bì guān] A point of Stomach Meridian of Foot-*yangming*. Location: Directly below the superior spine of the ilium, at the lateral side of the sartorius muscle at the level with the external genitalia. Regional anatomy: At the straight muscle of thigh. The branches of the lateral femoral circumflex artery and vein are in the deeper. The muscular branches of the lateral cutaneous nerve of thigh and the femaral nerve are distributed. Indications: Lumbago, coldness and pain in the knee and legs, foot *qi*, abdominal distension, neurocutaneous inflammation. Puncture: 3—4. 5 cm perpendicularly. Moxibustion: 3—5 moxa cones or 5—10 minutes with warming moxibustion.

big *zhuang* moxibustion 大壮灸 [dà zhuàng jiǔ] I. e., moxibustion with big moxa cone.

Bihuan 鼻环 [bí huán] An extra point. Located at the conjunction between the highest point of the outward protruding spot of anal nasi and face. Indications: Facial deep-rooted sore, brandy nose. Puncture: 1—1. 5 cm horizontally or prick to cause little bleeding with a triangular needle.

bijiao 鼻交 [bí jiāo] I. e., *bi jiao an zhong.*

Bijiaoanzhong 鼻交颏中 [bí jiāo è zhōng] An extra point. Called Bijiao in Science of Chinese Acupuncture. Located by "pressing from the midpoint of the two eyebrows downward along the nose to the depression slightly above the highest nosal bone." Puncture: 0. 9—1. 5 cm horizontally. Indication: Epilepsy, opisthotonos, sudden apoplexy, dreaminess, somnonence, jaundice.

Bijian 臂间 [bì jiān] An abbreviation of Shouzhanghoubijian Point.

Biliu 鼻流 [bí liú] An extra point, located at the opening of the nostril, above Kouhelia (LI 19), in the middle of the right nostril. Indications: Apoplexy, facial paralysis, stuffy nose, nasal discharge, reduced smelling, rhinites, traingualr neuralgia, spasm of masseter. Punctured: 1—1. 5 cm obliquely.

biliary fever 胆热 [dǎn rè] The febrile syndrome of the gallbladder. The main symptoms are distress of the chest and hypochondrium, bitter taste, dry throat, regurgitation of acid, dizziness, blurred vision, deafness, intermittent fever and chills, jaundice, etc.

Binao 臂脑 [bì nǎo] I. e., Binao (LI 14).

Binao (LI 14) 臂臑 [bì nào] A point of Large Intestine Meridian of Hand-*yangming*, also termed Touchong, Jinchong. Location: On the line connecting Quchi (LI 11) and Jianyu (LI 15), 21 cm above Quchi (LI 11) at the inferior edge of the deltoid muscle. Regional anatomy: At the lower end of the deltoid muscle. There are the branches of the posterior humoral circumflex artery and vein and the deep humoral artery and vein. Indications: Scrofula, contracture of the neck, pains in the shoulder and arm, ocular troubles. Puncture: 2. 5—4. 5 cm perpendicularly or obliquely. Moxibustion: 3—5 moxa cones or 5—10 minutes with warming moxibustion.

Binfeng (SI 12) 秉风 [bǐng fēng] A point of

Small Intestine of Hand-*taiyang*, the confluence of hand-*yangming*, hand-*taiyang*, hand-*shaoyang* and foot-*shaoyang* meridians. Location: Directly above Tianzong (SI 11) in the centre of the superior fossa of the spine of scapula. Regional anatomy: In the trapezius muscle and the supraspinous muscle. There is the superior artery and vein of the scapula. The posterior branch of the superior supraclavicular nerve and the accessary nerve are distributed. The suprascapular nerve is in the deeper. Indications: Pain in the scapular region, soreness and numbness of the upper limb. Puncture: 1.5—3 cm perpendicularly. Moxibustion: 3—5 moxa cones or 5—10 minutes with warming moxibustion.

Bingu 膑骨 [bīn gǔ] An alternate term for Huangtiao (GB 30).

bingu 鬓骨 [bìn gǔ] Temple. The area lateral to the orbit and superior to zygomatic arc.

Bishizitou 臂石子头 [bì shí zǐ tóu] An extra point, located at the radial aspect of the flexor side of the forearm, 9 cm above the level with Taiyuan (LU 9). Indication: Jaundice. Moxibustion: 5—7 moxa cones.

bishu 臂俞 [bì shū] 1. The upper most part of the lateral aspect of the thigh where the prominence of femur exists, i.e., the greater trochanter; 2. The acetabulum of the hip joint.

Bitong 鼻通 [bí tōng] I. e., Shangyingxiang (EX-HN 8).

bitterness-relieved pillets 救苦丹 [jiù kǔ dān] The drug used for moxibustion.

Biwuli 臂五里 [bì wǔ lǐ] I. e., Shouwuli (LI 13).

bixingu 蔽心骨 [bì xīn gǔ] I. e., Jiuwei.

Biyan 髀厌 [bì yàn] 1. Referring to the hip joint; 2. referring to Huantiao (GB 30).

Bizhu 鼻柱 [bí zhù] Referring to nose bridge.

Bizhun 鼻准 [bí zhǔn] 1. Referring to the end of nose, also called Zhuntou; 2. Suliao (GV 25).

Bladder 膀胱 [páng guāng] An ear point below the lower crus of antihelix, superior to

Large Intestine.

bladder blockage 胞痹 [bāo bì] A blockage syndrome affecting the bladder characterized by such manifestations as distension and tenderness of the hypochondrium, dysuria, etc.

Bladder Meridian of Foot-*taiyang* (**BL**) 足太阳膀胱经 [zú tài yáng páng guāng jīng] One of the twelve meridians. Called *pang guang zu tai yang zhi mai*. The course: Starting from the inner corner of eye, ascending to the forehead, crossing at the vertex. One branch runs from the vertex to the superficial corner of ear. The vertical one enters into the brain from the vertex, turns back to run by the spine and reaches at the middle waist, enters into the waist and runs along the sinew by the spine to connect with the kidneys and finally disappears in the bladder. The branch at the waist descends from the middle waist, runs by the spine, passes through the hip, enters into the cubital fossa. Another branch at the back descends respectively from the scapular area, passes through the hip joint, then descends along the lateroposterior thigh, joins at the popliteal fossa. Then, it passes through the gastrocnemius muscle, emerges from the posterior lateral ankle, reaches the medial side of the small toe along the tubercurosity of the 5th metatarsal bone (to connect with Kidney Meridian of Foot-*shaoyin*).

blepharoptosis 上胞下垂 [shàng bāo xià cuí] Drooping and inability to raise the upper eyelid.

blister-caused method by application of drugs 敷药发泡法 [fū yào fā pào fǎ] A kind of moxibustion. To make use of certain drugs that are stimulative to the skin to apply the point, so as to get the therapeutic effect, similar to moxibustion. In Zi Sheng Jing it was called 'spontaneous moxibustion.' The prescription is garlic, *ranuncu lus japonicus*, *thumb*, arisaema tuber, castor seed, clematis root (pounded into paste), or white

mustard seed, mylabus (ground into powder, mixed with water). The patient feels
scorching pain and gradual blistering in the
area where the drug is applied. The blistering action of mylabus is strongest while
that of galic is mild. If the duration of the
applied drug is short, congestion and hotness rather than blistering will result. For
treating asthma, Danzhong(CV 17), Dazhui
(GV 14) and Feishu (BL 13) can be applied. For malaria, Neiguan (PC 6) and
Dazhui (GV 14) can be applied. For tonsilitis, Hegu (LI 4) can be applied. For prolonged labor, Yongquan (KI 1) can be applied. After blistering, induce drug application. Attention should be paid to preventing
from being infection.

blockage of five storing viscera 五脏痹 [wǔ
zàng bì]A blockage syndrome, which is refractory to prolonged treatment, progresses
to affect the five storing viscera, and thus,
includes the symptom complex of one of
the five storing viscera.

blockage syndrome 闭证 [bì zhèng] Pain,
swelling and stiffness of muscles or joints,
etc. , due to an invasion of pathogenic cold,
wind, dampness, heat, etc. It is similar to
reheumatic arhritis, rheumatoid arthritis,
etc.

blood blockage 血闭 [xuè bì] A localized
numbness and pain due to a hidrance of circulation of *qi* and blood as caused by a del-
ficiency and weakness of *qi* and blood and
an invasion of pathogenic *qi*.

blood as the mother of *qi* 血为气母 [xuè wéi
qì mǔ] Blood is the material foundation to
produce *qi*, as the mother gives birth to a
child. That is, *qi* must rely on blood to develop its function.

blood collaterals 血络 [xuè luò] Also termed
xuemai. Referring to small veins and arteries. In clinic acupuncture for causing little
bleeding is generally called reducing collaterals.

Blood pressure lowering groove 降压沟 [jiàng
yā gōu] An ear point located at the upper

1/3 of the hollow groove at the lateral edge
of the protruding auricular concha on the
back of ear.

BL points 足太阳膀胱经穴 [zú tài yáng páng
guāng jīng xué] They are Jingming (BL
1), Zanzhu (BL 2), Meichong (BL 3),
Qucha (BL 4), Wuchu(BL 5), Chengguang
(BL 6), Tongtian (BL 7), Luoque (BL
8), Yuzhen (BL 9), Tianzhu (BL 10),
Dazhui (BL 11), Fengmen (BL12), Feishu
(BL 13), Pishu(BL 20), Weishu (BL 21),
Sanjiaoshu(BL 22), Shenshu (BL 23), Qi-
haishu (BL 24), Dachangshu (BL 25),
Guangyuanshu (BL 26), Xiaochangshu (BL
27), Pangguangshu (BL 28), Zhonglushu
(BL 29), Baihuanshu (BL 30), Shangliao
(BL 31), Ciliao (BL 32), Zhongliao (BL
33), Xialiao (BL 34), Huiyang (BL 35),
Fufen (BL 41), Pohu (BL 31), Gaohuang
(BL 43), Shentang (BL 44), Yishi (BL
45), Geguan (BL 46), Hunmen (BL 47),
Yangang (BL 48), Yishe (BL 49), Weicang
(BL 50), Huangmen (BL 51), Zhishi (BL
52), Baohuang (BL 53), Zhibian (BL 54),
Chengfu (BL 56), Chengshan (BL 57),
Weizhong (BL 40), Heyang (BL 55),
Chengjin (BL 56), Chengshan (BL 5),
Feiyang (BL 62), Kunlun (BL 60), Pucan
(BL 61), Shenmai (BL 62), Jingmen (BL
63), Jinggu (source point) (BL 64), Shugu
(stream-like point)   (BL 65), Tonggu
(spring-like point) (BL 66), Zhiyin (well-
like) (BL 67), 67 in total. (Fig 10)

bluish blindness 青盲 [qīng máng] A chronic
ocular trouble with a rather long course.
Visual defect progresses gradually, leading
to blindness without apparent abnormalities of the eyes. Similar to optic atrophy.

bluunt needle 锃针 [tí zhēn] One of the nine
ancient needles. Its body is thick and its tip
is short and sharp. It is often used for vascular and febrile diseases.

bo 膊 [bó] A collective term for the arm and
forearm.

body acupuncture 体针 [tǐ zhēn] A needling
technique for treating diseases by selecting

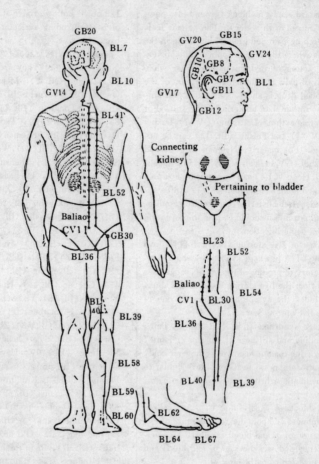

Fig 10

the meridian points or extra points, differing from some needling techniques of local selecting the point, e. g. , auriculo-acupuncture, scalp acupuncture, etc. In clinic there is the selection of the point-selection of body acupuncture, point-selection of auriculo-acupuncture, anesthesia of body acupuncture, anesthesia of auriculoacupuncture, etc.

body bone 体骨 [tǐ gǔ] I. e. , hip bone.

body position 体位[tǐ wèi]The position of the patient's body should take during selecting the point and administering the operation in acupuncture-moxibustion.

body fluids 津液[jīn yè]A collective term for body fluid. That flows outside the body is called 'jīn' while that stores within the body and has the nourishing action is called 'ye'.

body shape 身形[shēn xíng]Referring the external part of the body, often called together with the "limbs".

Bojing 膊井 [bó jǐng] An alternate term for Janjing (GB 21).

bone confluence 骨会 [gǔ huì] One of eight confluential points. The confluence of bone is Dazhu (BL 11), because Dazhu is located by the vertebra, and the vertebra is called *zhugu*. It can be used for treating disturbance of vertebrae, fever due to consumptive disease. Refer eight confluential points.

bone needle 骨针 [gǔ zhēn] A bone needle made of the beast's bone. It was found at Zhoukoudian, Beijing in 1933. According to the textual study it has existed approx. 100,000 years, which explained that at that time the ancients could make the bone needle and possibly use it for treatment of diseases.

bone unit method 骨度法 [gǔ dù fǎ] A main method to locate the meridian point, i. e., to measure the points at various portions by taking 'cun' recorded in Miraculous Pivot as the main reason.

Book of Bian Que's Experiences 扁鹊心书 [biǎn què xīn shū] A medical book written by Dou Cai in Southern Song Dynasty (1276—1279), three volumes. It mainly contains introduction to moxibustion techniques. The 1st volume describes the general rules of treatment and brings out, "In practicing medicine one should know the meridians well", "one must recognize Fuyang (BL 59)"and respectively described Yellow Emperors's moxibustion techniques, Bianque's moxibustion techniques and Dou Cai's moxibustion techniques; The 2nd and 3rd volumes introduced treatment of varieties of diseases and symptoms, and enumerated 22 points, such as Qihai (CV 6), Shimen (CV 5), and Guanyuan (CV 4). It was completed in 1146.

Boyang 脖胦 [bó yāng] An alternate term for Qihai (CV 6).

bundled needles 丛针 [cóng zhēn] Several filiform needles of the same length are bound together with the tips at the same level. It

may be used for superficial acupuncture on the surface of the skin.

brain 脑 [nǎo] Pertaining to the unusual organs, also called the sea of bone marrow, one of the 'four seas.' GV and foot-*taiyang* meridians all connect with brain. Foot-*yangming* meridian "runs along the ocular connection and enters and connects with the brain." Three yang meridians of foot, hand-*shaoyang* meridian and foot-*jueyin* meridian all connect with the ocular connection and communicate with the brain. It is also termed the residence of primordial mind.

Brain stem 脑干 [nǎo gàn] An ear point in the centre of the notch of the helix and tragus.

Brain point 脑点 [nǎo diǎn] An ear point at the top point of the centre of the upper zone.

branch meridians 经别 [jīng bié] See twelve branches meridians.

branch meridian of foot-*shaoyang* 足少阳经别 [zú shào yáng jīng bié] See collateral meridians of foot-*shaoyang* and foot-*jueyin*.

branch meridian of foot-*shaoyin* 足少阴经别 [zú shào yīn jīng bié] See collateral meridians of foot-*taiyang* and foot-*shaoyin*.

branch meridian of foot-*taiyin* 足太阴经别 [zú tài yīn jīng bié] See collateral meridians of foot-*yangming* and foot-*taiyin*.

branch meridian of foot-*jueyin* 足厥阴经别 [zú jué yīn jīng bié] See collateral meridians of foot-*shaoyang* and foot-*jueyin*.

branch meridians of foot-*shaoyang* and foot-*jueyin* 足少阳、足厥阴经别 [zú shào yáng zú jué yīn jīng bié] A pair of the branches of the twelve meridians. The foot-*shaoyang* meridian: Winding the hip, entering into the public region and joining foot-*jueyin* meridian, the branch enters into the hypochondrium, runs along the innter chest and pertains to the gallbladder, distributes itself over the liver, passes through the heart, ascends and runs by the esophagus, emerges from the middle mandible, distributes itself over the face, connects with the ocular connection (connective tissue posterior to the eye) and joins foot-*shaoyang* meridian at the outer canthus. The branch of foot-*jueyin* meridian splits from the dorsal foot, ascends to the pubic region and joins the branch of foot-*yangming* meridian to ascend.

branch meridians of foot-*taiyang* and foot-*shaoyin* 足太阳、足少阴经别 [zú tài yáng zú shǎo yīn jīng bié] A pair of twelve branches of meridian. The branch of foot-*taiyang* meridian: Enters into the cubital fossa, splits from the place 15 cm below sacrum and enters into the anus, pertains to the bladder, distributes itself over the kidneys, ascends along the sinew lateral to the spine, inwardly distributes itself over the heart. The vertical one ascends and emerges from the neck and connects with foot-*taiyang* meridian. The branch of foot-*shaoying* meridian: Splits from the centre of the cubital fossa, runs to join foot-*taiyang* meridians, and ascends to the kidneys, emerges from the 2nd lumbar vertebra, pertains to Girdle Vessel. The vertical one ascends and connects with the tongue proper, then emerges from the neck and joins foot-*taiyang* meridian.

branch meridian of foot-*taiyang* 足太阳经别 [zú tài yáng jīng bié] See branch meridians of Foot-*taiyang* and Foot-*shaoyin*.

branch meridians of foot-*yangming* and foot-*taiyin* 足阳明、足太阴经别 [zú yáng míng zú tài yīn jīng bié] A pair in the twelve meridians. The branch of foot-*yangming* meridians, ascends to the thigh, enters into the abdomen, pertains to the stomach, distributes itself over the spleen, and the esophagus (throat), and emerges from the mouth cavity, ascends to the root of nose, and the inferior eye, connects with the ocular connection (posterior to the eye ball), joins foot-*yangming* meridian. That of foot-*taiyin* meridian, ascends to the thigh, joins that of foot-*yangming* and ascends to-

gether, ascends and connects with the esophagus (throat), and finally passes through the tongue.

branch meridian of foot-*yangming* 足阳明经别 [zú yáng míng jīng bié] See branch meridians foot-*yangming* and foot-*taiyin*.

branch meridian of hand-*shaoyang* and hand-*jueyin* 手少阳、手厥阴经别 [shǒu shǎo yáng shǒu jué yīn jīng bié] A pair of the twelve branch meridians. The branch of hand-*shaoyang* meridian splits from the head, descends and enters into the supraclavicular fossa, runs downward over the upper, middle and lower energizer, and is distributed over the chest. The branch of hand-*jueyin* meridian enters into the chest 1 dm below the axilla, separately pertains to the upper, middle and lower energizer, ascends along the esophagus and emerges from the posterior ear, joins hand-*shaoyang* meridian at Wangu (GB 12).

branch meridians of hand-*taiyang* and hand-*shaoyin* 手太阳、手少阴经别 [shǒu tài yáng, shǒu shǎo yīn jīng bié] A pair of twelve branches of twelve meridians (corresponse), the branch of hand-*taiyang* meridian: Splitting from the scapula, entering into the axilla, running to the heart, and connecting with the small intestine. The branch of hand-*shaoyin* meridian: Entering into the space between the two tendons below the axilla, pertaining to the heart, upward running to esophagus, emerging from the face and joining the inner canthus (hand-*taiyang* meridian).

branch meridian of hand-*taiyang* 手太阳经别 [shǒu tài yáng jīng bié] See branch meridians of hand-*taiyang* and hand-*shaoyin*.

branch meridian of hand-*jueyin* 手厥阴经别 [shǒu jué yīn jīng bié] See the branch meridians of hand-*shaoyang* and hand-*jueyin*.

branch meridian of hand-*taiyin* 手太阴经别 [shǒu tài yīn jīng bié] See branches of hand-*yangming* and hand-*taiyin* meriolians.

branch meridian of hand-*shaoyang* 手少阳经别 [shǒu shào yáng jīng bié] See branch meridian of hand-*shaoyang* and hand-*jueyin*.

branch meridian of hand-*shaoyin* 手少阴经别 [shǒu shào yīn jīng bié] See branch meridians of hand-*taiyang* and hand-*shaoyin*.

branch meridians of hand-*yangming* and hand-*taiyin* 手阳明、手太阴经别 [shǒu yáng míng shǒu tài yīn jīng bié] A pair of branch meridians in the twelve branches of meridians. The branch meridian of hand-*yangming*: Splitting from Jianyu (LI 15), entering into the neck, descending to the large intestine, pertaining to the lungs; Emerging from the supraclavicular fossa, joining hand-*yangming* meridian. The branch meridian of hand-*taiyin*: Splitting from hand-*taiyin* meridian, entering into the axilla, running in front of *shaoyin* meridian, entering into the chest and running to the lungs, distributed over the large intestine; Emerging from the supraclavicular fossa, then joining hand-*yangming* meridian.

branch meridian of hand-*yangming* 手阳明经别 [shǒu yáng míng jīng bié] See branch meridians of hand-*yangming* and hand-*taiyin*.

Branchia 支气管 [zhī qì guǎn] An ear point in Lung Zone at 1/3 of the slightly medial side of Lung Zone.

Branchiectasis 支气管扩张 [zhī qì guǎn kuò zhāng] An ear point located at the lateral 1/3 of Lung Zone.

breaking of needle 断针 [duàn zhēn] Also called *zhe zhen*. During acupuncture the body of the needle is broken in the body, usually caused by injuries of the body of the needle, too strong power used in puncture or sudden change of the position by the patient. So, before acupuncture care should be taken of examining the needle and stress should be laid on preventing of it. For the severe case, it should be taken out by surgical operation.

breast carbuncle 乳痈 [rǔ yōng] The acute suppurative inflammation of the breast, i. e., acute mastitis.

brilliance of the spleen appears externally on the lips 脾其华在唇 [pí qí huá zhài chún] When the spleen functions normally, it provids an adequate source of *qi* and blood. It is brilliantly revealed on the lips.

bronze figure 铜人 [tóng rén] Referring to the bronze model marked with the meridians and points. It was made by Wang Weiyi in 1026. The bronze model is filled with the internal organs internally and is marked with the meridian points (holes) externally, through which the exterior and the interior of the model are communicated. It was made specially for acupuncture teaching.

Budig Point 不定穴 [bú dìng xué] Same with "where there is a pain there is a point", and Ashi Point. Also called Tianying Point.

Buyuan 补元 [bǔ yuán] An alternate term for Tianshu (ST 25).

burning needling 烧针 [shāo zhēn] One of ancient needling techniques, used for exereting pus in carbuncles.

Bulang 步郎 [bù láng] I. e., Bulang (KI 22).

Bulang (KI 22) 步廊 [bù láng] A point of Kidney Meridian of Foot-*shaoyin*. Location: 6 cm lateral to Zhongting (BN 16), at the thoracic midline in the 5th intercostal space. Regional anatomy: Below the greater pectoral muscle. There is the 5th intercostal artery and vein. The anterial cutaneous branch of the 5th intercostal nerve is distributed. The 5th intercostal nerve is in the deeper stratum. Indications: Cough, asthmatic breath, thoracalgia, vomiting, poor appetite, breast carbuncle. Puncture: 1—1. 5 cm obliquely (deep puncture is not advisable). Moxibustion: 3—5 moxa cones or 5—10 minutes with moxibustion.

Burong (ST19) 不容 [bú róng] A point of stomach Meridian of Foot-*Yangming*. Location: 6 cm lateral to Juque (CV, RN 14), 1. 8 dm above the umbilicus. Regional anatomy: At the straight muscle of abdomen. There are the branches of the 7th intercostal artery and vein and the branches of the hypergastric artery and vein. The branch of the 7th intercostal nerve is distributed. Indications: Stomachache, abdominal distension, vomiting, acid regurgitation, poor appetite, digestive ulcer, gastroptosis, colic pain. Puncture: 1. 5—3 cm perpendicularly. Moxibustion: 3—5 moxa cones or 5—10 minutes with warming moxibustion.

C

calculation of acupuncture anesthesia before the operation 针麻术前预测 [zhēn má shù qián yù cè] A term of acupuncture anesthesia. The clinical and experimental observation and anaylysis are made on the patient so as to estimate the effect of acupuncture anesthesia before hand. Besides the analysis on the types of diseases and the focus, the main observation is made on pain threshold, thigmesthesia, the pulse wave of the volume of the finger's vessel, etc., and differentation of the type of syndromes in traditional Chinese medicine and analysis of psychological factor are carried on. By prestimating before the operation the proper case can be conveniently selected and the corresponding measure can be adopted to improve the effect. In general, the favorable effect of acupuncture anesthesia will be obtained by those patients who can tolerate higher pain threshold, or whose pain threshold increase after acupuncture, whose value of touch threshold increased after acupuncture, whose amplitude of pulse wave of the finger was enlarged after acupuncture or that became smaller after a certain volume of pain stimulation was given. The patients' psychological factor, such as the patient's motion, exerts a certain influence upon acupuncture anesthesia. But, it can not play a decisive role.

can-drafting method 拔筒法 [bá tǒng fǎ] I. e., cupping technique.

Caoxiedai Point 草鞋带穴 [cǎo xié dài xué] I. e., Jiexi (ST 41).

Caoxi 曹溪 [cáo xī] An alternate term for Fengfu (GV 16).

cardiac connection 心系 [xīn xì] The frenum of the heart with other storing viscera.

cardiopulmonary stratum 心肺之部 [xīn fèi zhī bù] The division in acupuncture, referring to the superficial stratum (skin and muscle).

cardiac yang 心阳 [xīn yáng] Functional activities of the heart. It is related to the ebb and flow of coldness and heat. If cardiac activities are diminished and accompanied with cold symptoms, it is called deficiency of cardiac yang. If they are excessive and accompanied with heat symptoms, it is called excess of cardiac yang.

calcaneus 跟骨 [gēn gǔ] Same as in Western medicine.

cardiac ying 心营 [xīn yíng] Ying liquids of the heart. It is a component of blood. All of its physopatology are closely related to cardiac blood.

cardiac qi 心气 [xīn qì] Functional activities of the heart.

cantharides 斑蝥 [bān máo] A drug for applying to cause blistering. The dried insect body of Mylabris Phalerata Pallas or Mylabris cichorii L., poisonous. It has the action of strong stimulation to the skin and blistering action. If the area where it is applied is too large, poisonous symptoms such as vomiting, headache, and hypertension appear, it is applied on the point for causing blistering to treat rheumatic blockage and pain, malaria, etc.

cardiac blockage 心痹 [xīn bì] A blockage syndrome, which is refractory to prolonged treatment progresses to involve the heart and thus, includes the symptoms of palpitation, asthma, dry throat, restlessness, easiness to get astonished, etc.

Cardia 贲门 [pēng mén] An ear point at the lower edge of the crus of helix at the crossing point of the middle and medial 1/3 between Mouth and Stomach.

casing-pipe cutaneous needle 套管式皮肤针 [tào guǎn shì pí fū zhēn] A kind of cutaneous needle, cylinder-shaped, with a spring at the upper end, several small needles extend from the small holes at its bottom when it is pressed. It is used for superficially puncturing the skin for treatment. It suits the infants or the one fearing acupuncture.

central *qi* 中气 [zhōng qì] A collective term for the functioning of the spleen and stomach; Sometimes it specifically refers to the functioning of the spleen.

cereal channel 谷道 [gǔ dào] Referring to anus.

Cervical vertebra 颈椎 [jǐn zhuī] An ear point at the protruding spot of the starting part of the antihelix.

***changyang* 昌阳 [chāng yáng]** An alternate term for Fuliu (KI 7).

***changyang* meridian 昌阳之脉 [chāng yáng zhī mài]** Referring to the branch meridian of foot-*shaoyin* meridian at the leg.

cheek 腮 [sāi] Lateral to the mouth, its anterior portion of the cheek forming the wall of the oral cavity.

Changshan 肠山 [cháng shān] An alternate term for Changshan (BL 57).

Changfeng 肠风 [cháng fēng] 1. A name of disease, referring to diarrhea; 2. An extra point located 3 cm lateral to the spinal process of the 2nd lumbar vertebra. Moxibustion: 5 moxa cones. Puncture: 1.5—3 cm perpendicularly.

Changjie 肠结 [cháng jié] I.e., Fujie (SP 14).

Changrao 肠绕 [cháng rǎo] An extra point, just the same with that of Guilai (ST 29) in the location. Indication: Constipation. Moxibustion: with the moxa cone of which the number is the same with that of the patient's age.

Changyi 肠遗 [cháng yí] An extra point. "For constipation, do moxibustion on the point 6 cm to Zhongji (CV 3), called Changyi with the number of moxa cone same as that of the patient' age." (Prescriptions with a Thousand Gold)

Changku 肠窟 [cháng kū] Alternate term for Fujie (SP 14).

Changliao 长髎 [cháng liáo] An alternate term for Erheliao (LI19).

Changping 长平 [cháng píng] 1. An alternate term for Zhangmen (LR 13); 2. I.e., the extra point, Changgu.

***chan* collateral meridians 缠络 [chán luò]** The name of the collateral meridian. Refer collateral meridians.

Changgu 长谷 [cháng gú] An extra point. Also called Xunji, Changping, Xunji, Xunyuan. Located 7.5 cm lateral to Shenque (CV 8). Puncture: 3—4 cm perpendicularly. Moxibustion: 5—7 moxa cones or 10—15 minutes with warming moxibustion.

Changjia 长颊 [cháng jiá] An alternate term for Kouheliao (LI 19).

Chahua 插花 [chā huā] An extra point located at the face, 4.5 cm directly above the hairline of the two corners of the forehead. Indications: Facial deep-rooted sore, migraine. Puncture: 1—1.5 cm horizontally. Moxibustion: 1—3 moxa cones or 3—5 minutes with warming moxibustion.

Changqiang (GV1) 长强 [cháng qiáng] A GV point, the connecting point of GV where the *shaoyin* meridians knots. Also termed Qizhiyinxi, Juegu, Weilu, Xiongzhiyinshu. Located 1.5 cm below the tip of coccyx o at the midpoint between the tip of occcy and anus. Regional anatomy: In the anal tail, there are the branches of the ana artery and vein. The posterior branch of the coccygeal nerve and the anal nerve are distributed. Indications: Diarrhea, dysentery, constipation, hematuria, hemorrhoids, mania, epilepsy, stiff spine, itch in the pubic region, pains in the lumbar, sacral and coccygeal spine. Puncture: Strictly adhering the anterior coccyx, obliquely (perpendicularly puncture would easily injure the rectum), 3 cm. Moxibustion: 3—7 moxa cones or 5—15 minutes with warming moxibustion.

Changxi 长溪 [cháng xī] An alternate term for Erheliao (LI 19).

Chengman (ST 20) 承满 [chéng mǎn] A point of Stomach Meridian of Foot-*yangming*. Location: 6 cm lateral Shangwan (CV 13), 15 cm above the umbilicus. Regional anatomy: In the straight muscle of abdomen. There are the branches of the 7th intercostal artery and vein and the superior epigastric artery and viein. The branch of the 7th intercostal nerve is distributed. Indications: Stomachache, abdominal distension, vomiting, spitting blood, anorexia, firmness and pain below the hypochondrium, borborygmus, asthmatic breath. Puncture: 3—4.5 cm perpendicularly. Moxibustion: 3—5 moxa cones or 5—10 minutes with warming moxibustion.

Cheng Danan (1899—1957) 承淡安 [chéng dàn ān] A contemporary acupuncture expert, born at Jiangyin, Jiangshu Province. After the founding of the People's Republic of China, he was the member of China Science Academy and the Chancellor of Jiangshu Provinical School of Traditional Chinese Medicine. He had been ingaged in acupuncture medical care, teaching and experimental researching over 30 years, and was the chief representative of those that created China Acupuncture Research Institute, Special School of Chinese Acupuncture, Acupuncture Hospital, printed and published the magazine of acupuncture. He once went eastward to Japan to have a textual study on acupuncture medicine. His main works are Treatment of Science of Chinese Acupuncture, Science of Chinese Acupuncture, Essence of Acupucture and Notes to Expounding of Fourteen Meridians, which made certain contributions to popularizing and promoting the development of acupuncture medicine.

Chengguang (BL 6) 承光 [chéng guāng] A point of Baldder Meridian of Foot-*taiyang*. Location: At the midline of head, 7.5 cm into the frontal hairline, then 4.5 cm lateral to it or 4.5 cm posterior to Wuchu (BL 5). Regional anatomy: In galea aponeurotica.

There is the frontal artery and vein and the anastomotic branch of the temporal artery and vein and the occipital artery and vein. The lateral branch of the frontal nerve and the anastomotic branch of the greater occipital nerve are distributed. Indications: Headache, vertigo, vomiting, anxiety, blurred vision, stuffy nose with plenty of nasal discharge, febrile disease with no sweat. Puncture: 1—1.5 cm horizontally. Moxibustion: 1—3 moxa cones or 3—5 minutes with warming moxibustion.

Chengfu (BL 36) 承扶 [chéng fú] A point of Bladder Meridian of Foot-*taiyang*, also termed Rouxi, Yinguan, Pibu. Location: At the inferior edge of the greatest gluteal muscle, at the midpoint of the transverse crease of hip. Regional anatomy: At the inferior edge of the greatest gluteal muscle, between the semimembranous muscle and the biceps muscle of thigh. There is the inferior gluteal artery and the branch of the deep gluteal artery. The inferior cutaneous nerve of hip and the posterior cutaneous nerve of thigh are distributed. The sciatic nerve passes through the deeper stratum. Indications: Stiffness and pain in the lumbar spine, pain in the thigh. Puncture: 3—6 cm perpendicularly. Moxibustion: 3—5 moxa cones or 5—10 minutes with warming moxibustion.

Chengshan (BL 57) 承山 [chéng shān] A point of Blandder Meridian of Foot-*taiyang*, also termed Yufu, Rouzhu, Changshan. Location: Between the belly of the gastricnemius muscle of leg, at the end of the depression of the '人' suture when the tip of foot is straightened by force and the heel is lifted upward. Regional anatomy: At the muscle tendon to which the belly of the gastrocnemius muscle removes. There is the small vein in the superficial stratum and the posterior artery and vein of tibia are in the deeper. The medial cutaneous nerve of calf is distributed. The tibial nerve is in the deeper. Indications: Pains in the waist and back, pain in the leg, charley horse, hemorrhoids, constipation, foot *qi*, epistaxis, epilepsy, hernia, abdominal pain. Puncture: 3—4. 5 cm perpendicularly. Moxibustion: 3—4 moxa cones or 5—10 minutes with warming moxibustion.

Chengming 承命 [chéng mìng] An extra point. Located at the medial side of leg, 9 cm above Taixi (KI 3), posterior to the medial ankle. Indications: Epilepsy, Puffiness of lower limbs. Puncture: 1. 5—3 cm perpendicularly. Moxibustion: 3—7 moxa cones or 5—15 minutes with warming moxibustion.

Cheng **bone** 成骨 [Chéng gǔ] Referring to the place where the small head of fibula approaches the tibia.

Chengling (GB 18) 承灵 [chéng líng] A point of Gallbladder Meridian of Foot-*shaoyang*, the confluence of Foot-*shaoyang* meridain and Connecting Vessel of Yang. Location: Directly above the midline of eye, 12 cm into the hairline, i. e. , 4. 5 cm posterior to Zhengying (GB 17). Regional anatomy: In galea aponeurotica. There are the branches of the occipital artery and vein, and the branch of the greater occipital artery and vein. The branch of the greater occipital nerve is distributed. Indications: Headache, vertigo, ocular pain, rhinitis, epistaxis, obstruction of the nose with plenty of nasal discharge.

Check and Notes to Systematic Classic of Acupuncture 针灸甲乙经校释 [zhēn jiǔ jiá yǐ jīng jiào shì] A book written by Shandong College of Traditional Chinese Medicine, published by People's Health Press in 1979.

Chengjin (BL 56) 承筋 [chéng jīn] A point of Bladder Meridian of Foot-*taiyang*, also termed Ruichang, Zhichang. Location: In the centre of the belly of the gastrocnemius muscle of leg, at the midpoint of the line connecting Heyang (BL 55) and Chengshan (BL 57). Regional anatomy: In the gastrocnemius muscle of leg. There is the small

sephanous vein in the superficial stratum and the posterior artery and vein of tibia in the deeper. The medical cutaneous nerve of calf is distributed. The tibial nerve is in the deeper. Indications: Pain in the legs, soreness and heaviness of the knees, contracture of the waist and back, hemorrhoids, cholera cramp. Puncture: 3—4. 5 cm perpendicularly. Moxibustion: 3—5 moxa cones or 5—19 minutes with warming moxibustion.

Chengqi (ST 1) 承泣 [chéng qì] A point of Stomach Meridian of Foot-*Yangming*, the confluence of Motility Vessel of Yang, CV and Foot-*yangming* meridians, also termed *Xixue*, *Mianliao*. Location: Directly below the midline of eye, between the eyeball of the infraorbital edge. Regional anatomy: In the orbicular muscle of eye. There are the branches of the infraorbital nerve. The inferior branch of the oculomotor nerve and muscular branch of the facial nerve are distributed. Indications: Tremor of eyelids, congestion, swelling and pain in the eyes, lacrimation, night blindness, deviated mouth and eyes. Puncture: Advise the patient to close the eyes, and make the eyeballs upward and slightly fix them, then puncture slowly with the tip of needle along the infraorbital region 1. 5—3 cm. (It is not advisable to puncture deep.)

Chengjiang (CV 24) 承浆 [chéng jiāng] A CV point, the confluence of Foot-*yangming* neridian and CV, also termed *Tianchi*, *Xuanjiang* and *Cuijiang*. Location: At the midline of the face, in the centre of mentolabial sulcus. Regional anatomy: Between the orbicular muscle of mouth and the mentolabial muscle. There is the labial branch of the labial artery and vein. The branches of the facial nerve and of the mentolabial nerve are distributed. Indications: Deviated mouth and eyes, tense lips, swollen face, swollen gum, toothache, hemorrhage of the gums, salivation, emaciation, epilepsy, incontinence of urine. Puncture: 0. 9—1. 5 cm obliquely. Moxibustion: 5—10 minutes with warming moxibustion.

Chenjue 臣觉 [chén jué] An extra point located "At the edge of the upper corner of the scapula, at the end of the middle finger when the two hands are folded." Puncture: 1.5—3 cm obliquely. Moxibustion: 3—5 moxa cones or 5—10 minutes with warming moxibustion.

China Acupuncture Science 中华针灸学 [zhōng huá zhēn jiǔ xué] Originally called Outline of Secrets of Acupunture, compiled by Zhao Erkang. It contains acupuncture, moxibustion, meridian-points and treatment. In the part of meridian-point, detailed textual studies were made on indications of each point besides illustrations; In the part of treament, the therapeutic principles were expounded for the therapeutic method of each disease, and ancient acupuncture empirical prescriptions were selected for reference, published in 1953.

Chinese Acupuncture Science 中国针灸学 [zhōng guó zhēn jiǔ xué] Compiled by Cheng Anru, published by People's Public Health Press in 1955. It is the revised edition of the author's Lecture Notes to Chinese Acupuncture Science, containing acupuncture science, moxibustion science, meridian points science and treatment science, mainly dealing with meridian points and treaments. Diseases and symptoms were compared with those of Western medicine. The past and present achievements were combined for reference.

Chinese honey locust 皂角 [zào jiǎo] One of the interposing things used for moxibustion.

Chinese mugwort 艾 [ài] The drug used for moxibustion, also termed *bintai*, the dried leaves of Artemisia argyi levl. et Vant. (Fig 11)

Chimai (TE 18) 瘛脉 [chì mài] A point of Triple Energizer Meridian of Hand-*shaoyang*, also termed Zimai. Location: At the centre of the styloid process at the

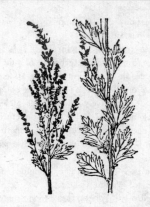

Fig 11

junction of the middle 1/3 and lower 1/3 of the helix line. Regional anatomy: There is the posteroaural artery and vein. The posterior auricular branch of the greater articular nerve is distributed. Indications: Headache, tinnitus, deafness, blurred vision, infantile convulsion, vomiting. Puncture: 1—1.5 cm horizontally. Moxibustion with 1—3 moxa cones or 3—5 minutes with warming moxibustion.

Chizhiwuli 尺之五里 [chí zhī wǔ lǐ] I. e., Shouwuli (LI 13).

Chize (LU 5) 尺泽 [chí zé] A point of Lung Meridian of Hand-*taiyin*, the sea-like (water) point of the meridian. Location: At the radial side of biceps muscle of arm of the transvers crease of the cubital fossa, select it with the elbow slightly flexed. Regional anatomy: At the radial side of biceps muscle of arm and the starting part of the branchial radial muscle. There is the cephatic vein and the radial artery and vein. The lateral cutaneous nerve of foream and the radial nerve are distributed. Indications: Cough, asthmatic breath, hemoptysis, tidal fever, distension and fullness of the chest, spitting suppurative blood, vomiting, sore throat, infantile convulsion, spasm and pain in the elbow and arm. Puncture: 1.5—3 cm perpendicularly. Moxibustion: 5—10 minutes with warming moxibustion.

Chicken-craw-like puncture 鸡足针法 [jī zú zhēn fǎ]A needling technique of puncturing one needle in the centre of the affected regioin once and left and right obliquely, twice respectively, which resembles the chicken's craw. Refer *Hegu* puncture.

china needle 瓷针 [cí zhēn] To puncture the skin to cause little bleeding with a piece of china.

Chitou 池头 [chí tóu] I. e., Shetou, another name of Wenliu (LI 7).

Chongdao 冲道[chōng dào]An alternate term for Guanyuan (CV 11).

Chonggu 崇骨[chóng gǔ]An extra point, also termed Taizhu, Zhuding. Located between the spinal processes of the 6th and 7th cervical vertebrae. Indications: Common cold, cough, malaria, stiff neck, pertussis, epilepsy, bronchitis. Puncture: 1—1.5 cm perpendicularly. Moxibustion: 5—7 moxa cones or 10—15 minutes with warming moxibustion.

Chongmen (SP 12) 冲门 [chōng mén] A point of Spleen Meridian of Foot-*taiyin*, the confluence of foot-*taiyin* and foot-*jueyin* meridians.

Chuan ncedle 篡针[chuàn zhēn]The needling instrument in ancient China.

Chuanglong 窗聋[chuáng lóng] I. e., Classified as another name of Tianchuang (SI 16).

Chuanglong 窗笼 [chuāng lóng] 1. Referring to the aurical region; 2. An alternate term for Tianchuang (SI 16).

Chuanghuang 窗簧 [chuāng huáng] The wrong form of Chuanglong.

Chuanshijiu 传尸灸 [chuán shī jiǔ] The extra point located 9 cm above Jiexi (ST 41) at the anterior spine of the tibia at the extending side of the leg.

Chuanxi point 喘息穴[chuǎn xī xué]An extra point, also termed Dingchuan, Zhichuan. Located 1.5—3 cm lateral to the spinal process of the 7th thoracic vertebra, where

tenderness is obvious. There is the transverse cervical and deep cervical artery and vein. The medial lateral branch of the posterior branch of the 8th cervical nerve is distributed. Indications: 1. 5—3 cm perpendicularly. Moxibustion: 3—5 moxa cones or 5—15 minutes with warming moxibustion.

Chunli point 唇里穴 [chún lǐ xué] An extra point located at the midpoint of the mucoid membrane of the lower lip, opposite to Chengjiang (CV 24). Indications: Juandice, pest, closejaw, foul mouth, swelling and pain in the face and cheek as well as gingivitis, stomachitis. Puncture: 0.3—0.6 cm perpendicularly or to prick to cause blittle bleeding. (Fig 12)

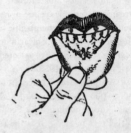

Fig 12

Chongmai point 冲脉穴 [chōng mài xué] 1. A confluential point of Vital Vessel. According to Systematic Classic of Acupuncture, the Vital Vessel (Chongmai) crosses Huiyin (CV 1), Yinjiao (CV 7), Qichong (ST 30) of foot-*yangming* meridian. Henggu (KI 11), Dahe (KI 12), Siman (KI 14), Zhongzhu (TE 3), Huangshu (KI 6), Shanggu(KI 17), Shiguan(KI 18), Yidu (KI 19), Tonggu (KI 20) and Youmen (KI 21); 2. referring to Gongsun (SP 4), "Gongsun is communicated with Vital Vessel, on the eight confluential points."

Chongyang (ST 42) 冲阳 [chōng yáng] 1. A point of Stomach Meridian of Foot-*yangming*, the source point of the meridian, also called Huiyan. Location: At the pulsation of the dorsal artery of foot, directly opposite to the interspace of the 2nd metatarsal bone at the highest point of the dorsal foot or 4 cm below Jiexi (ST 41). Regional anatomy: At the medial long extensor muscle of the toe, reaching at the short extensor muscle of the great toe. There is the dorsal artery and vein of foot and the dorsal vein network of foot. The superficial and deep peroneal nerves and the medial dorsal cutaneous nerve of foot are distributed. Indications: Stomachache, abdominal distension, deviated mouth and eyes, swollen face and toothache, weakness of foot, swollen dorsal foot, easiness to be frightened and mania. Puncture: 1—1.5 cm perpendicularly. (avoid the artery). Moxibustion: 3—5 minutes with moxa cone; 2. Another name of Yingxiang (LI 20); 3. Quchi (LI 11).

chopstick-like needle 箸针 [zhǔ zhēn] Referring to puncture with a bamboo chopstick used for causing little bleeding and fire needle.

Chronic blockage 远痹 [yuǎn bì] A blockage syndrome refractory to prolonged treatment.

chronic infantile convulsion 慢惊风 [màn jīn fēng] The infantile convulsion with gradual onset. It is manifested by slightly cyanotic complexion, listlessness, somnolence, slow intermittent convulsion of four limbs, seaphoid abdomen, cold clammy limbs, shallow breath, deep, small and weak pulse, etc.

Chuanbi 穿鼻 [chuān bí] I. e., Shangyingxiang (EX-HN 8).

Chuaichang 踹肠 [chuài cháng] I. e., Chuaichang, an alternate term for Chengjiang (CV 24).

Clavicle 锁骨 [suǒ gǔ] An ear point located at the lower end of the saphoid fossa at the level with Heart.

cloth-interposed moxibustion 实按灸 [shí àn jiǔ] A kind of moxibustion with a moxa stick contrary to hovering moxibustion. After igniting a moxa stick, press it on the point that is interposed by several strata of

cloth or paper, to make heat penetrate through the skin and muscle; and again ignite it to press it after fire disappears and heat is reduced. Each point can be pressed several or over ten times. (Fig 13)

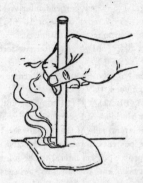

Fig 13

Classified Classic 类经 [lèi jīng] A medical book written by Zhang Jiebing in Ming Dynasty (1368—1644), 32 volumes in total. The book divided Plain Questions and Miraculous Pivot into health preservation, yin-yang, visceral symptoms, pulse indications, meridians, *biao-ben*, flavor, treatments, diseases, acupuncture, *qi* movement, etc., and noted them comparatively minutely. Later he continued to write Supplementary Illustrations (11 volumes) and Appendix (4 volumes), which were completed in 1642 and is an important reference book for research on Internal Classic.

Classic of Man's Mirror 人镜经 [rén jìng jīng] A medical book. The complete name is Classic and Treatment of Viscera Compiled by Wang Zongquan in Ming Dynasty (1368—1644), 8 volumes. Compiled according to the sequence of the four meridians, collecting ancient literatures with the prescriptions and drugs and illustrations. Later Qian Lei added the Appendix, and Zhang Jingying added the Continuous Appendix and brought out the new concepts of the *chanluo*, *xiluo* and *sunluo*, etc.

Cigong 慈宫 [cí gōng] 1. An alternate term for Chongmen (SP 12); 2. An extra point, located 7.5 cm lateral to the midpoint of symphysis pubis. Indications: Diarrhea, dysentery, irregular menstruation. Puncture: 1.5—3 cm perpendicularly. Moxibustion: 5—7 moxa cones or 10—15 minutes with warming moxibustion.

Chiya 齿牙 [chǐ yá] An alternate term for Jiache (ST 6).

Cimen 次门 [cì mén] An alternate term for Guanyuan (CV 4).

Ciliao (BL 32) 次髎 [cì liáo] A point of Bladder Meridian of Foot-*taiyang*. Location: On the lateral side of the medial sacral crest in the posterior foramen of the 2nd sacrum, approx. 2.5 cm lateral to the inferior edge between the pseudospinal process of the 2nd sacral vertebra. Regional anatomy: There are the posterior branches of the lateral sacral artery and vein. The posterior branch of the 2nd sacral nerve is distributed. The 2nd posterior sacral foramen is below. Indications: Lumbago, leukorrhea, irregular menstruation, dysmenorrhea, spermatorrhea, impotence, abnormal micturition and defecation. Puncture: 3—4 cm perpendicularly. Moxibustion: 3—7 moxa cones or 5—15 minutes with warming moxibustion.

Cirrhosis Zone 肝硬化区 [gān yìn huà qū] An ear point located appearing in the centre of Hepatomegaly Zone.

cixue bagua 刺血拔罐 [cì xué bā guàn] An alternate term for *ciluo baguan*.

Classified Collection of Yellow Emperor's Internal Classic 黄帝内经明堂类成 [huáng dì nèi jīng míng táng lèi chéng] A medical book also called Huangdi Neijing Mingtang, written and noted by Yang Shangshan in Sui and Tang dynasties (581—907A. D.). It is mainly to classify and note *Mingtang* Points in ancient China under the guide line of the twelve meridians and eight extra meridians. One volume for the twelve meridians, another for the eight extra

meridians, 13 volumes in total. Only one volume dealing with Lung Meridian of Hand-*taiyin* has been preserved. It is a book dealing with a textual study on the points according to the meridians during the early period.

Classic of Experiences of Acupuncture on Treatment 针灸资生经 [zhēn jiǔ zī shēng jīng] A book written by Wang Zhizhong in Southern Song Dynasty (1127—1274), divided into 7 volumes. The 1st records the points on the whole body; The 2nd one generally describes acupuncture-moxibustion techniques; The 3rd—7th ones respectively describes selection and treatment of diseases and symptoms of various specialties. It collects acupuncture literatures in the previous dynasties, has a textual study on the points of the human body, and adds some extra points. It stresses the introduction to moxibustion techniques, and advocates accessary treatment of formulary drugs, records acupuncture treatment for 195 diseases, appended with a lot of therapeutic experiences. The original was once corrected by Wei Shijie and published in 1220.

Collected Book of Acupuncture 针灸集书 [zhēn jiǔ jí shū] A book written by Yang Xun in Ming Dynasty (1368—1644), completed in 1515. The 2nd volume of the Korean edition is still preserved.

Collection of Acupuncture 针灸集成 [zhēn jiǔ jí chéng] A book compiled by Liao Runhong in Qing Dynasty (1644—1911), 4 volumes. Originally called *Mian Xue Tang Zhen jiu Ji cheng*. The first two volumes are called Collection of Acupuncture, the second two volumes are called Detailed Collection of Acupuncture. It was first published in 1874.

Collection of Gems in Acupuncture 针灸聚英 [zhēn jiǔ jù yīng] A book written by Gao Wu in Ming Dynasty (1368—1644), also called *Zhenjiu Jiying Fahui*, divided into 4 volumes. The 1st volume records the viscera, meridians and *shu* points; the 2nd selection of points and treatment of various diseases; the 3rd acupuncture-moxibustion techniques; the 4th varieties of rhythmed articls. The whole book-is based on Internal Classic and Difficult Classic, combines with clinical practice. It was completed in 1529.

code of the name of the point 穴名代号 [xué míng dài hào] Referring to denoting the names of the meridian points with abbreviation and the numbers of sequence. In general, the points are denoted by the name of meridian plus the number order. It has been widely used in acupuncture books and journals in Europe and USA. As the sequence of the meridian points' arrangement is somewhat different, they must be further unified, and their unification should be further searched.

cold from within the body 寒从中生 [hán cóng zhōng shēng] The pathologic changes of the substancial cold caused by the impairment of visceral functions.

cold blockage 寒闭 [hán bì] A blockage syndrome caused by a relative excess of pathogenic cold with characteristics of agonizing and well-localized pain of the limbs and the body, relief by heat and aggreviation by cold.

cold induces contraction 寒则气收 [hán zé qì shōu] The damaging effects of pathologic cold may induces closure of the papillae and blood vessels, resulting in pathogenic manifestations of contraction and retraction.

cold injures the structure while heat injures *qi* 寒伤形热伤气 [hán shāng xíng rè shāng qì] The external pathogenic cold injures mostly the external structure of the body first, producing symptoms of headache, chilly sensation, aching of the limbs, etc. The external pathogenic heat tends to dissiate yang *qi* of the body, producing symptoms of profuse sweating, fatigue, weakness, etc.

collateral meridians 络脉 [luò mài] The branch splitted from the meridian. They are

fifteen collateral meridians, grandson collateral meridians, blood collateral meridians, floating collateral meridians, etc., recorded in Internal Classic.

collateral meridian of hand-*taiyin* 手太阴络脉 [shǒu tài yīn luò mài] One of the fifteen collateral meridians. Its point is Lieque (LU 7), starting from 4.5 cm above the wrist, between the skin and muscle, entering into the palm together with hand-*taiyin* meridian, distributed over *Yuji* (dorsopalmar boundary), splitting and running over hand-*taiyin* meridian. In case it is excess, feverish sensation in the palms occurs, in case it is deficiency, enuresis and frequent urination result.

collateral meridian of hand-*shaoyang* 手少阳络脉 [shǒu shào yáng luò mài] One of the fifteen collateral meridians. Its point is Waiguan (TE 5). It outwardly winds the arm and joins the hand-*jueyin* meridian. "Spasmodic elbow occurs in case it is in excess; the elbow can not flex and extend in case it is in deficiency." (Miraculous Pivot)

collapse syndrome 脱证 [tuō zhèng] The pathologic manifestations of the terminal stage of a disease due to extreme loss of yin, yang, *qi* and blood, such as profucse sweat, cold and clammy limbs, mouth opened and eyes closed, incontinenece of stool and urine, barely palpable pulse, etc. Acupuncture point prescription: Shuigou (GV 26), Suliao (GV 25), Shenque (CV 8), Guanyuan (LI 1), Zusanli (ST 36).

collateral meridian of hand-*jueyin* 手厥阴络脉 [shǒu jué yīn luò mài] One of the fifteen collateral meridians. Its name is Neiguan (PC 6). It emerges between the two tendons, 6 cm above the wrist, ascends along the meridian and connects with the pericardium, disappears at the cardiac connection. According to Miraculous Pivot, in case it is overactive, cardialgia may result; in case it is weak anxiety may result.

collateral meridian of foot-*taiyin* 足太阴络脉

[zú tài yīn luò mài] One of the fifteen collateral meridians. The name of its point is Gongsun (SP 4). It splits from the area 3 cm posterior to the 1st segement of the great toe, runs to foot-*yangming* meridian. One branch ascends to the abdomen, decentralizes over and connects with the intestine and abdomen.

collateral meridian of foot-*jueyin* 足厥阴络脉 [zú jué yīn luò mài] One of the fifteen collateral meridians. The name of its point is Ligou (ST 45). It splits from the place 5 cm above the medial ankle, runs to foot-*shaoyang* meridian. One branch runs along the meridian to the testes, knots at the penis.

collateral meridian of foot-*yangming* 足阳明络脉 [zú yáng mīng luò mài] One of the fifteen collateral meridians. The name of its point is Fenglong (ST 40). It splits from the place 1 cm above the lateral ankle, runs to foot-*taiyin* meridian. One branch ascends along the lateral side of tibia and distributes itself over the head and nape, meets *qi* in various meridians. Its lower part distributes itself over the Adam's Apple.

collateral meridian of foot-*taiyang* 足太阳络脉 [zú tài yáng luò mài] One of the fifteen collateral meridians. The name of its point is Feiyang (BL 58). It splits from the place 21 cm above the lateral ankle, running to foot-*shaoyin* meridian.

collateral meridian of foot-*shaoyang* 足少阳络脉[zú shào yáng luò mài]One of the fifteen collateral meridians. The name of its point is Guangming (GB 37). It splits from the place above the lateral ankle, runs to foot-*jueyin* meridian and its lower part spreads over and connects with the dorsal foot.

collateral puncture 络刺 [luò cì] It refers to letting little bleeding by puncturing the collateral meridian, contrary to puncturing the meridian.

collateral meridian of hand-*shaoyin* 手少阴络

脉 [shǒu shào yīn luò mài] One of the fifteen collateral meridians. Its point is Tongli (HT 5), spliting and ascending from the point 3 cm above the wrist, entering into the heart along the meridian, connecting with the tongue proper, pertaining to the ocular connection. Its branch runs to hand-*taiyang* meridian. According to Miraculous Pivot, in case it is overactive, obstruction and discomfort at diaphragm results, in case it is weak, aphasia results.

collateral meridian of hand-*taiyang* 手太阳络脉 [shǒu tài yáng luò mài] One of the fifteen collateral meridians. Its point is Zhizheng (SI 7). It joins the hand-*shaoyin* collateral meridian at the place 1.5 dm above the wrist; its branch ascends along the elbow, and connects with Janyu (LI 15). According to Miraculous Pivot, "In case it is overactive, debility of elbow may occur; in case it is weak, wart may appear."

collateral meridean of hand-*yangming* 手阳明络脉 [shǒu yáng mīng luò mài] One of the fifteen collateral meridians. The name of its points is Pianli (LI 6). Its collateral splits from 9 cm above the wrist. One branch runs to hand-*taiyin* meridian; the other ascends along the arm to the corner of mandible, and distributes itself over teeth; the other enters into the ear and meets the assembled vessel. "In case it is overactive, dental carrier and deafness result; in case it is weak, cold teeth would result."(Miraculo)

collateral *shu* 络俞 [luò shū] Referring to the point of the floating colateral meridian, used for letting little bleeding.

combination of the five *shu* points 五腧配穴法 [wǔ shū pèi xué fǎ] One of point-combined methods. The method of appling the combination of the well-like, spring-like, stream-like, river-like and sea-like points, including combination of the five *shu* points for their main indications, maternal-offspring, reinforcing-reducing, reducing south and reinforcing north, midnight-noon ebb-flow.

Compilation of Textual Study on the Points a-long the Meridians 循经考穴编 [xún jīng kǎo xué biān] A book, two volumes. Origi-nally it was a copy. Its contents are in se-quence of the Fourteen Meridians, appen-ded with the contents of the eight extra meridians of illustrations of the viscera.

congmao 丛毛 [cóng máo] The place proximal to the terminal phalanx of the big toe.

Constipation point 便秘点 [biàn mì diǎn] An ear point located near the middle segment of the lower crus of the helix, superomedial to Sciatic point.

contrary treatment 反治 [fǎn zhì] The remedy coincides with the false symptoms of the disease, contrary with remedy for the heat symptoms. Actually it is directed to the cold nature of the disease itself.

contralateral puncture 交经缪刺 [jiāo jīng miù cì] The needling technique by selecting the point on the right side of the body for the trouble on the left side and that at the left for that on the right.

confusion of mind by phlegm 痰迷心窍 [tán mí xīn qiào] The pathologic changes of un-consciousnes and mental confusion as caused by phlegm. The main symptoms are disorientation, coughing with rales, coma, chest distress, whitish glossy coating of tongue, slippery pulse, etc.

constipation 便秘 [biàn mì] It denotes that the patients stools are dry, firm and can hardly be excreted.

confluence of emptying viscera 腑会 [fǔ huì] One of the eight confluential points. "The confluence of emptying viscera is Zhong-wan (CV 12). It is therefore called because Zhongwan (CV 12) is the anterior referred point of the stomach which holds food and is the head of the six emptying viscera. In clinic it can be used for treating gasstroen-testinal disorders.

congestion, swelling and pain of the eyes 目赤肿痛 [mù cì zhǒng tòng] An acute symptom of various ocular troubles, popularly called

red eyes or fire eyes.

cone-shaped needle 角针 [jiǎo zhēn] Made of plastic, bakelite or metal, cone-shaped, re-sembling a small moxa cone. Its height and diameter to the buttum are all 0.3 cm. While using it, press the tip of it on the point, and make its buttum at the level with the skin, then fix it with ruberrized cloth. Its usage is similar to subcutaneous needle.

convulsive symptom complex 痉证 [jìn zhèng] A disease mainly manifested by stiff neck and back, lockjaw, contracton of four limbs and opisthotonons. Acupuncture point prescription: Baihui (GV 20), Fengfu (GV 16), Dazhui (GV 14), Quchi (LI 11), Yongquan (KI 1), Taichong (LR 3) for the case due to injury of yin by high fever, Quze (PC 3), Laogong (PC 8), Weizhong (BL 40), Xingjian (LR 2). For the case due to invasion of heat in *Ying* and blood.

Connecting Vessel of Yang 阳维脉 [yáng wéi mài] One of the eight extra vessels, parallel with Connecting Vessel of Yin. It ascends below the lateral malleolous and travels a-long the lateral aspect of the lower limb, the lateral aspect of the abdomen and the chest to the shoulder and the posterior part of the cheek, and terminates in the vertex of the head. When it is diseased, there may appear such symptoms as chilliness and fever. (Fig 14)

contralateral puncture 巨刺 [jù cì] One of nine needling techniques. When a disease occurs on one side (left or right) of the body, the points on the opposite side (right or left) are punctured. It is mainly indicated in: 1. the unilateral side; 2. Affection of a meridian. In clinic sequela of apaoplexy, sciatica, etc., are treated by selecting crossing punc-ture of the point on the healthy side.

cold needling 冷针 [lěng zhēn] Different from warming needling, referring to simple acupuncture.

cold moxibustion 冷灸 [lěng jiǔ] Contrary to hot moxibustion, also called "non-heat mo-xibustion". It generally refers to the moxi-

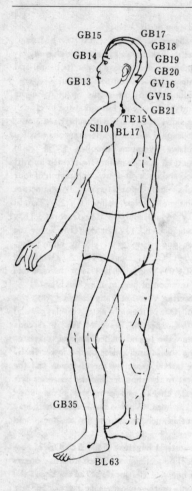

GB15 GB17
GB14 GB18
GB13 GB19
GB20
GV16
GV15
GB21
TE15
SI10 BL17

GB35

BL63

Fig 14

bustion treatment by applying the drugs but without any heat source.

cold syndrome 寒证 [hán zhèng] The symptoms and signs caused by an invasion of pathogenic cold, or a deficiency of yang *qi* and excess of yin *qi* leading to hypofunction and reduced metabolism of the body, for example, abnormal temprature, pale complexion, listlessness, curling up to sleep, intolerance to cold, epigastric and abdominal pain relievable by hot compress, no thirst, or thirst with predilection for hot drinks, loose, stools, copious pale urine, pale toungue with whithish mucoid coating, deep slow pulse, etc. It is frequently seen in chronic and hypofunctional diseases.

collateral *qi* 络气 [luò qì] Referring *qi* flowing in the collateral meridians, contrast to meridianal *qi*.

Collection of Selecting Dates for Acupuncture-Moxibustion 针灸择日编集 [zhēn jiǔ zé rí biān jí] A book jointly compiled by Quan Xunyi and Quan Yisun in Ming Dynasty (1368—1644). It mainly records the data concerning acupuncture in the acupuncture books before Ming Dynasty and compares them and ascertains whether acupuncture can be administered or not according to the heavenly stems and earthly branches. It was completed in 1447.

Collection of Digest of Acupuncture Classic 针经摘英集 [zhēn jīng zhāi yīng jí] A book compiled by Du Siyuan in Yuan Dynasty (1271—1368), originally recorded in the 3rd volume of *Jishen Bacui*. It adapted nine ancient needling techniques, measurement of *shu* points, reinforcing and reducing methods, as well as therapeutic methods of 69 diseases. It is mostly from the predecessors' acupuncture books with descriptions and prescriptions. It was published in 1315.

cool like a clear sky night 透天凉 [tòu tiān liáng] An acupuncture manipulation, contrary to setting the mountain on fire. The synthetical application of reducing manipulation of acupuncture. The operation is carried on according to the superficial, middle and deep strata (first insert the needle into the deep stratum and swiftly lift and slowly thrust the needle or twirl the needle) with the number of times of six. Then withdraw the needle to the middle stratum and the superficial, and operate it just the same. It is called one time after finishing the operation sequentially from the deep to the middle to the superficial. It can also be inserted into the deep and repeated several times. Some of the patients can generate cool sensation, and it suits febrile diseases. (Fig 15)

collateral points 络穴 [luò xué] The fifteen collateral meridians have one each, totally 15, plus the big collateral point of stomach, Xuli, there are toatlly 16, of which the collateral points of the twelve meridians have the action of communicating *qi* and blood in the superficial and deep meridians. They are clinically used for treating the superficial disease that has got deep and the deep disease that gets superfical and the simultaneous disease of the superficial and deep regions; CV, GV and the big collateral point of spleen have the action of communicating and regulating *qi* and blood in the anterior, posterior and lateral parts of the trunk. It can be clinically used for treating diseases or symptoms of the abdomen, back and hypochondriac region.

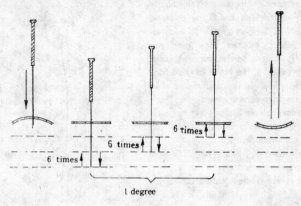

Fig 15

Collateral Points on the Upper limbs		Collateral Points on the Lower Limbs		Collateral Points on the Trunk
Deep	Supperficial	Deep	Superficial	
Hand-*Taiyin* Liegue (Lu 7)	Hand-*yangming* Fianli (LI 6)	Foot-*Taiyin* Gongsun (SP 4)	Foot-*yangming* Fenglong (ST 40)	CV Collateral Jiuwei (CV 15)
Hand-*shaoyin* Tongli (HT 5)	Hand-*Taiyang* Zhizhen (SI 7)	Foot-*shaoyin* Dazhong (KI 4)	Foot-*Taiyang* Feiyang (BL 58)	GV Collateral Changqiang (GV1)
Hand-*Jueyin* Neiguan (PC 6)	Hand-*shaoyang* Waiguan (TE, 5)	Foot-*Jueyin* Ligou (LR 5)	Foot-*shaoyang* Guangming (GB 37)	Big collateral Dabao (SP 21)

collateral meridian of same yin 同阴之脉 [tóng yīn zhī mài] The branch collateral of foot-*taiyang* meridian at the leg. The collateral of the same yin is located at the lower end of fibula.

collateral of pericardium 心包络 [xīn bāo luò] The external membrane is called the pericardium, the collaterals appending to it is called the collateral of pericardium, the function of which is to externally protect the heart, and carry on the function instead of the heart. The hand-*jueyin* meridian "pertains to the pericardium collateral", while the hand-*shaoyang* meridian distributes itself over the pericardium". In clinic, mental confusion, etc. caused by high fever are called pathogenic *qi* entering into the pericardium. Its back-*shu* point is Jueyinshu (BL 14) and its anerior-referred point is Danzhong (CV 17).

Comprehensive Notes to Yellow Emperor's Internal Classic 黄帝内经太素 [huáng dì nèi jīng tài sù] A medial book briefly termed *Taisu* compiled and noted by Yang Shangshan during the Sui and Tang dynasties (581—907 A. D.), originally 30 volumes. Twenty three volumes have been preserved. It is the handed-down book during the early period of the noted Internal Classic. It has preserved the original face of Internal Classic to certain extent.

concave bronze mirror 阳燧 [yáng suì] The concave bronze mirror used for getting fire, used to ignite mugwort.

connecting collateral 系络 [xì luò] The name of the collateral meridian.

connecting *qi* and communicating the meridian 接气通经 [jiē qì tōng jīng] The time needed for applying acupuncture manipulation was speculated according to the times of respiration according to different lengths of the meridians in ancient China. For example, three yang meridains of hand are 1. 6 m in length, the time for needling must be 9 breaths; Three yang meridians of foot are 2. 4 m in length, the time for needling must be 14 breaths, to make it exceed the length of the meridian 1. 2 m, so as to make meridian *qi* flow freely and connected.

confluence of vessel 脉会 [mài huì] One of the eight confluential points. Taiyuan (LU 9) is called the confluence of vessel because it is the source point of hand-*taiyin* meridian and is located at the *cunkou*, artery and all vessels meet at the lung. It is clinically used for treating cardialgia, retarded pulse, no -pulse symptoms, etc.

Conception Vessel (CV) 任脉 [rèn mài] One of the eight extra meridians. The course: Starting from the inner small abdomen ascending from the public region along the central part of the abdomen, passing through the throat, mandible, connectting with the lower lips, entering into the infeirior parts of the two eyes. Then ascending to connect with GV, and foot-*yangming* meridian, communicating with Vital Vessel, and joining the three yin meridians anteriorly (Fig 16)

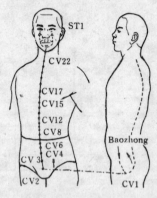

Fig 16

confluential points 交会穴 [jiāo huì xué] The *shu* point where the two or over two meridians pass through, briefly called *hui xue*. Most of them are distributed over the head, face, and trunk. In general one yang meridian and the other mridian converse the yin one and the other meridian converses; the yang one converses GV, the yin one converses CV, Vital Vessel, Girdle Vessel, Motility Vessel of Yin and Connecting Vessel of Yang all converse with the fourteen meridians. Their therapeutic actions are comparatively wide, e. g. , the confluential point of three yin meridians can treat the diseases or syndromes concerning spleen meridian, kidney meridian and liver meridian.

Complete Acupuncture-Moxibustion 针灸全生 [zhēn jiǔ quán shēng] A book compiled by

Xiao Fuan in Qing Dynasty (1644—1911), two volumes, also called *Tongren Mingtang Zhenjiu*. It first records the illustrations and rhythmed articles of the meridian points and the points of the fourteen meridians of the whole bldy and then records the selection of acupuncture for various diseases and symptoms. It is simple and essential in contents and was completed in 1824.

Compendium of Acupuncture-Moxibustion 针灸大成 [zhēn jiǔ dà chéng] A book compiled by Yang Jizhou in Ming Dynasty (1368—1644). It was divided into 10 volumes. The first volume collects the original of Internal Classic and Difficult Classic concerning acupuncture-moxibusion theories, and notes them; The 2nd and 3rd ones, collects rhythmed acupuncture articles and test papers; The 4th deals with acupuncture techniques; The 5th deals with five *shu* points, mid-night-noon ebb-flow and eight miraculous turtle methods; The 6th and 7th ones deal with meridians, meridian points and extra points; The 8th, various syndromes treated by acupuncture; The 9th deals with famous doctors' acupuncture techniques and Yang's general line of treating symptoms and medical records (1556—1580); The 10th appended with Chen's Infantile Massage Classic. It generalizes the achievements of acupuncture science before Ming Dynasty (1368—1644), and was treanslated into foreign languages, and spread widely. It is a famous book of acupuncture science and was first published in 1601.

Complete Book of Acupuncture-Moxibustion 针灸大全 [zhēn jiǔ dà quán] A book compiled by Xu Feng in Ming Dynasty (1368—1644), also called *Zhenjiu Jiefa*, *Zhenjiu Jiefa Daquan*. It chiefly collects the rhythmed acupuncture articles of various schools, divided into six volumes. The 1st volume contains the rhythmed articles of famous acupuncture experts; The 2nd notes *Biao You Fu*; The 3rd, Meridian Points of Different divison in Rhythim; The 4th deals with eight methods flow; The 5th deals with gold needle and midnight-noon ebbflow; The 6th contains miscelllaneous descriptions of acupuncure-moxibustion. It was completed in the fifteen century and exerts a great influence upon the development of acupuncture-moxibustion.

composition of the points of the meridians with the same names 同名经配穴法 [tóng míng jīng pèi xué fǎ] One of the point-composed methods. Referring to the simultaneous application of the points pertaining to the meridians of hand and foot with the same name. E. g. , the hand-*taiyin* and foot-*taiyin* meridians, the hand-*yangming* and foot-*yangming* meridians, etc. , which are connected one another, and have the cooperative action in treatment. E. g. , for toothache, Hegu (LI 4) of the hand-*yangming* meridian is selected. It originated from the theory of the connection of the hand and foot meridians with the same name together with selection of the point from the connected meridians. The latter refers that the points of the meridians with the same name can be used each other i. e. , for the disorder of the foot meridian the point of the hand meridian is selected and that of the hand meridian, that of the foot meridian is selected. But, the former refers that the points of the meridians with the same name can be used cooperatively.

contrary selection 气反 [qì fǎn] It refers that the location of the point selected is contrary to that of disease, "*Qifan* means to select the point at the lower part of the body for the disease at the upper; to select the point at the upper for the disease at the lower; to select the point on the lateral side for ther disease on the central. " (Internal Classic)

Connecting Vessel of Yin 阴维脉 [yīn wéi mài] One of the eight extra vessels, parallel with Connecting Vessel of Yang. Starting from Zubin (KI 9) of foot-*shaoyin* meridian, the gap-like point to it, which is located in the 15 cm above the medial ankle; Ascending along the medial aspect of thigh, again ascending to enter into the lower abdomen, joining foot-*taiyin*, foot-*jueyin* and foot-*shaoyin* meridians at Fushe(SP 13), ascending continuously to join foot-*taiyin* meridian at Daheng (SP 15), foot-*jueyin* and Fuai (SP 16), running along the hypochondrium to meet foot-*jueyin* meridian at Qimen (LR 14); Ascending to the diaphragm, running by the throat, and finally meeting CV at Tiantu (CV 22) and Lianguan (CV 23). (Fig 17)

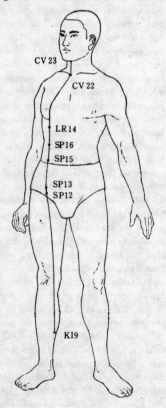

Fig 17
Connective Compilation of Meridians 经络汇

编 [jīng luò huì biān] A book written by Qu Liang during Ming and Qing dynasties. (1368—1911). It was based on Textual Study on Meridians and its contents are arranged according to the sequence of the fourteen meridians and connect with and describe the viscera, meridians and their points. And it is also appended with the figures of the viscera, meridians, and the rhythmed articles and the treatise on the eight extra vessels. It was completed in 1626.

couple puncture 偶刺 [ǒu cì] One of the tewelve needling techniques used for treating precordial pain(angina pectoris). It consists of palpating the painful areas of the chest and the corresponding area of the back, puncturing these areas obliquely with one needle each. But, care must be taken to avoid perpendicular and deep acupuncture causing damages to the viscera. In clinic for the disorders of the internal organs the anterior referred points of the chest and abdomen and back *shu* points are used cooperatively.

cough 咳嗽 [ké sòu] One of the commonly seen clinical symptoms of the respiratouy system. It may be caused by external affection and internal injury, cough due to external affection. 1. 1)Wind-cold type;Liequee, 2) Wind-heat type: Chize (LU 5), Kongzui (LU 6); 2. Deficiency syndrome, Dingchuai (EX-B1), Gaohuang (BL 43), Feishu (BL 13), Taiyuan (LU 9).

cow-hide tinea 牛皮癣 [niú pí xuǎn] A skin disease with lesions resembling the thick and hard skin of the neck of a cow.

crossing puncture 缪刺 [miù cì] When pathogenic *qi* invades the collateral meridians, crossing puncture should be used to reduce collateral meridians by adopting the left point for the right trouble and the right for the left. It differes from cotralateral puncture which involves puncturing the meridians. In clinic for acute tonsilitis Shangyang (LI 1) and Shaoshang (LU

11) on the opposite side are selected to be pricked to cause little bleeding, etc.

crossing selection of points 交叉取穴 [jiāo chā qǔ xué] One of point-selected methods. Also called *dui che qu xue* (selecting the point from the opposite side). There are two ways: 1. Left-right cross, i.e., the disease or pain on certain side of the body is treated by selecting the point on other side. 2. Left-right and upper-lower cross, i.e., the disease or pain in the left upper limb is treated by selecting the point at the right lower limb, those at the left lower limb, the right upper limb. (Fig 18)

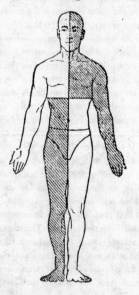

Fig 18

Chuishou 垂手 [chuí shǒu] An alternate term for Fengshi (GB 31).

Chuiju 垂矩 [chuí jù] An alternate term for Zhongju.

Chuijiang 垂浆 [chuí jiāng] An alternate term for Chengjiang (CV 24).

Cuishisihua 崔氏四花 [cuī shì sì huā] I.e., Shihua.

cupping technique 拔罐法 [bá guàn fǎ] Also called *xi bei fa*, *xi tong fa*. To apply various methods to drain air in the cup to form the negative pressue and to make it closely absorb on the body surface, so as to treat disease. To cause local congestion or stagnant blood through absorbing it can play a role in promoting blood circulation, promoting *qi* flow, relieving pain, and subsiding swelling. In clinic it is also divided into fire cupping technique. It is used for treating cough, pneumonea, asthma, headache, pains in the chest and hypochondrium, wind-damp blockage and pain, sprains, lumbago, stomachache, furuncle, carbuncle and snake-bites. (draining poisonous liquid). (Fig 19

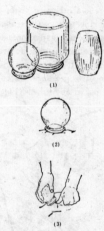

(1)

(2)

(3)

Fig 19

cup-absorbing 吸杯法 [xī bēi fǎ] I.e., cupping technique.

cup-pushed technigue 推罐法 [tuī guàn fǎ] A kind of cupping technique. Also termed *la guan fa*, *zhou guan fa*. After the cup absorbs the skin, move the cup by pushing and pulling it to enlarge the area to be selected. While applying it, first paint lubricant things such as vasilin, etc., on the opening of the cup or the therapeutic location. After making the cup absorb the skin for a while, hold the body of the cup with the hand and push and pull it to and fro 6— 8 tomes segement by segement till local redness occurs. It is frequently used at the back and waist, suitable for rheumatic pain and gastroentestinal disorders, etc.

Cunping 寸平 [cùn píng] An extra point, located 3 cm at the centre of the transverse crease of the dorsal hand, 1.5 cm lateral to the radial side. Indications: Heart failure, shock. It has the action of reviving yang and regulating the meridians. Puncture: 1 cm perpendicularly.

cupping technique by drawing *qi* 抽气拔罐法 [chōu qì bá guàn fǎ] A kind of cupping technique. Use a specially-made cup of which there is a ruberized piston at its bottom and connected with the absorbing instrument to form negative pressure, so as to make it absorb the skin for treating disease and pain. It is stronger in absorbing and the negative pressure can be regulated and measured at any time. (Fig 20).

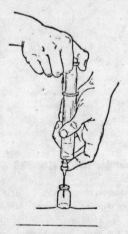

Fig 20

cutting therapy 割治法 [gē zhì fǎ] To cut certain skin at certain area and open and remove a small amount of subcutaneous fat to give the local area a proper stimulation

for treating diseases. There is cutting therapy at *Yuji*, cutting therapy at Shangzhong, etc. It can be used for treating chronic bronchitis, asthma, infantile indigestion, malnutrition, ulcer, neurosis. Before the treatment strict sterilization should be done lest the injury should occur and attention should be paid to the nursing of the wound.

cutaneous regions of six meridians 六经皮部 [liù jīng pí bù] For details see cutaneous regions.

cun **spot** 寸口 [cùn kǒu] The location at both wrists, medial to the head of the radius, where the pulse diagnosis is performed.

cutaneous needle 皮肤针 [pí fū zhēn] It developed on the basis of the arrowhead needle in ancient China, varied in the small-hammer type, the broom type, and the cylinder type. It is also respectively termed the seven-star needle (seven needles), plum needle (five needles) and bound needle (the number is not limited) according to the number of the needle. It is also termed the infantile needle as its stimulation is mild.

cutaneous region 皮部 [pí bù] 1. The cutanious regioins of the whole body divided according to the meridians. The division of the skin accords with the meridian. The region that the twelve meridians pertain to is divided into the twelve. The regions that the six meridians of hand and foot correspond with one another are the regions of the six meridians. Their names are as follows. 2. An alternate term for Chengfu (BL 36). (Fig 21)

cupping after puncturing the collateral meridian 刺络拔罐 [cì luò bá guàn] One of cupping techniques, also called *ci xue ba guan*. To superficially puncture the skin and then administer cupping, so as to absorb little blood. Frequently used in internal injury by over sprains, strains, rheumatic pain in the shoulder, back of waist and leg. It is not advisable to use it for the disease and symptom tending to bleeding, and at the area

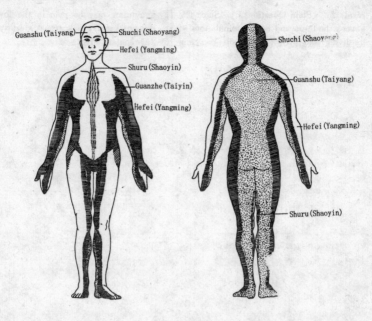

Fig 21

where the big vessel is located.

cupping *qi* 火罐气 [huǒ guàn qì] Referring to cupping technique.

cup-pushed technique 拉罐法 [lā guàn fǎ] See *tui guan fa*.

cyprus-tuber paste 香附饼 [xiāng fù bǐng] A kind of medicinal paste for moxibustion. Fresh cyprus-tuber paste ground as power, juice of fresh jinger shaped according to the size of the affected area. Indications: Srofula, redness and swelling due to invasion of wind-cold to the meridian.

CV points 任脉穴 [rèn mài xué] 1. The points pertaining to Conception Vessel. They are Huiyin (CV 10) (confluence of GV and Vital Vessel), Qugu (CV, RN 2) (confluence of foot-*jueyin* meridian), Zhongji (CV 3) (confluence of three yin meridians of foot), Guanyuan (CV 4) (confluence of three yin meridians of foot), Shimen (CV 5), Qihai (CV 6), Yinjiao (CV 7) (confluence of Vital Vessel), Shenque (CV 8), Shuifeng (CV 9), Xiawan (CV 10) (confluence of foot-*taiyin*), Jianli (CV 11) and Zhongwan (CV 12) (confluencek of hand-*taiyang*, hand-*shaoyang* and foot-*yangming* merdians), Shangwan (CV 13) (hand-*yangming* and hand-*taiyang* meridian), Juque (CV 14), Jiuwei (CV 15), Zhongting (CV 16), Danzhong (CV 17), Yutang (CV 18), Zigong (CV 19), Huangai (CV 20), Xuanji (CV 21), Tiantu (CV 22) (confluence of Connecting Vessel of Yin), 24 in total; 2. referring to Lieque (LU 7).

CV collaterals 任脉络 [rèn mài luò] One of the fifteen collateals. Its point is Weiyi (Jiuwei, CV, RN 15) and distributes itself over the abdomen. If it is *shi* (excess), pain in the abdominal skin occurs; If it is *xu* (deficiency), itching in the abdominal skin occurs. " (Miraculou Pivot).

CV diseases 任脉病 [rèn mài bìng] "If CV is diseased, male internal stasis and severe hernias may result; Female leukorrhea may result. " (Plain Questions) "Since CV govens the fetus and is the foundatioin of its living and growing, its diseases and symptoms may be pain in the lower abdomen, hernia, leukorrhea, sterility, etc. " (Miraculaus Pivot)

D

Danzhong（CD 17）膻中［dàn zhōng］A CV point, the anterior referred point of the pericardirm, the confluence of *qi* of the eight confluential points, also termed Yuaner, Shangqihai. Location: At the midline of the chest, at the interspace at the level with the 4th intercostal space. Regional anatomy: At the sternal bone proper, there are the anteriorly perforating branches of the mamary artery and vein. The anteior cutaneous branch of the 4th intercostal nerve is distributed. Indications: Cough, spitting purulent blood, asthmatic breath, chest blochage, cardialgia, palpitation, anxiety. Puncture: 1—1.5 cm horizontally. Moxibustion can be done. (Fig 22)

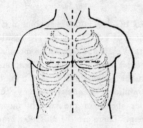

Fig 22

dantian 丹田［dān tián］It is located where one concentrates the mind on the upper 2/3 of the line joining the umbilicus and symphesis pubis. It is also called lower *dantian*. The epigastrium is called middle *dantian*. The gallbadder is called upper *dantian*.

damp blockage 湿痹［shí bì］A blockage syndrome caused by a relative excess of pathologic dampness and characterized by heavy feeling and numbnes of the limbs and body with well-localized swelling and pain.

Damen 大门［dà mén］An extra point, located on the midline of the head, 1 dm above the posterior hairline, i. e. , 3 cm above Naohu

（GV17）. Indication: Hemiplegia. Puncture: 1.5 cm horizontally. Moxistion: 3—5 moxa cones or 5—10 minutes with warming moxibustion.

Danshu（BL 19）胆俞［dǎn shū］A point of Bladder Meridian of Foot-*taiyang*, the back-*shu* point of the gallblaer. Location: 4.5 cm lateral to Zhongshu (GV, DU 7) between the 10th and 11th thoracic vertebrae. Regional anatomy: At the broadest muscle of back and the longest muscle. In the ilio-costal muscle. There are the medial branches of the dorsal branches of the 10th intercostal artery and vein. The medial cutaneous branch of the posterior branches of the 10th thoracic nerve is distributed. The lateral branch of the postrior branch of the 10th thoracic nerve is in the deeper. Indecations: Jaundice, bitter mouth, dry tongue, sore throat, vomiting, hypochondriac pain, poor appetite, pulmonary tuberculosis, tidal fever, swelling below the axilla. Puncture: 1.5—2.5 cm obliquely. (It is not advisable to puncture deep). Moxibustion: 3—5 moxa cones or 5—15 minutes with warming moxibustion.

Dannang Point 胆囊穴［dǎn náng xué］An extra point, located at the most obvious tender part directly below Yanglingquan (GB 34), in the long muscle of fibula and the long extensor muscle of toe. The lateral cutaneous nerve of calf, the superficial calf and the branch of the anterior artery are distributed. Indications: Acute and chronic cholecystits, biliary ascariasis, numbness or paralysis of the lower limb. Puncture: 3—4.5 cm perpendicularly.

'Dark-green dragon sways its tail' 青龙摆尾［qīng lóng bǎi wěi］An acupuncture manipulation, one of the four meridian-flying and *qi*-walking manipulations, symetrical to the 'white tiger shakes its head'. (Fig 23)

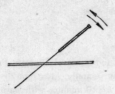

Fig 23

dan and *jie* 担截 [dān jié] An acupuncture term. There are several explanations. 1. *Dan* refers to selecting the two points, *jie* refers to selecting only one point. 2. *Dan* refers to the thrusting method, reducing manipulation, *jie* refers to pressing method and reinforcing manipulation.

dampeness and heat in large intestine 大肠湿热 [dà cháng shí rè] The pathologic changes due to simultaneous accumulation and retention of damp and thermal *qi* in the large intestine. The main symptoms are frequent purulent and bloody stools, abdominal pain, tenesmus, scanty dark urine, yellowish and glossy coating of tongue, slippery and rapid pulse, etc. It is often seen in bacillary dysentery, amebic dysentery, acute enteritis, etc.

Dazhui (CGV14) 大椎 [dà zhuī] 1. A point of Governor Vessel, the confluence of three yang meridians and Governor Vessel, also called Bailao. Location: On the posterior midline, between the spinal process of the 7th cerviacal vertebra and that the 1st thoracic vertebra. Select it in the depression at the inferior edge of the highest protrusion of the posterior nape. Regional anatomy: Passing through the supraspinal ligament and interosseous ligament. There is the branch of the cervical transverse artery. The posterior branch of the 8th cervical nerve and the medial branch of the posterior branch of the 1st thoracic nerve are distributed. Reaching deep at the spinal cord. Indications: Febrile diseases, malaria, cough, asthmatic breath, steamiong of bones, stiffness and pain in the nape, pains

in the shoulder and back and stiffness in the lumbar spine, opisthonos, infantile convulsion, mania, epilepsy, heatstroke, cholera, vomiting, jaundice, wind rash. Puncture: 1. 5—3 cm perpendicularly. Moxibustion: 3—7 moxa cones or 5—15 minutes with warming moxibustion; 2. The 7th cervical vertebra. (Fig 24)

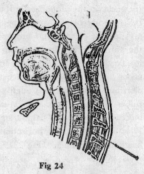

Fig 24

Dahe (KI 12) 大赫 [dà hè] A point of Kidney Meridian of Foot-*shaoyin*. The confluence of Vital Vessel and foot-*taiyin* meridian, also called Yinwei, Yinguan. Location: 1. 5 cm lateral to Zhongji (RN 3), 1. 2 dm below the umbilicus. Regional anatomy: At the anterior sheath of the straight muscle of abdonen. There are the muscular branches of the inferior epigastric artery and vein. The branches of the inferacostal nerve and the ililhypogastric nerve are distributed. Indications: Pain in the pubic region, prolapse of uterus, spermatorrhea, leukorrhea, dysmenorrhea, irregular nenstruation, infertility, diarrhea, dysentery. Puncture: 3—5 cm perpendicularly. Moxibustion: 3—5 moxa cones or 5—10 minutes with warming moxibustion.

Dachui 大馈 [dà chuí] I. e., Dazhui (GV, DU 14).

Daheng (SP 15) 大横 [dà héng] A point of Spleen Meridian of Foot-*taiyin*, the confluence of foot-*taiyin* meridian and Connecting Vessel of Yin. Also called Shenqi. Location: 12 cm lateral to the abdominal midline at the level with the umbilicus. Regional anatomy: Passing through the membrane of the external oblique muscle of abdomen, the internal oblique muscle of abdomen and transverse muscle of abdomen. There are the 10th intercostal artery and vein. The 10th intercostal nerve is distributed. Indecations: Diarrhea due to asthenia, constipation, pain in the lower abdomen. Puncture: 3—5 cm perpendicularly. Moxibustion: 5—7 moxa cones or 10—15 minutes with warming moxibustion.

Daju (ST 27) 大巨 [dà jù] A point of stomach Meridian of Foot-yangming, also termed Yemen. Location: 6 cm lateral to Shimen (CV 5) below the umbilicus. Regional anatomy: In the straigt muscle of abdomen. There are the branches of the 11th intercostal artery and vein. The inferior artery and vein of the abdominal wall are on its lateral side. The branch of the 11th intercotal nerve is distributed. Indications: Distension in the lower abdomen, nocturnal emission, prospermia, hernia, difficulty in urination, obstruction of the intestine, palpitation and insomnia. Puncture: 3—4 cm perpendicularly. Moxibustion: 5—7 moxa cones or 10—20 minutes with warming moxibustion.

Dazhongji 大中极 [dà zhōng jí] An alternate term for Guanyuan (CV 4).

Dacang 大仓 [dà cāng] I. e., Taicang. Referring to Zhongwan (CV 12).

Dabao (SP 21) 大包 [dà bāo] A point of Spleen Meridian of Foot-taiyin, the big collateral of spleen. Location: On the axillary line in the 7th intercostal space, or selected on the middle of the line connecting the centre of axilla and Zhangmen (LR 13). Regional anatomy: At the seratus anterior muscle. There are the thoracic and dorsal artery and vein and the 6th intercostal artery and vein. The terminal branches of the 7th intercostal nerve and long thoracic nerve are distributed. Indications: Pain in the chest

and hypochondrium, asthmatic breath, general ache, weakness of the four limbs. Puncture: 1. 5 cm obliquely or 5—10 minutes with warming moxibustion.

Dadun (LR 1) 大敦 [dà dūn] A point of Liver Meridian of Foot-jueyin. The well-like point (wood) of the meridian, also called Shuiguan. Location: On the lateral side of the great toe, 0. 3 cm lateral to the corner of the toenail. Regional anatomy: There are the dorsal planter artery and vein. The dorsal planter nerve from the superficial-deep peroneal nerve is distributed. Indications: Prolapse of uterus, hernia, withdrwal of genitalia, pain in the pubic region, irregular menstruation, metrorrhagia, hematuria, uroschesis, enuresis, dysuria, mania, epilepsy, pain in the lower abdomen. Puncture: 0. 3—0. 6 cm obliquily or prick to cause little bleeding. Moxibuston: 3—5 moxa cones or 5—10 minute with warming moxibustion.

Dashu 大腧 [dà shū] I. e., Dazhu (BL 11).

Daxi 大溪 [dà xī] I. e., Taixi (KI 3).

Dazhu (BL 11) 大杼 [dà zhù] A point of Bladder Meridian of Foot-taiyang, the confluence of hand-taiyang and foot-taiyang meridiains, also connected by Governor Vessel. The bone confluence of eight confluent points. Locadtion: 4 cm lateral to Taodao (DU 13) between the spinal processes of the 1st and 2nd thoracic vertebrae. Regional anatomy: Passing through the trapezius muscle, rhomboid muscle, superoposterior musculus serratus and longest muscle. There are the dorsal branches of the 1st intercostal artery and vein. The medial cutaneous branch of the posterial branch of the 1st thoracic nerve is distributed. The lateral branch of the posterior branch of the 1st thoracic nerve is in the deeper. Indications: Cough, headache, fever, stuffy nose, stiffness of the neck and nape, pain the in scapular region, sore throat. Puncture: 2 cm obliquely. Moxibustion: 3—5 moxa cones of 5—10 minutes with warming moxibustion.

Dazhijieli 大指节理 [dà zhǐ jié lǐ] I. e. , the transverse crease of the metarcar-pophalangeal joint of thumb.

Dazhijiehengwen 大指节横纹 [dà zhǐ jié héng wén] An extra point, located on the palmar side of the thumb, at the midpoint of the transverse crease of the metacarpopha-langeal joint.

Dagukong 大骨孔 [dà gú kǒng] I. e. , dà gú kǒng.

Dagukong 大骨空 [dà gú kǒng] An extra point located on the dorsal side of the thumb, at the midpoint of the transverse crease of the thumb. Select it by flexing the thumb. Indi-cations: Ocular pain, nebula, cataract, con-gestion and ulceration of lid margin, epis-taxis, vomiting and diarrhea. Moxibustion: 3—5 moxa cones. (Fig 25)

'dark-green dragon shakes its tail' 苍龙摆尾 [cāng lóng bǎi wěi] Same as *qin long bai wei*.

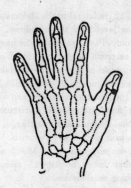

Fig 25

'dark-green turtle explores the point' 苍龟探穴 [cāng guī tàn xué] An acupuncture ma-nipulation, symetrical to 'red phoenix'. That is to insert the needle into a proper depth, then withdraw it to the subcuta-neous region. (Fig 26)

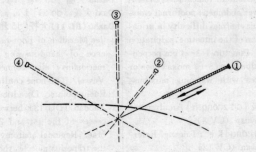

Fig 26

Dantian 丹田 [dān tián] 1. An alternate term for Shimen (CV5); 2. Guanyuan (CV4); 3. Qihiai (CV6).

Dachangshu (BL 25) 大肠俞 [dà cháng shū] A point of Bladder Merdian of Foot-*taiyang*. The back *shu* point of the large in-testine. Location: 4cm lateral to the place between the 4th and 5th lumbovertebral spinal process. Regional anatmy: Between the iliocostal muscle and the longest mus-

cle. There are the posterior branches of the 4th lumbar artery and vein. The posterior bronch of the 3rd lumbar nerve is distribut-ed. Indicadtions: Borborygmus, abdominal distension, diarrhea, dysentery, pain in the lumbar spine. Puncture: 3—5 cm perpendi-cularly. Moxibustion: 5—15 minutes with warming moxibustion.

Daying (ST 5) 大迎 [dà yíng] A point of stom-ach Meridian of Foot-*yangming*. Also called Suikong. Location: In the depression 4 cm anterior to the corner of the mandible. When the mouth is closed, it appears at the edge of the mandible, i. e. , at the anterior edge of masseter, where the pulsation of the artery can be felt. Regional anatomy: At the anterior edge of the muscle, the facial artery and vein are in front of it. The facial and buccinator nerves are distributed. Indications: Swelling cheek, close-jaw, toothache, deviated mouth and eyes, facial puffiness, dislocation of the jaw, scrofula, pain in the neck, tremor of the corner of the mouth. Puncture: 0. 7 cm perpendicularly, avoiding the artery or 1. 5—3 cm horizontally or 5—10 minutes with warming moxibustion.

Dachong 大冲 [dà chōng] I. e. , Taichong (LR 3).

Daimai point 带脉穴 [dài mài xué] 1. The confluential point of Girdle Vessel. According to Wang Bin's record, Girdle Vessel crosses foot-*shaoyang* meridian at Daimai (GB 26, Wushu (GB 27) and Weidao (GB 28). 2. referring to Zulinqi (GB 41), one of the eight confuencial points.

Damuzhitou 大拇指头 [dà mǔ zhǐ tóu] An extra point, also called Muzhi-jianduan, Dazhitou. "For administering moxibustion Damuzhitou of the two hands with 7 *zhuang* on each hand. " (Prescriptions Worth a Thousand Gold).

Dazhong (KI 4) 大钟 [dà zhōng] A point of Kidney Meridian of Foot-*shaoyin*, the connecting point of the meridian. Location: Slightly posterior and 1. 5 cm inferior to Taixi (KI 3) at the midpoint of the line connecting the posteroinferior medial ankle with the level of tendon Achilles. Regional anatomy: There is the medial branch of calcaneus of the posterior tibial artery. The medial cutaneous nerve of leg and the medial nerve of calcancus of the tibial nerve are distributed. Indications: Coughing up blood, asthmatic breath, idiocy, somnolence, stiffness and pain in the lumbar

spine, pain in the heel, irrgular menstruation. Puncture: 1. 5 cm perpendicularly. Moxibustion: 3—5 moxa cones or 5—10 minutes with warming moxibustion.

Daquan 大泉 [dà quán] 1. I. e. , Taiyuan (LU 9); 2. The extra point, located at the end of the plica of the anterior axilla. Indications: Pains in the shoulder and arm, pains in the chest and hypochondrium. Puncture: 2—3 cm perpendicularly.

Dangyang 当阳 [dāng yáng] An extra point located 3 cm in the hairline directly above the pupil (when the eyes look straight forward.), i. e. , 1. 5 cm posterior to Toulinqi (GB 15). Indications: Headache, vertigo, common cold, stuffy nose, congestion, swelling and pain in the eyes. Punctured: 1—1. 5 cm horizontally. Moxibustion: 1—3 moxa cones or 3—5 minutes with warming moxibustion.

Dangrong 当容 [dāng róng] An extra point. According to Textual Study on Illustuatioin of Meridian Points of Acupuncture, it is Taiyang (EX-HN 5). At the level with the depression at the lateral aspect of the protuberance of the zygomatic bone at the outer canthus.

Daling (PC 7) 大陵 [dà líng] A point of Pericardium Meridian of Hand-*jueyin*. The stream-like (earth) and source point of the meridian or called Guixin. Location: At the midpoint of the transverse crease of the wrist joint, between the long palmar muscle and radial flexor muscle of wrist. Select it by making the hand in supine position. Regional anatomy: Between the long palmar muscle and radial flexor muscle of wrist, there is the network of the palmar artery and vein of wrist. The palmar cutaneous branch of the central nerve is distributed. The sterm of the cental nerve is in the deeper. Puncture: 1. 5 cm perpendicularly. Moxibustion: 3—5 minutes with warming moxibustion.

Dadu (SP 2) 大都 [dà dū] A point of Spleen of Foot-*taiyin*, the spring-like (fire) point of the meridian it pertains to. Location: On the medial side of the great toe, at the dorso-ventral boundary of foot at the anterior edge of the metatarsophalangeal joint. Regional anatomy: The terminal spot of the abductor muscle of the toe beneath it. There are the branches of the medial planter artery and vein. The proper planter digital nerve of the medial planter nerve. Indications: Febrile diseases with no perspiration, abdominal distension, stomachache, vomiting, diarrhea, constipatioh, indigestion, puffiness and sweating of the trunk and limbs, insomnia, anxiety. Puncture: 1. 5 cm perpendicularly. Moxibustion: 3—5 *zhuang* with moxa cone of 5—10 minutes with warming moxibustion; 2. An extra point, one of Baxie (EX-UE 9). The eight points of Baxie between the bone juncture of the dorso-ventral boundary of the fingers are 4 on each hand. Dadu (two) is one of them, located at the dorso-ventral boundary of hand between the thumb and index finger. Select it with a fist formed. Seven moxa cones may be used for moxibustion on it. Or it may be punctured 0. 7 cm deep. Indications: Persistent severe headache and toothache.

Darong 大容 [dà róng] I. e. , Tianrong (SI 17).

Dazhijumao 大趾聚毛[dà zhǐ jù máo]An extra point or Dadun (LR 1). Located on the dorsal side of the great toe, in the toe hair at the metatarsal bone. Indication: Apoplexy, headache, vertigo, hernia, testitis. Puncture: 0. 3—0. 6 cm perpendicularly. Moxibustion: 3—5 moxa cones or 5—10 minutes with warming moxibustion.

Daimai (GB 26) 带脉 [dài mài] Gallbladder Meridian of Foot-*shaoyang*, the confluence of foot-*shaoyang* meridian and Girdle Vessel. Location: At the lateral waist, directly below Zhangmen (LR 13), at the free end of the 11th rib at the level with the umbilicus. Regional anatomy: There is the external oblique muscle of abdomen, the internal

oblique muscle of abdomen, the transverse muscle of abdomen, and the infracostal artery and vein. The infracostal nerve is distributed. In dications: Irregular menstruation, leukorrhea, amenorrhea and abdominal pain, hernia, lumbago, abdominal distension, paralysis. Puncture: 1. 5—3 cm perpendicularly. Moxibustion: 3—5 moxa cones or 5—10 minutes with warm needling.

deficiencies of both *qi* and yin 气阴两虚 [qì yīn liǎng xū] Symptoms due to exhaustion of yin liquids and yang *qi*.

deficinecy of *qi* resulting in fullness of the middle energizer 气虚中满 [qì xū zhōng mǎn] Symptoms due to the impairment of the normal functions of the spleen, resulting in distension and fullness of the abdomen.

deficiency of splenic yin 脾阴虚 [pí yīn xū] The pathologic condition in which the digestive and absorptive functions of the spleen and stomach are affected by their shortage of yin fluid, accompanied with febrile symptoms. The main syndromes are emaciation, dry lips and mouth, polydipsia, impaired appetite,constipation,thin and dry coating of tongue, faint and rapid pulse, etc.

deficiency of *qi* 气虚 [qì xū] The pathological manifestations caused either by generalized weakness or by hypofunction of one viscus, such as pallor, shortness of breath, malaise, low voice, sweating on slight exertion, etc.

deficiency of spleni *qi* 脾气虚 [pí qì xū] The pathologic changes of hypofunction of the spleen. The main manifestations are symptoms of its decreased digestive and absorptive functions.

deficiency syndrome 虚证 [xū zhèng] The manifestations due to the insufficcient antipathogenic *qi* in the human body, weakened resistance to disease and impaired physiologic functions including deficiencies of blood, *qi*, yin and yang, etc.

defensive *qi* 卫气 [wèi qì] Derived from *qi* of grains together with nutritional *qi*, distributed over the superficial part of the meridian to have an action of protecting the body.

deficiency and excess 虚实 [xū shí] Two of the eight guiding principles of diagnosis for differentiating the virulence of pathogenic *qi* and the adequacy of the body resistance to disease.

deficiency of splenic yang 脾阳虚 [pí yáng xū] The pathologic manifestations of the decline of splenic functions together with the cold syndrome. The main symptoms are distention, chilliness and pain of epigastrium, anorexia, loose stools, chronic diarrhea or chronic dysentery, cold limbs, pale tongue with whitish coating, empty and slow pulse, etc.

deficiency of *qi* resulting in cold manifestations 气虚则寒 [qì xū zé hán] The cold symptoms caused by hypofunction of the viscera and decreased metabolism.

deficiency pulse 虚脉 [xū mài] 1. A general term for various kinds of weak pulse; 2. the rough, week and empty pulse, indicating the deficieney syndrome.

deep pulse 沉脉 [chén mài] The pulse which can not be detected with a light pressure but can by a heavy press. It usally indicates the interior syndrome.

depletion of yin 亡阴 [wáng yīn] Pathologic manifestations of an excessive exhaustion of yin fluid due to high fever, profuse perspiration, severe vomiting and diarrhea, etc.

descent of *qi* in the middle energizer 中气下陷 [zhōng qì xià xiàn] pathological manifestations due to visceroptosis as a result of relatively severe deficiency of gastrosplenic *qi*. The main symptoms are anorexia, loose stools, abdominal distension aftere eating, short breath, lassitude, perspiration, sallow complexion, heavy and dragging feeling in the abdomen, frequent urinaton, prolapse of uterus, prolaspse of rectum, gastroptosis,

renoptosis and even universal viscroptosis.

deep-rooted sore 疔疮 [dīng chuāng] An acute suppurative inflammatory lesion of the body surface, which progresses rapidly and is fulmulating and dangerous. It is small in size but deep-rooted like a nail, thus the name.

deaf-mutism 聋哑 [lóng yǎ] Two different symptoms. It is called deafmutism that mutism is caused by deafness.

delayed labor 滞产 [zhì cǎn] It denotes that the whole stage of labor of the parturient who is near delivery. It often occurs when the uterus contracts abnormally, the head of fetus and the parturient's pelvic do not match or the position of the fetus is abnormal.

disease of Motility Vessel of Yang 阳跷病 [yáng qiāo bìng] Contrary to Motility Vessel of Yin, Motility Vessel of Yang relates to consciousness or activities of sleep and of limbs and trunk. "If Motility Vessel of Yang is diseased, yin chronicity and yang acuteness may appear. There is the sympotm of paralysis, resulting in stress of the extensor muscle of lower limbs and strephexopodia.

diseases of Bladder Meridian of Foot-*taiyang* 足太阳膀胱经病 [zú tài yáng páng guāng jīng bìng] The chief diseases and symptoms are headache, ocular pain, stuffy nose, epistaxis, stiff neck, pains in the spine and back, lumbago, hemorrhoids, inabitlity of the hip joint to flex, stiffness of the cubital fossa, pains in the calf and leg, malaria, mania, swelling and pain in the lower abdomen, uroschesis, enuresis.

Dingchuan (EX-BU) 定喘穴 [dìng chuàn xué] An extra point, also termed Chuanxi Point.

Dividing Line of Meridians 经脉分野 [jīng mài fēn yě] A book compiled by Zhen Zilu in Ming Dynasty(1368—1644). In the book the course and distribution of the meridians were respectively described according to different locations. Later it was supplemented as Complete Book of Meridains by Xu Shizhen. Its contents were absorbed by Supplementary Illustrations of Classified Classic.

diaphragm 募原 [mù yuán] Also called *moyuan*, chiefly referring to the source of diaphragm, also generally referring to the area where pathogenic *qi* stagnates.

deficiencies of pulmonary and renal yin 肺肾阴虚 [fèi shèn yīn xū] The pathologic changes due to deficiencies of both pulmonary and renal *qi*. The main symptoms are asthmatic attacks, short breath, spontaneous sweating, weakness, cold torso and limbs, cough with copious sputum, etc.

deficiency of yin induces internal heat 阴虚则内热 [yīn xū zé nèi rè] The heat manifestations due to extreme exhaustion of yin fluid with fluctuating fever, hot palms and soles, nocturnal sweating, malar flush, red tongue and rapid faint pulse, etc.

deficiency of gastric qi 胃气虚 [wèi qì xū] The pathologic manifestations due to the weak receiving function of the stomach. The main symptoms are anorexia, dyspepsia, epigastric distress, even vomiting immediately after eating, etc.

deficiency of renal yang 肾阳虚 [shèn yáng xū] The pathologic manifestations due to the impairment of the renal function with the accompanying cold symptom. The main symptoms are chilliness, cold limbs, lumbago, spermatorrhea, premature ejaculation, impotence, frequent nocturia, pale tongue, deep and formicant pulse, etc.

deficiency of gastric yin 胃阴虚 [wèi yīn xū] The pathologic manifestations due to the deficiency of gastric acquous essence with accompanying febrile symptoms. The main symptoms are dry mouth and lips, preferene for cold drinks, anorexia or ravenous appetite, constipation, scanty dark urine, red tongue with thin and dry coating, soft and rapid pulse, etc.

deficiency of renal yin 肾阴虚 [shèn yīn xū] The pathologic manifestations due to insuf-ficiency of yin fluids of the kidney. The main symptoms are lumbago, lassitute, dizziness, tinnutus, spermatorrhea and premature ejaculation, dry mouth and sore throat, malar flush, hot palms and soles, afternoon fever, red tongue with little coating, faint and rapid pule, etc.

deepest vital vessel 伏冲之脉 [fú chōng zhī mài] Referring to one of vital vessels that runs deeply in the spine. "If the desease is at the deepest vital vessel, heaviness and pain in the body may result. "

deficiency of the gallbladder 胆虚 [dǎn xū] a syndrome due to hypofunction of biliary *qi*, often manifested as fright, anxiety, palpitation, suspicions, insomnia, sighing, etc.

decentralized Pulse 散脉 [sǎn mài] The pulse which is scattered and disordered to gentle touch and disappears when heavily pressed. It is chiefly seen in the critical cases of collapse of *qi* and blood.

decentralized points 散俞 [sǎn shū] The points used to cause little bleeding.

decentralized puncture 散刺 [sǎn cì] One of needling techniques to puncture the point and its surrounding areas superficially.

Difficult Classic 难经 [nàn jīng] A medical book, originally named Emperor's Eighty-One Difficult Classic written by Qin Yueren (Bian Que) during the Warring States Periods (770—221 B. C.). In the book eighty one questions were discussed in the form of questions and answers. It is an important work after Internal Classic, of which diagnostic techniques, twelve meridians, eight extra veels, five *shu* points, and application of reinforcing and reducing manipulations were expounded. Some of the contents can not be seen in Internal Classic that has been preserved. In the aspect of meridians, it was brought out that moving *qi* between the kidneys below the umbilicus is the "foundation of the viscera and the root of the twelve meridians"; besides the twelve meridians, eight extra vessels were specially described. The eight confluential points, such as Zanghui, Fuhui, Qihui, Xuehui, Maihui, Guhui, and Suihui were also put forth. In the aspect of acupuncture treatment, the point-selected method of "reinforce its maternal in case deficiency and reduce its offspring in case excess" was brought out, as well as "acquiring *qi*" of acupuncture, reinforcing and reducing manipulations, which have exerted a great influence upon the development of acupuncture science in latter generations.

Dingshanghuimao 顶上回毛 [dǐng shàng huí máo] An extra point; circling or explained as Baihui (GV 20), located at the midpoint of the hair on the vertex. Indications: Infantile fright and epilepsy, prolapse of anus, hemorrhoids with bleeding. Moxibustion: 3—7 *zhuang* of moxa cone, or 10—15 minutes with warming moxibustion.

Dingshangxuanmao 顶上旋毛 [dǐng shàng xuán máo] I. e., Dingshanghuimao.

Dingmen 顶门 [dǐng mén] I. e., Xinhui (GV 22).

decentralized collateral meridian 结脉 [jié mài] The blood collateral scattering at the popliteal fossa.

dian 颠 [diān] Referring to the vertex.

Diaphragm 膈 [gé] An ear point on the crus of helix to form a right line with the interspace between Mouth and Esophagus.

Dianshang 巅上 [diān shàng] An alternate term for Baihui (GV 20).

diagnosis in accordance with the eight guiding principles 八纲辨证 [bā gāng biàn zhèng] The eight guiding principles—yin, yang, exterior, interior, cold, heat, deficiency, and excess are clinically utilized for anlysis, deduction, and diagnosis of diseases.

disorders of *qi* mechanism 气机不利 [qì jī bú lì] Symptoms due to disturbances of visceral function.

dispersing and discharging functions of the liver 肝主疏泄 [gān zhǔ shū xié] These functions are closely related to the changes of the emotions, normality of digestive activities, and flow of *qi* and blood. If all

these are disturbed, such symptoms as depression of hepatic *qi*, dyspepsia, pain in the hypochondrium, epigastric pain, irregular menstruation, dysmenorrhea, etc. will be produced.

diagnosis according to symptoms and signs rather than pulse 舍脉从证 [shě mài cóng zhèng] In the clinical examination when the pulse does not accord with the symptoms and sings while the latter actually reflect the condition of the illness, the diagnosis is made according to the latter rahther than of the former.

distension 鼓胀 [gǔ zhàng] The disease and symptom complex characterized by abdominal distension, sallow skin, varicosity of veins, etc.

disturbance of the regulation between water and fire 水火不济 [shuǐ huǒ bú jì] Here, water refers to renal water; while fire to cardiac fire. When renal water is deficient or cardiac fire blazes, there is a loss of control by either of them. Disturbance of the equilibrium of the physiologic dynamics of both would result in symptoms and signs like anxiety, insomnia, spermatorrhea, etc.

disturbance of heart by phlegmatic fire 痰火扰心 [tán huǒ lǒng xīn] Evil fire and heat in combination with 'phlegm' causes mnetal disturbance. The main symptoms are mental confusion, delirium, mania and excitability, spitting sputum and saliva, red tongue with yellowish and glossy coating, slippery and rapid pulse, etc.

distraction of the lungs by phelgm and damp 寒痰阻肺 [hán tán zhǔ fèi] The pathologic manifestations due to accumulation and retention of patholgenic damp and phlegm in the lungs. The main symptoms are fever, cough with copious whitish sputum, fullness and distress of chest and hypochondirium, rough or whitish and slippery coating of the tongue, stringy and smooth pulse, etc.

disharmony between heart and kidney 心肾不交 [xīn shèn bù jiāo] The pathologic manifestations due to abnormalities of the physiologic relationship between cardiac yang and renal yin. The main symptoms are dyspnea, insomnia, palpitation, frequent dreams, spermatorrhea, etc.

diagnosis according to pulse rather than symptoms and signs 舍证从脉 [shě zhèng cóng mài]In the clinical examination, when the pulse does not accord with the symptoms and signs while the pulse reflects the actual condition of the illness, the diagnosis should be made according to the pulse rather than symptoms and sings.

diseases caused by change of meridians 所生病[suǒ shēng bìng]A term used in meridian diseases. It refers to the reluvent diseases or symptoms appearing when the meridion changes abnormally. The points of this meridian can treat the diseases or symptoms in this aspect.

disharmony of gastric *qi* 胃气不和 [wèi qì bù hé]The pathologic manifestations of abnormality of gastric *qi*, e.g., epigastric distress, indigestion, nausea and vomiting, etc.

diseasesy of Connecting Vessel of Yin 阴维病 [yīn wéi bìng]If Connecting Vessle of Yin is diseased, chills and fever and cardialgia may result.

diseases of Girdle Vessel 带脉病 [dài mài bìng] As Girdle Vessel restrains various merdians, its disorders are distension and fullness of the waist and abdomen, luekorrhea, pains in the umbilical abdomen and lumbar spine, atrophy and softness of the lower limbs.

Diwei 地卫 [dì wèi] I.e., Dicheng, another name of Yongquan (KI 1).

diseases of Liver Meridian of Foot-*jueyin* 足厥阴肝经病[zú jué yīn gān jīng bìng]The chief diseases and symptoms are hypochondriac pain, full chest, hernia, swelling of the lower abdomen, dry throat, dull complexion, headche, vertigo, vomiting, diarrhea, enuresis, uroshchesis.

diseases of Motility Vessel of Yin 阴跷病 [yīn qiāo bìng] Contrary to Motility Vessel of Ying. It relates to sleep and activities of the limb and trunk. "If Motility Vessel of Yin is diseased, the symptoms such as epilepsy induced by terror, and paralysis may result, accompanied by stress of the flexor muscle of the lower limb and strephenopodia, etc."

diseases of Vital Vessel 冲脉病 [chōng mài bìng] "If Vital Vessel is diseased, adverse flow of *qi* and contraction of the genital organ may appear." It is closely related to the genital disorders, such as irregular menstruation, metrorrhagia, adverse flow of *qi* to the heart, etc.

diseases of Connecting Vessel of Yang 阳维病 [yáng wéi bìng] According to Chassic of Difficulty, they are mainly chills and fever, cardialgia, amnesia, trance.

distal and proximal 主应 [zhǔ yìng]In selecting the acupuncture points, that distal to the affected area is regarded as the major one while that proximal to the affected area, the auxiliary.

distal-proximal combination of points 远近配穴法 [yuǎn jìn pèi xué fǎ] One of point-combined methods. It refers that the piont distal to the affected area and that proximal are used in combination, i.e., the distal selection of the point and the proximal selection of the point are combined. E.g., for stomachache trouble Neiguan (PC 6) and Zusanli (ST 36) are selected distally, and Zhongwan (CV 12) `proximally; for toothache, Hegu (LI 4) and Neiting (ST 44) are selected distally and Jiache (ST 6) proxymally.

distal selection 远取 [yuǎn qǔ] A brief term for selecting the point from the distal area.

Direct Acupuncture-Moxibustion 针灸直指 [zhēn jiǔ zhí zhǐ] A book compiled by Xu Chuanpu in Ming Dynasty(1368—1644). It was collected into Orthodox Medicine, Ancient and Modern and arranged in the 7th volume. Its contents are adapting the part concerning acupuncre in Internal Classic, describing reinforicing and reducing manipulations, by acupuncfure, number of *zhuang* of moxa cone, moxibustion technique, prohibitions as well as rhythmed articles of acupuncture.

distal puncture 远道刺 [yuǎn dào cì] One of nine needling techniques. According to Miraculous Pivot, *Fushu* originally referring to the lower joinning points on three yang meridians of foot are used for troubles of six emptying viscera. In its broadest sense, it can be called distal puncture that the points of the four limbs are selected for treating diseases and symptoms of the head, face, trunk and viscera.

distal selection of points 远隔取穴 [yuǎn gé qǔ xué] I. e. , *yuan dao qu xue*.

Diji 地箕 [dì jī] I. e. , Diji (SP 8).

Diji (SP 8) 地机 [dì jī] A point of Spleen Meridian of Foot-*taiyin*, the gap-like point of the merician, also termed Pishu. Location: 10 cm directly below Yanglingquan (GB 34), 18 cm below Neixiyang (EX-LE 4) at the leg. Regional anatomy: In the soleus muscle. There is the great saphenous vein and the branch of ᵗhe highest artery of tibia in the deeper. The cutaneous nerve at the medial aspect of leg is distributed. There is the tibial nerve in the deeper. Indications: Abdominal distension and pain, anorexia, diarrhea, difficulty in urination, edema, irregular menstruation, dysmenorrhea, spermatorrea, lumbago, dysuria. Puncture: 3—4 cm perpendicularly. Moxibustion: 3—5 moxa cones or 5—10 minutes with warming moxibustion.

Dihe 地合 [dì hé] An extra point located at the highest point of the forward protuberance of the middle mandible. Indications: Deep-rooted sore at the head and face, toothache. Puncture: 1—1. 5 cm obliquely.

Dichong 地冲 [dì chōng] An alternate term for Yongquan (KI 1).

Dicang 地苍 [dì cāng] The wrong form of Dicang (ST 4).

Dishen 地神 [dì shén] An extra point located at the midpoint of the transverse crease of the metacarpophalangeal joint on the palmar side of the thumb and the midpoint of the transverse crease of metatarsophalangeal joint of the metatarsal side of the big toe, 4 in total.

Dicang (ST 4) 地仓 [dì cāng] A point of Stomach Meridian of Foot-*yangming*, the confluence of foot-*yangming* meridian and Motility Vessel of Yang. Locatioin: 12 cm lateral to the lateral side of the corner of mouth. Regional anatomy: There is the facial artery and vein. The branch of the facial neve and the branch of the infroaoccipital nerve are distributed. The terminal branch of the nerve of the buccinator muscle is the deeper. The needle passes through the orbicular muscle of mouth and reaches at the bucinator muscle. Indications: Deviated mouth, salivation, tremor of eyelids, looseness of the legs, toothache, swollen cheek. Puncture: 1. 5—3 cm obliquely or horizontally. Moxibustion: 5—10 minutes with warming moxibustion.

Diwu 地五 [dì wǔ] Referring to Diwuhui (GB 42).

Diwuhui (GB 42) 地五会 [dì wǔ huì] A point of Gallbladder Meridian of Foot-*shaoyang*. Location: 3 cm above Xiaxi (GB 43) at the end of the toe, at the edge of the medial side of extensor muscle of the small leg between the 4th and 5th metatarsal bones. Regional anatomy: Passing through the medial aspect of the long extensor muscle of toe, reaching the dorsal interosseous muscle. There is the network of the artery and vein of the dorsal foot, and the dorsal artery and vein of the 4th metatarsal bone. The branch of the medial cutaneors nerve of the dossal foot is distribured. Indications: Headache, congestion, swelling and pain in the eyes, tinnitus, breast carbuncle, swelling of the dorsal foot, fullness, hypochondriac pain, sowollen axilla. Puncture: 1—2 cm perpendiculrly. Moxibustion: 1—3 moxa cones or 3—5 minutes with warming moxibustion.

direct moxibustion 直接灸 [zhí jié jiǔ] A kind of moxibustion with moxa cone. It is also called *zhao fu jiu*, *zhao ru jiu*, *ming jiu* that the moxa cone is put directly on the point for administering moxibustion. While administering moxibustion, apply a little vaselin or garlic juice on the skin, put the moxa cone on it and ignite it; Till the moxa cone burns near the skin, gently pad or touch the surrounding point with the two hands to relieve pain. After one moxibustion, repeat the moxibustion according to the previously method. In general, one time of moxibustion is done for one point; and 3—9 for one time of moxibustion. It is called suppurative moxibustion that if the moxa cone used is large, let it scorch the skin to cause suppuration. It is often used for treating asthma, chronic gastroentestinal trouble, emaciation, etc. It pertains to warm-heat moxibustion that if the maxa fire is got red before it burns the skin, and the patient feels scorching, change moxa cone till the local skin becomes tidal red.

Dou Hanqing 窦汉卿 (1196—1280) [dòu hàn qīng] A famous acupuncture expert in Jin and Yuan dynasties (1271—1368). The works he wrote are Guide book of Acupuncture Classic, Secret Talk about Bronze Figure of Acupuncture.

dorso-palmar (**dorso-ventral**) **boundary** 赤白肉际 [chì bái ròu jì] I. e. , *bai rou ji*. Referring to the boundary between the palmar (planter) surface and the dorsal surface.

dotting puncture 点刺 [diǎn cì] A kind of needling technique. To insert the needle swiftly and withdraw it immediately. The puncture is superficial and the duration is short, usually used for puncturing the well-like point or puncturing collateral meridians.

dorsal foot 足跗 [zú fū] The dorsum of the foot.

Douzhou 斗肘 [dǒu zhǒu] An extra point. Located at the highest point of the laterosuperior condyle of humurus, lateral to Quchi

(LI 11). Indicatioins: Neuralgia in the elbow, paraplegia, neurasthenia. Moxibustion: 5—7 moxa cones or 10—15 minutes with warming moxibustion.

dorsop almar (**dorso-ventral**) **boundary** 白肉际 [bái ròu jì] The boundary between the palmar side (ventral) and the dorsal side of hand and foot. It is so called because the skin of the palmar surface is comparatively pale.

drug-cup method 药筒法 [yào tǒng fǎ] I. e. , drug-boiled and cupping method. To boil the drug cup hot and cup the point with it for a long time and then take it off till the point is warm.

drug-boiled cupping method 煮药拔罐法 [zhǔ yào bā guàn fǎ] A kind of water cupping. The cupping therapy is carried on after the bamboo cup is boiled with Chinese druy fluid.

dry phlegm 燥痰 [zào tán] Thick mucoid phlegm of small quantity or with blood streaks, commonly accompanying dry manifestations.

drug ion point penetrated method 药物离子穴位透入法 [yào wú lí zǐ xué wèi tòu rù fǎ] An abbreviation of *zhi liu dian yao wu li zi sue wei tou ru fa*.

dry stagnation 燥结 [zào jié] Pathogenic heat becomes stagnant in the stomach and intestines, and impairs the gastrointestinal fluid, resulting in such symptoms as afernoon tidal fever, abdominal distension and pain, constipation, urine of deep color and small amounts with yellowish and dry coating of the tongue, rapid pule, etc.

dryness-heat 燥热 [zào rè] 1. The pathogens with dry and heat characteristics; 2. the dry-heat syndromes. The clinical manifestations are congestion of the eyes, pain and swelling of the gums, thirst, dryness of the throat and nose, epistaxis, dry cough, hemoptysis, deep-coloured urine, constipation, red tongue with dry and yellowish coating, rapid pulse, etc.

Duichong 兑冲 [duì chōng] An alternte term

for Shenmen (HT 7).

Duigu 兑骨 [duì gǔ] 1. An alternate term for Quanliao (ST 18); 2. Referring to processs stylodeus ulnae; 3. Referring to Shenmen (HT 7).

Duiduan (GV 27) 兑端 [duì duān] A GV point. Location: At the tip of the upper lip, at the conjunction between the skin and the mucoid membrane of the upper lip. Regional anatomy: At the orbicular muscle of mouth. There is the labial artery and vein. The branch of the buccinator muscle of the facial nerve and the branch of the infraorbital nerve are distributed. Indications: Coma, syncope, mania, hysteria, deviated mouth and emaciatioin-thirst disease, stomatitis, tremor of lips, toothache, closejaw, stuffy nose. Puncture: 0.6—1.5 cm obliquely. Moxibustion is prohibited.

Duyin 独阴 [dú yīn] An extra point. Located at the midpoint of the transverse crease of the metatarsal joint of the palmar side of foot. Indication: Spitting blood, dystocia, dead fetus, retention of placenta, hernia of the small intestine, irregular menstruation. Puncture: 0.3—0.6 cm perpendicularly. Moxibustion: 3—5 moxa cones or 5—10 minutes with warming moxibustion. (Fig 27).

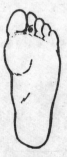

Fig 27

dun **moxibustion** 顿灸 [dùn jiǔ] Referring to administering moxibustion once with the speculated number of *zhuang*. Contrary to repeated moxibustion.

Dueodenum 十二指肠 [shí èr zhǐ cháng] An ear point located at the upper edge of the crus of helix, opposite to Cardia.

Duosuowen 多所闻 [duō suǒ wén] An alternate trm for Tinggong (SI 19).

Duoming 夺命 [duó mìng] An extra point, also termed Xiaomo, Xinxing. Located at the midpoint of the line connecting Jianyu (LI 15) and Chize (LU 5) in the biceps muscle of arm. Indications: Syncope, pain in the upper arm, erysipelas. Puncture: 1.5—3 cm perpendicularly.

Duji 督脊 [dū jǐ] An extra point, located at the midpoint of the line connecting the spinal process of the 7th thoracic vertebra and the end of coccyx. Indications: Epilepsy. Moxibustion: 3—5 moxa cones or 5—10 minutes with warming moxibustion.

Dushu (BL 16) 督俞 [dū shū] A point of Bladder Meridian of Foot-*taiyang*, also termed Gaogai. Location: 4.5 cm lateral to Lingtai (GV 10) between the spinal processes of the 6th and 7th thoracic vertebrae. Regional anatomy: At the trapezius muscle and the broadest muscle of back and the longest muscle. There is the medial branch of the dorsal lateral branch of the 6th intercostal artery and vein, and the descending branch of the cervical transverse artery. The dosal scapular nerve and the medial cutaneous branch of the posterior branch of the 6th thoracic vertebra are distributed. The lateral branch of the posterior branch of the 6th thoracic nerve is in the deeper. Indications: Cardialgia, abdominal pain, abdominal distension, borborygmus. Puncture: 1.5—2.5 cm obliquely. (It is not advisable to puncture deep). Moxibustion: 3—5 moxa cones or 5—15 minutes with warming moxibustion.

dysmenorrhea 痛经 [tòng jīng] A common disease in gynecology with mainly hypogastric and lumbar pain prior to, during or after the menstrual period.

dysentery 痢疾 [lì jí] An acute infection commonly seen in the summer and the autumn, with the cardinal symptoms of abdominal pain and small amounts of mucoid bloody stools, and tenesmus, including bacillary dysentery, amebic dysentery and some other intestinal diseases.

E

e 颊 [é] The root of nose.

ear meridian 耳脉 [ěr mài] The name of the meridian during the early period, similar to hand-*shaoyang* meridian.

Earshang 耳上 [ěr shàng] 1. The name of the extra point, located 3 transverse finger-*cun* directly above the tip of the ear; 2. An alternate term for Ershangfaji.

ear acupuncture 耳针 [ěr zhēn] Referring to treatment of diseases by puncturing the reactive points of the auricle. In treatment of diseases by puncturing or moxibustioning the ear points, there was only the decentralized record in the past. But its clinical application has developed rapidly in modern times. The reactive points of the auricle, which are characterized by being tender and lower in resistance and relating to certain viscera are of value in diagnosis besides being applied in treatment of diseases. During puncturing them the points must be selected accurately and sterilized strictly lest infection should result. They can also be stimulated by medicinal press or embedment of the subcutaneous needle. The distribution of the reactive points on the auricle can be seen from the following chart and picture. (Fig 28)

Ear apex 耳尖 [ěr jiān] An ear point located 1/2 alove the lateral side of the trugus.

Ear 耳 [ěr] An ear point superolateral to Zone$_5$.

earth stratum 地部 [dì bù] The depth of the point, referring to the deep stratum, between the tendon and bone, also called *dicai*.

earthworm-excreted mud 蚯蚓泥 [qiū yǐn ní] The mud excreted by the earthworm, one of the things for interposing moxibustion.

earthly branches 地支 [dì zhī] Also termed the twelve branches, i. e., *zi*, *chou*, *yin*, *mao*, *chen*, *ji*, *wu*, *wei*, *shen*, *we*, *hai*, the names for recording the date and hour. Corresponding with the ten stems, it is called the branches and stems, respectively called the heavenly stems and the earthly branches.

Easy-learned Acupuncture 针灸易学 [zhēn jiǔ yì xué] A book written by Li Shouxian in Qing Dynasty (1644—1911) collects the records on the origin of acupuncture, manipulations and indications, introduces acupuncture methods and the 2nd records and describes the points of the fourteen meridians and extra points. It was published in 1798.

eclipta 旱莲 [hàn lián] One of the drugs applied for cold moxibustion.

eczema 湿疹 [shi zhěn] A common skin disease. It varies due to different affected locations. E. g., that occurs at the face is called infantile eczema, that occurs at the ear is called ear sore, that occurs at the scrotum is called scrotum wind, that occurs at the cubital and popliteal fossas is called four-curve wind, etc.

eclampsia 妊娠痫证 [rèn shēn xián zhèng] During the 3rd trimester of pregnancy or during labor, the patient may suddenly be seized by fainting and coma, convulsions of the limbs with jaw slightly closed, eyes fixed, frothy salivation, and even opisthotonos. The patient, then, regains consciouness gradually. This may recur repeatedly from time to time.

edema 水肿 [shuǐ zhǒng] It refers to retention of body fluids that spread over the skin, causing puffiness of the head, face, eyes, four limbs, abdomen, even the whole body.

Effective Method of Puncturing *Ding* 疔疗捷法 [cì dīng jié fǎ] A book written by Zhang Jing in Qing Dynasty (1644—1911), one volume, first describing treatment, then the illustration of the points of the whole body, and finally the rhythmed article of treating deep-rooted sore, published in 1876. Later it was collected in Chen Xiuyuan's 72 Medical Books; 2. A look written by an unknown person, inscribed as Sun Dezang's family-stored book, one vol-

ume. It contains differentiation of deep-rooted sores and the manipulation to treat them, various illustrations of deep-rooted cores and the points used for selection of the points in the rhythmed article.

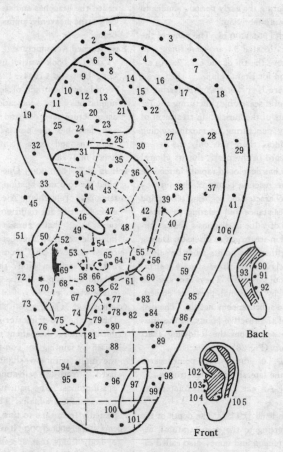

Fig 28

1. Tonsil$_1$ 2. Ear apex   3. Liver yang$_1$ 4. Finger   5. Toe   6. Heel   7. Helix$_1$ 8. Ankle   9. Point for lowering blood pressure   10. Upper segement of rectum   11. External genitalia$_2$ 12. Uterus   13. Hepatitis point   14. Knee joint   15. Hip point   16. Urticaria area   17. Wrist   18. Liver yang$_2$ 19. External genitalia$_1$ 20. Asthma point   21. Shenmen   22. Knee   23. Guanyuan   24. Sciatic   25. Sympathetic   26. Hip   27. Abdomen   28. Elbow   29. Helix$_2$ 30. Lumbosacral vertebrae   31. Bladder   32. Urethra   33. Lower segment of rectum

34. Large intestine   35. Kidney   36. Pancreas gallbladder   37. Shoulder   38. Chest
39. Thoracic vertebra   40. Mammary gland   41. Tonsil$_2$ 42. Liver   43. Small intestine
44. Appendix   45. External ear   46. Diaphragm   47. Dueodenum   48. Stomach   49. Esophagus
50. Throat   51. Tip of tragus   52. Lower abdomen   53. Mouth   54. Cardia   55. Spleen
56. Cervical vertebra   57. Scapular joint   58. Trachea   59. Clavicular bone   60. Neck
61. Brain stem   62. Brain point   63. Point for relieving asthma   64. Lung   65. Heart
66. Lung   67. Triple energizer   68. Upper abdomen   69. Bronchus   70. Internal nose   71.
External nose   72. Adrenal gland   73. Hypertension   74. Ovary   75. Endoctine   76. Eye$_1$
77. Parotid gland   78. Testes   79. Subcortex   80. Forehead 81. Eye$_2$ 82. Taiyang
83. Occiput   84. Nape   85. Helix$_4$ 86. Tonsil$_2$ 87. Lower jawbone   88. Tongue   89.
Upper jawbone   90. Upper back   91. Middle back   92. Lower back   93. Groove for lowering
blood pressure   94. Toothache point   95. Anesthesia point   96. Eye   97. Cheek   98. Helix$_5$
99. Internal ear   100. Tonsil$_4$ 101. Helix$_6$ 102. Ear Apex   103. External ear   104.
Adrenal gland   105. Testes   106. Helix$_3$

Ear Points

Division	Name of Point	Location
Lobre	Upper Pallate	At the lower 1/4 of the lateral line of Zone$_2$
	Lower pallate	At the medial 1/3 of the upper line of Zone$_2$
	Upper jaw	At the centre of Zone$_3$
	Lower jaw	At the midpoint of the transverse line of Zone$_3$
	Eye	At the centre of Zone$_5$
	Ear	Laterosuperior to Zone$_5$
	Internal Ear	Slightly above the centre of Zone$_6$
	Thyloid	At the lateral 1/3 of the boundary line of Zone$_3$ and Zone$_4$
	Tonsil	In the centre of Zone$_8$
	Cheek	Surrounding the boundary line of Zone$_5$ and Zone$_6$
	Tongue	Slightly above the interspace between the upper and lower jaws
antitrageus	parotid	At the highest point of the middle zone
	Pingchuan	Approx. 0. 2 cm anteroposterior to Thyloid point
	Testis	Approx. 0. 2 cm posteroinferior to Thyloid point
	Brain point	At the top of the upper zone
	Occiput	At the edge of the cartilege of the antitragus opposite to the upper zone and brain spot
	Temple	At the edge of the cartilege of antitragus between Occiput and Temple in the centre of the upper zone
	Taiyang	At the edge of the cartillege of antitragus between Occiput and Temple
	Vertex	Approx. 0. 15 cm below Occiput
	Lower zone of cortex	At the medial aspect of the lower zone
	Exciting point	At the midpoint between Testes and Lung Spot

Continued

Division	Name of Point	Location
Scaphoid Fossa	Clavicle	At the lower end of the scaphoid fossa, at the level with Heart Point
	Finger	At the lower edge of the upper end of the scaphoid fossa
	Shoulder Joint	Divid the scaphoid fossa between the clavicle and Finger into the four equivalent parts, in the 1st division above the Clavicle
	Shoulder	In the 2nd equivalent division above Clavicle
	Elbow	In the 3rd equivalent division above Clavicle
	Wrist	In the 4th equivalent division above Clavicle
	Nephritis point	Lateroinferior to Clavicle
	Appendix point	There are totally 3 points: One is slightly above Finger, another is above Shoulder, the last is below Clavicle
	Urticaria point	Between Finger and Wrist
antihelix antihex	Cervical vertebra	At the protruding part of the starting point of the antihelix
	Sacral vertbea	At the protruding part of the upper and lower parts of antihelix, which divides the interspace between Cervical Vertebra and Sacral Vertebra into the 2
antihelix antihex	Thoracic vertebra	In the 1st equivalent area above Cervical Vertebra
	Lumba vertebra	In the 2nd equivalent area above Cervical vertebra, slightly medial
	Neck	Between Cervical Vertebra and Thoracic Vertebra, slightly medial
	Chest	Between Thoracic Vertebra and Lumbar Vertebra, slightly medial
	Abdomen	Between Lumbar Vertebra and Sacral Vertebra
	External Abdomen	At the lateral side of anthelix approx. at the level with Kidney
	Heat Point	Between Scral-Coccygeal Vertebra and lumbago point Approx. at the level with Hip Point
	Thyloid	Laterosuperior to Cervical Vertebra, at the level with Neck
	Mammary Gland Point	Above Thoracic Vertebra, formed an equi lateral triangle together with Thoracic Vertebra
	Ke	At the terminal part of a helix near the scaphoid fossa
	Lumbago point	0. 2 cm inferomedial to Sacrococcyx Vertebra
Upper Crus of antihelix	Toe	At the end of the terminal part of anthelix, slightly lateral
	Heel	At the end of the terminal part of antihelix, slightly medial
	Ankle Joint	Below Toe and Heel, forming a triangle
	Knee	At the starting part of the upper crus of antihelix
	Hip Joint	In the middle between Sacral Vertebra and Toe
	Knee Joint	In the middle between Hip Joint and Toe

Continued

Division	Name of Point	Location
Lower Crus of antihelix	Hip	At the medial aspect of the starting part of the lower crus of antihelix
	Sympathetic	At the end of the lower crus of antihelix
	Sciatic nerve	Between Hip and Sympathetic
Triangular Fossa	Uterus	At the most depressive point of triangular fossa
	Shenmen	At the palce of 1/2—1/3 near the upper crus of antihelix
	Pelvic cavity	At the point of the upper crus of antihelix and the lower one
	Point for loweling blood preasure	At the end of the upper crus of antihelix
	Asthma point	Approx. 0.2 cm lateral to uterine
	Guguan	At the upper edge of the lower crus of antihelix, forming a triangle with Sciatic and Hip
	Constipation Point	Near the middle segment of the lower edge of antihelix, mediosuperior to Sciatic, to form a horizontal line
	Hepatitis point	At the midpoint between Asthma point and Shenmen
Orus of Helix	Diaphragm	At the crus of helix, forming a right line with Mouth and Esophagus
	Erzhong	Lateral to Diaphragm, forming a right line with Esophagus and Cardia
Surrounding Crus of Helix	Mouth	Between the crus of helix, laterosuperior to antianthrum auris
	Esophagus	At the inferior edge of the crus of helix, at the middle and medial 1/3 boundary line between Mouth and Stomach
	Cardia	At the inferior edge of the crus lateral 1/3 boundary line between Mouth and Stomach
	Stomach	At the merging place of the crus of helix
	Duodenlum	At the superior edge of helix, opposite to Cardia
	Small intestine	At the superior edge of the crus of helix, opposite to esophagus
	Appendix	Between Large Intestine and Small Intestine
	Large intestine	At the superior edge of the crus of helix, opposite to Mouth
Cymba Conchae	Bladder	Below the lower crus of antihelix, above Large Intestine
	Kidney	Below the lower crus of antihelix, below Pelvic Cavity
	Urehtral Duct	Between Bladder and Kidney
	Prostate	Medial to Bladder inferior to Sympathetic point
	Liver	Posterosuperior to Stomach
	Pancrititis point	At the lower 2/3 between Dueodenlum and pancreas
	Panccreas, gallbladder	Between Liver and Kidney
	Cirrhosis Point	Among Kindey, Pancsreas-Gallbladder and Small Intestine

Continued

Division	Name of Point	Location
Cavity of Concha	Heart	At the most depressive part of the centre of cavity of concha, the reflex light area
	Spleen	Lateroinferior to Stomach Area Point
	Lung	At the surrounding Heat
	Branchus	At 1/3 of internal side of Lung Area
	Tuberculosis Point	At the centre of Lung Area
	Bronchiectasis Point	Lateral 2/3 of Lung Area
	Trachea	At the point where the external auditory canal is at the level with Heart
	Hepatomegaly Area	At the place where the crus of helix disappears, an area above and below the external stomach
	Cirrhosis Area	In the centre of Hepatomegaly Area, appearing like a loap
	Triple Energizer	Between Inner Nose, Endocrine and Lung
	Hepatitis Point	Slightly below the interspace between Stomach and Spleen
	Ear Trouble	At the point where the notch of upper tragus crosses the opening of the external auditory canal
	New Eye Point	Between Esophagus, Cardia and Lung
Tragus	Inner Nose	At the lower 1/2 of the medial side of tragus
	Throat	At the upper 1/2 of the medial side of tragus
	Adrenal Gland	At the lower 1/2 of the lateral side of tragus
	Tip of Tragus	At the upper 1/2 of the lateral side of tragus
	External Nose	At the anterior edge of the cartilege of tragus, forming an equilateral triangle together with Tip of Tragus and Adrenal Gland
Notch of upper Tragus	Endocrine	Approx. 0.2cm at the medial side of the notch between the tragi
	Ovary	Anteroinferior to infrocortex
	Eye_1	Anteroinferior to the notch between tragi
	Eye_2	posteoinferior to the notch between tragi
	Point for hightening blood preasure	Between Eye_1 and Eye_2
Cavity of Councha	External Ear	In the depression annterior to the notch of Tip of tragus
	Heart Point	In the depression above the Tip of tragus
	Brain stem	In the centre of the notch of the helix and tragus
	Houya	Anteroinferior to Brain Stem
	Toothache point	At the medial side of Brain Stem, opposite to Houya

Continued

Division	Name of Point	Location
Helix	External Genitalia	At the helix at the level with Sympathetic Point
	Urethra	At the helix at the level with Bladder Point
	Lower portion of Rectum	At the helix at the level with Large Intestine Point
	Anus	In the middle between Lower Segment of Rectum and Urethra
	Ear apex	At the tip of the upper end of auricle when the helix is flexed toward the tragus
	Hemorrhoid Point	At the medial aspect of tip of ear, above Jianyadian
	$Tonsil_1$	Lateral to the tip of ear, forming a right angle together with Tonsil in Lobre Zone
	$Tonsil_2$	On the helix between Tonsil of Lobre and $Tonsil_1$
	$Tonsil_3$	On the helix between Tonsil of Lobre and $Tonsil_2$
	$Liver\text{-}yang_1$	At the superior edge of the node of helix
	$Liver\text{-}yang_2$	At the lower edge of the node of helix
	Helix 1, 2, 3, 4, 5, 6	Lun_1 is below the node of helix, Lun_2 is at the lower edge of Tonsil of Lobre, of which is divided into the four equivalent parts, namely, Lun_2, Lun_3, Lun_4 and Lun_5 from upper to lower
	Lesser Occipital Nerve	At the medial side 0.2 cm to the superior edge of the node of helix
Back of Ear	Upper portion of the back	At the back, near the superior edge of the protruding auricular concha
	Middle portion of the back	At the ear back, at the comparatively higher protruding part of auricular concha
	Lower portion of the back	At the ear back near the lower edge of the protruding auricular concha
	Groove for Lowesing blood preasure	At the upper 1/3 of the depressive groove at the lateral edge of protruding auricular concha
	$Spinal\ Cord_1$	At the most superior edge of the ear root
	$Spinal\ Cord_2$	Anterior to the mastoid process, at the inferior edge of the ear root
	Ermigen	At the crossing point of the ear back and the midpoint of the mastoid process (equal to the ear root at the level with Diaphram Point)
Other	Upper Abdomen	Below the medial edge of the opening of the external auditory canal
	Lower Abdomen	Above the medial edge of the opening of the external auditory canal

Egen 蛾根 [é gēn] An extra point located at the medial edge of the mandible, 3 cm anteroinferior to the corner of the mandible. Indications: Acute /chronic tonsilitis, laryngopharyngitis. Puncture: 1.5—3 cm perpendicularly.

egg-interposing moxibustion 鸡子灸 [jī zǐ jiǔ] A kind of indirect moxibustion, i. e., to administer moxibustion by puting half a ripened egg (get rid of its egg yellow) covering the swelling and posionus area.

eight matters for attention before acupuncture 荣备回避八法 [róng bèi huí bì bā fǎ] According to prescriptions with Extraordinary Effects: Wind—if it is windy, order the patient to be punctured in a place where the wind can be avoided. Cold—if it is cold, order the patient to be in a warm place and drink some hot beverages. Summer-heat—if it is very hot in summer, order the patient to wash his or her face with fresh water and sit in a windy and cool place for a while. Damp—before acupuncture order the patient to take something pungent and dry in nature. Yin—if yin *qi* is serious and the patient's *qi* and blood can not flow, order the patient first to take some drugs of warmly tonifying nature. Dryness—if it is dry, order the patient to be in a windy and cool place and take some drugs of unobstructing *qi* and blood. Car—if the patient comes to the hospital by car let the patient rest a while and let his or her *qi* and blood be at ease. Horse—if the patient comes to the hospital by riding a horse, let him or her have a rest.

eight empirical points for foot *qi* 脚气八处负 [jiǎo qì bā chù xué] Referring to the eight empirical moxibustion points for treating foot *qi*. "At initial stage of foot *qi*, moxibustion should be done immediately first on Fengshi (GB 31), then Futu (ST 32), and then Dubi (ST 35), Xiyan (EX-LE 5) (double), Zusanli (ST 36), Shangjuxu (ST 37), Xiajuxu (ST 36), and finally Jugu …" (Prescriptions Worth a Thousand Gold).

eight miraculous turtle techniques 灵龟八法 [líng guī bā fǎ] One of the ancient theories to select acupuncture points. The eight points in the eight extra meridians are related to the day and the hour in terms of Heavenly Stems and Earthly Branches to select the appropriate acupuncture points.

eight-wood fire 八木火 [bā mù huǒ] The fire due to the burning of the eight kinds of woods. (pine, cypress, bamboo, tangerine, elm, trifoliate orange, mulberry and jujube). In ancient China it was not advisable to use it to ignite mugwart for moxibustion.

eight depressions 八虚 [bā xū] The depression of the bilateral elbow, axilla, femur and knee. An abnormal reaction may appear if the five storing viscera are diseased, cardial and pulmonary troubles are reflected at the elbow and arm; The hepatic trouble at the axilla, the splenic trouble at the femur, the renal trouble at the knee. These portions are the vital pathways for circulation of *qi* and blood. If pathogenic *qi* retains there the meridian will be injured, appearing the symptoms such as difficulty in flexion and extension.

eight confluences 八会 [bā huì] 1. The *shu* points where the viscera, *qi*, blood, sinew, vessels, bones and marrow are confluent;

Eight Confluences	Name of Point
Emptying Viscera	Zhongwan (CV12)
Storing Viscera	Zhongmen (LR 13)
Tendon	Yanglingquan (GB 34)
Marrow	Juegu
Blood	Geshu (BL 17)
Bones	Dazhui (GV 14)
Vessels	Taiyuan (LU 9)
Qi	Danzhong (CV 17)

2. Referring to eight points where the eight

meridians are communicated with the eight points at the four limbs; 3. an extra point, located 1. 5 cm below Yangxi (LI 5). Indications: Mania, cataract, myopia, hypertension, apoplexy, oval trouble. Moxibustion: 3—5 moxa cones.

eight guiding principles 八纲 [bā gāng] The eight guiding principles for diagnosis, namely, yin, yang, exterior, interior, cold, heat, deficiency, and excess.

eight joints 八溪 [bā xī] A collective term for the eight joints—two elbow joints and two wrist joints of the upper limbs, two knee joints and the two ankle joints of the lower limbs.

Eighty-one Difficult Classic 八十一难经 [bā shí yī nàn jīng] A medical book originally called Huang Di's Eight-one Difficult Classic.

eight extra vessels 奇经八脉 [qí jīng bā mài] The eight vessels that have different actions besides the twelve meridians. They are Connecting Vessel of Yang, Connecting Vessel of Yin, Motility Vessel of Yang, Motility Vesel of Yin, Vital Vessel, Govornor Vessel, Conception Vessel, and Girdle Vessel.

eight confluential points 八脉交会八穴 [bā mài jiāo huì bā xué] Also termed *liuzhu baxue*, *jianjing baxue*, *bamai baxue*. Referring to the eight pairs of the points at the four limbs, which are communicated with the eight extra vessels, i. e., Gongshun (SP 4), Neiguan (PC 6), Houxi (SI 3), Shenmai (BL 62), Lingqi, Waiguan (TE 5), Lieque (LU 7) and Zhaohai (KI 6). Indicadtions: Varieties of diseases and symptoms of various parts of the head and body. Their actions are from the meridians they pertain to the eight extra vessels. (Chart)

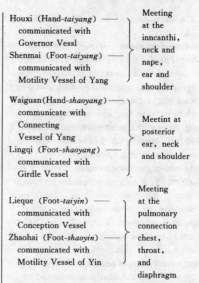

Neiguan (Hand-*jueyin*) communicated with Connecting Vessel of Yin
Gongsun (Foot-*taiyin*) communicated with Vital Vessel
} Meeting at the heart, chest and stomach

Houxi (Hand-*taiyang*) communicated with Governor Vessl
Shenmai (Foot-*taiyang*) communicated with Motility Vessel of Yang
} Meeting at the inncanthi, neck and nape, ear and shoulder

Waiguan(Hand-*shaoyang*) communicate with Connecting Vessel of Yang
Lingqi (Foot-*shaoyang*) communicated with Girdle Vessel
} Meetint at posterior ear, neck and shoulder

Lieque (Foot-*taiyin*) communicated with Conception Vessel
Zhaohai (Foot-*shaoyin*) communicated with Motility Vessel of Yin
} Meeting at the pulmonary connection chest, throat, and diaphragm

Eight Confluential Points In Rhythm 八脉交会八穴歌 [bā mài jiāo huì bā xué gē] A rhythmed acupuncture article. It contains the combination of the eight confluential points, i. e., "Gongsun (SP 4) and Chongmai…

eight diagrams 八卦 [bā guà] 1. The eight basic diagrams in Classic of Change, formed with two kinds of symbols "-"(yin)and "—" (yang). 2. *Bagua*, the old name of the massage point. It is now called *Bafeng*. A collective term for eight points surrounding the palm. It is near the small head of the 3rd metacarpal bone. If moxibustion is done on them, they can smooth the chest, eliminate phlegm and relieve thoracic depression and can also treat asthmatic breath and profuse sputum, and anorexia.

eight usages 八法 [bā fǎ] 1. The usages of the eight confluential points, mainly referring to eight methods of the miraculous turtle and the eight *feiteng* methods; 2. Referring to the eight acupunefure manipulations.

eight vessels 八脉 [bā mài] The eight extra vessels.

eight *yindu* points 阴独八穴 [yīn dú bā xué]

The extra points. I. e., Bafeng (EX-LE 10).

eight manipulations 下手八法 [xià shǒu bā fǎ] The eight manipulations applied in the course of the acupuncture operation, including pinching, fingernail pressing, rotatory kneading, springing, shaking, kneading-closing, searching and twirling.

eight *feiteng* The point-combined methods 飞腾八法 [fēi téng bā fǎ] The point-combined method according to time.

eight mid-night-noon methods 子午八法 [zǐ wǔ bā fǎ] A collective term for midninght-noon ebb-flow needlings and eight needlings of the miraculous turtle.

eight-*qi*-flow points 流注八穴 [liú zhù bā xué] I. e., the eight points of eight meridians.

eight points of eight vessels 八脉八穴 [bā mài bā xué] I. e., *bamai jiaohui baxue.*

***ejiao* 额角** [è jiǎo] Referring to the node of the forehead.

***elu*额颅** [è lú] Referring to the hairline at the forehead.

elbow-flexed and palm-prone position 屈肘俯掌位 [qū zhǒu fǔ zhǎng wèi] See sitting position.

elbow-flexed and palm-supine position 屈肘仰掌位 [qū zhǒu yǎng zhǎng wèi] See sitting potsition.

Elbow 肘 [zhǒu] An ear point in the 3rd equivalent zone superior to clavicle.

electroacupuncture apparatus 电针机 [diàn zhēn jī] An electric therapeutic appratus by making use of the wave to strengthen the acupuncture action on the point. It has many kinds, such as beebuzzing electroacupuncture apparatus, electrotube electroacupuncture apparatus, semiconductive electroacupuncture apparatus, etc. The first one is the one that makes the direct current become the pulse the direct current by making use of the principle of the vibration of the electric bell, which passes through the inductive coil to produce the inductive current. The electric wave generated is very

narrow, just like the needle, and suits electroacupuncture. Yet it has the weaknesses of unstable output, electric volume difficult in regulating its frequencies, and increased electric volume and high noise. At present it has been rarely used. The second one is the one that varieties of vibrations are generated by making use of the electronic tube. Its strength is various vibaration in waves, bulky and poor shock proof. At present it has not been used frequently. The 3rd one is made of the semiconductive elements. Because of being not limited by the varieties of elctric source, it is safe, economic in electricity, small in volume, light in weight, and anti-shock. At present, it has been used frequently in China.

electroacupuncture therapy 电针法 [diàn zhēn fǎ] The therapeutic method by acupuncture in combination with current stimulation. It was seen in the lst of 1934's Acupuncture Magazine and has seen widely used in recent years. That is in the course of needle retention during acupuncture, connect the pulse current transmitted from the electroacupuncture apparatus with the grouped points concerned (two points as a group), the pulse current varies in two-way pulse current (intermittent vibration current), square wave, etc.

electric heat moxibustion 电热灸 [diàn rè jiǔ] A kind of moxibustion technique. In modern times moxibustion with moxa cone is replaced by making use of electric heat. First connect the current with a specially-made electric moxibustion apparatus. When it reaches at a certain temperature, do dotting moxibustion or ironing moxibustioin to and fro at the selected area. It is used for rheumatic brochage and pain, etc.

electric examination of the point 穴位电测定 [xué wèi diàn chè dìng] In modern times the specificity of the point has been researched from the electric phenomenon of skin. One is to examine the change of skin resistance on the condition of extraordinarily adding the current; the other condition is to induce the current and examine the change of electric potential without adding the current. The skin resistance is usually examined by adopting the meridian point examination apparatus. Some points of which their resistance is low but their volume of electric conduction is high are called the "good conductive point." Most of their positions accord with the points. It was found by the examination of the skin potential that some points of which the potential is high is to to certain extent related to the visceral functions, which are called the "active points of skin", the number of which is more than that of the points and some points accord with the points. Viewing from the result of the examination, the skin potential of the whole tends to gradually increase but its resistance tends to gradually decrease from the four limbs to the head and face. The face is the place where the potential is higher or the resistance is lower. The flourishing and decline of *qi* and blood in various meridians can be analysed from the volume of electirc conduction. Refer examination on the meridian points.

elongated needle 芒针 [máng zhēn] In modern times, it is made of stainless steel, the body of the needle being as thready and long as the awn of wheat. Its length varies with 15 cm, 21 cm, 4. 5 dm, used for deep puncture and transverse horizontal puncture.

eleven meridians 十一脉 [shí yī mài] Referring to foot-*shaoyang*, foot-*yangming*, foot-*shaoyin*, foot-*taiyin*, foot-*jueyin*, hand-*taiyin*, hand-*shaoyin*, hand-*taiyang*, hand-*shaoyang* and hand-*yangming* meridians.

eleven heavenly-star points 天星十一穴 [tiān xīng shí yī xué] Eleven empirical effective points. They are Zusanli (ST 36), Quchi (LI 11), Hegu (LI 4), Weizhong (BL 40), Chengshan (BL 53), Kunlun (BL 60), Huantiao (GB 30), Yanglingquan (GB 34), Tongli (HT 5) and Lieque (LU 7).

emaciation-thirst disease 消渴 [xiāo kě]

Thirst, polydipsia, polyphagia, emaciation and polyurina as the main symptoms, often seen in diabetes, mellitus, diabetes insipidius, etc.

empirical point-selection 经验取穴 [jīng yàn qǔ xué] One of points-selected methods. To select the point concerned according to clinical experiences, usually referring to selection of the extra point, e. g., puncture Sifeng (EX-UE 10) for infantile malnutrition, Yiming (EX-HN 14) is selected for blurred vision.

epilepsy 痫证 [xián zhèng] A kind of mental abnormal disorder charaterized by sudden loss of consciousness, followed by convulsion of the limbs, frothy salivation, upward turning of the eyeball, or crying like a pig or sheep, being mentally normal as usual after regaining consciousness.

epiglottis 吸门 [xī mén] One of the seven vital portals.

epistaxis 鼻衄 [bí niù] Bleeding of the nasal cavity.

emptying viscera trouble treated by selecting sea-like points 治腑者治其合 [zhì fǔ zhě zhì qí hé] One of point-selected principles in Internal Classic. It implies that for treating the disorders of six emptying viscera the sea-like points of the six emptying viscera on three yang meridians of foot should be selected.

Endocrine 肾上腺 [shèn shàng xiàn] An ear point located the lower 1/2 of the lateral side of the tragus.

Erbai(EX-UE 2) 二白 [èr bái] An extra point, located 12 cm above the transverse crease of the wrist, each on either side of the flexor muscle of wrist. Two on each hand. Indication: Bleeding of hemorrhoids. Puncture: 1—2 cm perpendicularly or moxibustion is administered on it with 3—5 moxa cones or 5—10 minutes with warming moxibustion.

Erjian (LI 2) 二间 [èr jiān] A point of Large Intestine Meridian of Hand-*Yangming*. The spring-like (water) point of the meridian. Also termed *Jiangu*. Location: On the radial side of the index finger, in the depression anteroinferior to the metacarpophalangeal joint, at the dorso-palmar boundary. Select it by flexing the finger. Regional anatomy; There is the superficial flexor muscle and the deep flexor muscle of finger. The metacarpophalangeal proper artery and vein and the metacarpophalangeal nerve of the central nerve are distributed.

Ershanmen 二扇门 [ěr shàn mén] A massage point. It has the diaphoretic action when pinched and kneaded. Located on the ulnar side of the small head of the 3rd metacarpal bone or between the small head of the 4th metarcarpal bone and that of the 5th. Each hand has the two, located bilateral to the small head of the 3rd metacarpal bone.

Erzhishang 二指上 [ěr zhǐ shàng] An extra point, located in the depression at the posterior rim of the small head of the 2nd metatarsal bone and that of the 3rd. Indications: Edema, gingivitis. Puncture: 0. 3 cun. Moxibustion: 3—5 minutes with moxa stick.

Errenshangma 二人上马 [ěr rén shàng mǎ] A massage point. Also termed Shangma. Located between the small heads of the 4th and 5th metacarpal bones. It has a diuretic action, and can cure *lin* syndrome, refresh the mind, regulate *qi* and subdue something stagnant. According to Illustrations of Extra Points, it is located on the ulnar side of the dorsal hand, posterior to the small head of the 5th metacarpal bone or at the transverse crease of the distal side of the palm, opposite to the small finger on the dorsal side of Houxi (SI 3).

Ergu 耳骨 [ěr gǔ] An alternate term for Qugu.

erjian 耳尖 [ěr jiān] 1. An alternate term for Shuaigu; 2. An extra point, also termed Eryong, located at the tip of the ear. Select it by folding the ear. There is the ocular temporal nerve and the posterior ocular artey. Indications: Swollen and painful eyes, nebula, migraine or vertical headache,

deep-rooted sore at the face, high fever, acute conjunctivitis. Puncture: 0. 3 cm perpendicularly or to cause little bleeding with a triangular needle.

Erhoufaji 耳后发际 [ěr hòu fà jì] An extra point. Located at the inferior edge of the mastoid process of the posterior ear at the hairline. Indications:Goiter,scrofula. Moxibustion:3—5 moxa cones or 5—15 minutes with warming moxibustion.

Erchui 耳垂 [ěr chuí] An extra point. Located in the middle point anterior to the lobre. Indications: Mouth-shut deep-rooted sore. Puncture: 0. 3 cm perpendicularly or cause little bleeding with a triangular needle.

Erzhuixia 二椎下 [ěr zhuī xià] An extra point located at the posterior midline in the depression below the styloid process of the 2nd thoracic vertebra at the posterior midline. Indications:Mental trouble, epilepsy, malaria. Puncture: 0. 5—1 cun obliquely. Moxibustion: 3—5 moxa cones or 5—10 minutes of warming moxibustion.

Ermenqianmai 耳门前脉 [ěr mén qián mài] An extra point, located 3 cm above and below Ermen. Moxibustion: 3—7 moxa cones or 5—15 minutes with warming moxibustion.

Ermen (TE 21) 耳门 [ěr mén] 1. A point of Triple Energizer Meridian of Hand-*shaoyang*. Anatomy: There is the superfical temporal artery and vein. The branch of the ocular temporal nerve and the branch of the facial nerve are distributed. Indications: Tinnitus, deafness, *tin* ear, vertigo, toothache, pain in the neck, otitis media, inflammation of the mandibular joint. Puncture: With the mouth open, 1. 5—3 cm perpendicularly. Moxibustion: 1—3 moxa cones or 3—5 minutes with warming moxibustion. 2. an alternate term for Tinghui.

Ershangfaji 耳上发际 [ěr shàng fà jì] The name of the extra point, also termed Ershang, located directly above the tip of ear in the hairline. Indications: Goiter, epilepsy. Puncture: 0. 9—1. 5 cm horizontally.

Moxibustion: 3—5 moxa cones or 5—10 minutes with warming moxibustion.

Ershangjiao 耳上角 [ěr shàng jiǎo] The name of the location, referring to the superoposterior ear.

Eryong 耳涌 [ěr yǒng] An alternate term for Erjian.

ereca 槟榔 [bīng láng] One of interposing things for moxibustion. The seed of Areca techu L. Indication: Deafness. "Cut it sharp and make a hole on it and put a little musk on it, then insect it into the ear and burn it with moxa.

Ermigen 耳迷根 [ěr mí gēn] An ear point at the crossing point of the back of the ear and the midpoint of the mastoid process (equivalent to the root of ear at the level with Diaphragm) (Fig 29)

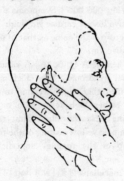

Fig 29

essence and blood are of the same origin 津血同源 [jīn xuè tóng yuán] It denotes that the liver and kidney are of same origin. The blood is stored in the liver and the essence in the kidney. The blood may nourish the esence while the latter may change into the former. They nourish each other with a very close relationship.

Essentials of Plain Questions and Difficult Classic Dealing with Acupuncture 针灸素难要旨 [zhēn jiǔ sù nàn yào zhǐ] A book written by Gao Wu in Ming Dynasty (1386-1644), also called *zhen jiu yao zhi*, *Zhen jiu*

Jie yao. It adopts from Internal Classic and Difficult Classic concerning the acupuncture literatures, and re-compiles them. It is divided into three volumes, and collects the original of nine needlings, needling techniques, reinforcing and reducing manipulations, meridians, *shu* points, etc. The purpose of which is to explore the origin of acupuncture academy.

Essential Compilation of Acupuncture 针灸纂要 [zhēn jiǔ chuàn yào] 1. A book written by an unknoun person, seen in Catarloque of Medical Books in Ming Dynasty (1368-1644), one volume, lost; 2. A book written by Qiu Maoliang, published by People's Health Press. It generally describes the brief history of acupuncture, mays of learning acupuncture, meridians, meridian points, needling techniques, treatment, prohibition, and cites the literatures. It is simple, direct, and convenient for reference study.

Esophagus 食道 [shí dào] An ear point at the edge of the crus of helix, at the crossing point of the middle and medial 1/3 between Mouth and Stomach.

Essentials of Meridians 经络枢要 [jīng luò shū yào] A book written by Xu Shizhen in Ming Dynasty (1368—1644). It contains the primary diseases, yin-yang, storing-emptying viscera, *ying* and *wei* (nutrition and defence), meridians, comon meridians (twelve meridians), extra meridians, Renying, Qikou, three modes, pulse feeling, clear and turbid, pathogenic *qi*, transmission and variation, 14 chapters in total. It cites the articles of various experts on meridians and expounded them. It was collected in the later compilation of Complete Book of Meridians written by You Chengzhong.

Essentials of Acupuncture Classic 针经节要 [zhēn jīng jié yào] A book compileed by Du Sijin in Yuan Dynasty (1271—1386), originally recorded in the lst volume of *Jisheng Bachui*. It mainly adopts part of Acupuncture Classic. It also deals with the figures of the points the twelve meridians flow over, the syndromes and symptoms of the twelve meridians and treatment and syndromes of the points of the twelve meridians (three chapters). It specially describes the diseases of the twelve meridians and the indications of 66 points, and was published in 1315.

Essentials of Experiences of Acupuncture 刺灸心法要诀 [cì jiǔ xīn fǎ yào jué] A book compiled by Wu Qian in Qing Dynasty (1644—1911), one of Golden Mirror of Medicine. It was written by mainly using the rhythmed article, in cooperation with illustrations and notes, popular and easy to be understood. It was completed in 1742.

evacuatioin puncture 大泻刺 [dà xiè cì] An acupuncture technique in Internal Classic. One of the nine needlings. It belongs to the category of surgery in traditional Chinese medicine.

Expounding of Fourteen Meridians 十四经发挥 [shí sì jīng fā huī] A medical book written by Hua Shou (Boren) in Yuan Dynasty (1206-1368), three volumes, published in 1341. It comparatively minutely noted and expounded the fourteen meridians described in Jinlan Meridians and other books, and supplemented the recording and description of the points pertaining to various meridians. There is its printing edition.

external moxibustion plaster 外灸膏 [wài jiǔ gāo] One of the formularized drugs for dressing. "External moxibustion plaster is indicative for all kinds of cold due to asthenia, diarrhea with red and white stool, or occasional pain in the abdomen, incontinence of the diarrhea. Auklandia root, prepared aconite root, cnidium fruit, Evodia rutaecarpa, pepper, and Sichuan aconite root 10 g each, are mixed with juice of fresh ginger and made as paste, then distribute it on a piece of paper, dress it on the umbilicus, and then cover it with clothe, and finally iron it with an iron." (Yang's Family Stored Prescriptions).

extra merdians 奇经 [qí jīng] An abbreviation of qi jing ba mai (eight extra vessels).

extra point 奇穴 [qí xué] I. e., the extra point.

extremely abnormal pulse 脉悬绝 [mài xuán jué] The pulse is very different from the normal, for instance, it may be three or four times faster than or one-half or even less the rate of the normal. It indicates a severe case.

extreme heat produces cold 热极生寒 [rè jí shēng hán] 1. Climatic changes from extremely hot weather into the cold one; 2. When the pathologic changes of the febrile syndrome evolves to its climax, pseudo-cold symptoms may appear instead.

excessive waste of cardiac nutrition 心营过耗 [xīn yíng guò hào] Symptoms due to the excessive loss of cardiac yin fluid. The clinical picture is the same as that of deficiency of cardiac yin.

exterior heat 表热 [biǎo rè] A variety of the external syndrome. The chief manifestations are rather slight aversion to wind and cold, rather high fever with or without sweating, headache, slight thirst, thin white or thin pale yellow coating of the tongue, or red tip of the tongue, superficial rapid pulse, etc.

external meridians 外经 [wài jīng] The external portion of the meridian that runs superficially, contrary to that of running over the storing viscera. The diseases or syndromes pertaining to the external portion of the body are generally called external meridian diseases or meridian syndromes, while those pertaining to the viscera, the diseases or syndromes of storing or emptying viscera.

examination of meridian points 经穴测定 [jīng xué cè dìng] It was found from contemporary study on the electric phenonmenon of skin that the skin resistance at the points is usually lower. The volume of electric conductivity of the point can be examined with a meridian-point examination apparatus. The flourishing and decline of *qi* and blood in various meridians can be predicted through analysing the volume of electric condustivity of the representative points of various meridians. The representive points are usually source points, and then the well-like, gap-like and back *shu* points. The examination is carried on under the quiet state, and attention is paid to various interupting factors. According the result of examination, the high and low and different numbers of electric conductivity of the point at the bilateral side are analysed. That 1/3 higher than that other point is the higher number while that 1/3 lower than that of other points is the lower number. The high number usually indicates that the disease pertains excess type while the lower number indicates that the disease pertains deficiency type. That of the different side indicates that the meridian is in the pathological change. This method should be synthetically analysed in association with the four diagnostic techques and eight guiding principles. Only in such a way can the correct conclusion be got.

Experiences of Moxi bustion with *Taiyi* Moxa-stick 太乙神针心法 [tài yí shén zhēn xīn fǎ] A medical book, compiled by Han Yifeng in Qing Dynasty (1616—1911), two volumes. The 1st volume deals with the symptoms, the 2nd the case records of acuncture treatment, appended with the origin in Qing Dynasty (1616—1911), accomplished in 1717.

excretion with no storage 泻而不藏 [xiè ér bù cáng] Referring to the physiologic functions of the six emptying viscera. In general they have the cavities with the functions of receiving, transporting, digesting and excreting food and water. Most of them open directly to the exterior and do not have the function of storing the refined material and are merely the paths for food and water.

extra points 经外穴 [jīng wài xué] I. e. , *jing wai qi xue*.

extra points 经外奇穴 [jīng wài qí xué] Briefly called *qi xue* or *jing wai xue*. Referring to the empirical and effective points besides *shu* points of the fourteen meridians. Of them some only have the locations and indications but have no names. They were nomencatured by latter generations. A few of them were classified into the meridian points, e. g. , Gaohuang(BL 43), Fengshi (GB 31), etc.

External nose 外鼻 [wài bí] An ear point located at the anterior edge of the cartillege of the tragus to form an equable triangle with the tip of Tragus and Adrenal Gland.

excessive dryness brings about dry symptoms 燥盛则干 [zào shèn zé gān] When *qi* becomes excessive, it would exhaust body fluids and bring about various pathologic manifestations of dry nature.

extra points 别穴 [bié xué] They are called the extra points that do not orginate from the Bronze Figure Marked with Points but are seen in various acupuncture books.

exterior cold 表寒 [biǎo hán] A variety of the exterior syndrome. The chief manifestations are severe aversion to wind and cold, low-grade fever with or without scaling, headache and stiff neck, soreness of the limbs and joints, thin white coating of tongue, superficial and taut or superficial and slow pulse, etc.

exterior syndrome 表证 [biǎo zhèng] The superficial and mild illness. The chief symptoms are chilly sensation, fever, headache, general aching, stuffy nose, running nose, cough, superficial pulse, thin coating of tongue, etc. It is usually seen in common cold, influenza, and the premonitory or early stages of various acute infectious diseases.

excess syndrome 实证 [shí zhèng] The manifestations due to the yang rampancy of pathogenic *qi* and intense struggle between the normal and the abnormal, including the external excess and internal excess syndromes.

excessive rise of hepatic yang 肝阳上亢 [gān yáng shàng kàng] Hepatic yang *qi* becomes excessive and causes symptoms in the upper part of the body. The main symptoms are vertigo, headache, flushed face, blurred vision, tinnitus, bitter taste, stringy and rapid pulse, etc.

external cold due to deficiency of yang 阳虚则外寒 [yáng xū zé wài hán] The cold manifestations that are aroused by shortage of yang *qi* and hypofunction of the viscera, e. g., chilliness, coldness of limbs, pale complexion, etc.

exterior excess 表实 [biǎo shí] A type of the exterior syndrome with characteristics of chills, no sweating, superficial and taut pulse besides the symptoms and signs of the exterior syndrome.

excess of *qi* induces fire 气有余便是火 [qì yǒu yú biàn shì huǒ] When yang *qi* becomes excessive, pathologic manifestations of various fire syndromes may be produced.

extreme cold produces heat 寒极生热 [hán jí shēng rè] 1. Climatic changes from the extremely cold weather into warm one; 2. When the pathologic changes of the cold syndrome evolves to its climax, pseudoheat symptom may appear instead.

external *fu* organs 外府 [wài fǔ] Referring to the six emptying viscera, contrary to the internal organs.

External ear 外耳 [wài ěr] An ear point located in the depression anterior to the intertragus notch.

exhaustion of *qi* associated with severe hemorrhage 气随血脱 [qì suí xuè tuō] Symptoms of severe depletion of *qi* due to profuse hemorrhage.

Excitant point 兴奋点 [xīn fèn diǎn] An ear point at the centre of Testicle and Lung point.

External genitalia 外生殖器 [wài shēng zhí qì] An ear point at the helix at the level with Sympathetic.

extending-holding hand 舒张押手 [shū zhāng yá shǒu] See needle-insertion by stretching the skin surrounding the inserted needle.

external pathogenic *qi* 表邪 [biǎo xié] The pathogen which invades the superficial portion of the body.

examining the point 审穴 [shěn xué] Referring to examining the point.

Eye₁ 目₁ [mù yī] An ear point anteroinferior to the intertragus notch.

Eye₂ 目₂ [mù ěr] An ear point posteroinferior to the intertragus notch.

Eye 眼 [yǎn] An ear point located at the centre of Zone₅.

eyes, the window of the liver 肝开窍于目 [gān kāi qiào yú mù] Some physiopathologic conditions of the liver may manifest as changes of the eyes.

F

facial needling 面针 [miàn zhēn] A therapeutic method by puncturing specific points at the face. It was reported in 1960. The points mainly accord with the inspecting location of the face (Fig 30).

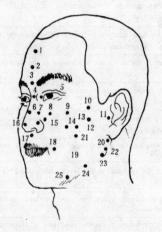

Fig 30

fanzhen 燔针 [fān zhēn] 1. Referring to warming needling; 2. Referring to fire needling.

Face-cheek 面颊 [miàn jiá] An ear point loca-

ted in the surrounding boundary line between Zone₅ and Zone₆.

faint pulse 微脉 [wēi mài] The pulse that is extremely faint and weak and barely palpable. It usually indicates the extremely deficiency syndrome.

failure after prolonged palpation 久持索然 [jiǔ chí suò rán] The pulse is hard to be felt even after prolonged palpations. It is a reflection of an extreme weak pulse.

failure of the stomach to propel downward 胃失和降 [wèi shí hé jiàng] It is normal for gasstric *qi* to function downwards. If it fails to do so as it should, various symptoms of retrogressive upward motion will occur such as belching, regurgitation of acid, nausea and vomiting, hiccup, anorexia, epigastric distension and pain, etc.

face, the mirror of the heart 心，其华在面 [xīn qí huá zhài miàn] The functional normality of th heart and the sufficiency of the blood may be exhibited as radiant facial complexion.

facial paralysis 面瘫 [miàn tān] It is acute in onset which is caused by muscular flaccidity of one side of the face, with no hemiplegia and mental confusion, frequently seen in youth and the aged.

Division	Name of Point	Location and Method of Point Selection
Forehead	1. Shoumian	At the centre of the forehead, at the junction of the upper and middle 1/3 of the midline between the two eyebrows to the anterior hairline.
	2. Throat	At the junction of the middle and lower 1/3 of the middle of the two eyebrows to the anterior hairline, i. e., at the midpoint of line connecting Shoumian and Lung Point.
	3. Lung	At the midpoint (Yitan, EX-HN 3) connecting the ends of the medial brains.
Nasal Zone	4. Heart	At the lowest point of the nose bridge, just at the midpoint (Shangen) of the line connecting the two inner canthi.

Continued

Division	Name of Point	Location and Method of Point Selection
Nasal Zone	5. Liver	Below the highest point of the nose bridge, at the crossing point of the midline of the nose and the line connecting the two zygomatic bones, i. e. , the midpoint between Heart Point and Spleen Point.
	6. Spleen	Above the tip of the nose, at the middle of the superior edge of Zhuntou at the tip of the nose.
	7. Gallbladder	Below the lateral edge of the nose bridge, bilateral to Liver Point, directly below the inner canthus at the inferior edge of the nose bridge.
	8. Stomach	Above the centre of ala nasi, bilateral to Spleen Point, directly below Gallbladder Point, at the crossing point of the two lines.
Ocular Zone	9. Yingru	Slightly above the inner canthus in the depression at the lateral edge of the nose bridge.
Mouth Zone	10. Bladder	Above the philtrum, at the junction of the upper and middle 1/3 of the philtrum (Renzhong).
	11. Guli	1. 5 cm lateral to the corner of the mouth, at the anastomotic place of the upper and lower lips.
Auricular one	12. Back	In front of tragus between the medial side of the tragus and the mandible joint.
Zygomatic Zone	13. Small intestine	At the medial edge of the zygoma, at the level with Liver Point and Gallbladder Point.
	14. Large intestine	At the zygomatic region directly below the outer canthus , at the inferior edge of the zygoma.
	15. Shoulder	At the zygoma, directly below the outer canthus, at the superior edge of the zygomative arc.
	16. Arm	Postero superior to the zygoma. Posterior to Shoulder point, at the superior edge of the zygomatic arc.
	17. Hand	Postero inferior to the zygoma, below Arm Point, at the inferior edge of the zygomantic arc.
cheek zone	18. Thigh	At the junction of the upper and middle 1/3 of the line connecting the lobre and the mandible corner.
	19. Knee	At the junction of the middle and lower 1/3 of the line connecting the lobre and the mandible corner.
	20. knee-cap	In the depression superior to the mandible corner.
	21. Tibia	Anterior to the mandible corner, at the superior edge of the mandible.
	22. Foot	Anterior to Tibia point, diredtly below the outer canthus, at the inferior edge of the mandible.
	23. Kidney	At the cheek, at the junction between the horizontal line of ala nasi and the vertical line directly from Taiyang Point.
	24. Umliti-	At the cheek, about 2 cm inferior to Kidney Point.

fearful and timid 心虚胆怯 [xīn xū dǎn qiè] Symptoms due to timidity and fear.

Fengguan 风关 [fēng guān] A point used for infantile massage. The palmar surface of the lst, 2nd and 3rd segments of the index finger are generally called three keypasses. The lst segment is called fengguan (wind pass), the middle, Qiguan (*qi* pass) and the 3rd, Mingguan (vital pass). Chiefly used for inspection, diagnosis and massage.

Fenglong (ST 40) 丰隆 [fēng lóng] A point of Stomach Meridian of Foot-*yangming*, the connecting point of the meridian it pertains to. Location: On the anterolateral side of the leg, 2.4 dm above the tip of lateral ankle, about 3 cm lateral to Tiaokou (ST 38). Regional anatomy: Between the long extensor muscle of toe and the short muscle of calf. There are the branches of the anteriotibial artery and vein. The superficial peroneal nerve is distributed. Indications: Profuse sputum, asthma, cough, thoracic pain, headache, dizziness, sore throat, difficulty in defecation, mania, epilepsy, atrophy of the lower limmbs. Puncture: 3—5 cm perpendicularly. Moxibustion: 5—7 moxa cones or 5—15 minutes with warming moxibustion.

Feichu 飞处 [fēi chù] An alternate term for Zhigou (TE 6).

Feiyang 飞扬 [fēi yáng] I. e., 飞阳 (Feiyang, BL58).

feiyang **collateral meridian** 飞阳之脉 [fēi yáng zhī mài] The collateral meridian of foot-*taiyang* meridian at the leg.

Feihu 飞虎 [fēi hǔ] An alternate term for Zhigou (TE 36).

Fengmen (BL 12) 风门 [fēng mén] A point of Bladder Meridium of Foot-*taiyang*, the confluence of GV and foot-*taiyang* meridian, also termed Refu. Location: 4.5 cm lateral to the inferior spinal process of the 2nd thoracic vertebra. Regional anatomy: Passing through the trapezius muscle. There is the medial branch of the dorsal branches of the 2nd intercostal artery and vein. The

medial cutaneous branch of the posterior branch of the 2nd thoracic nerve is distributed. The latral branch of the posterior branch of the 2nd thoracic nerve is in the deeper. Indications: Common cold and cough, fever, headache, vertigo, profuse nasal discharge, stuffy nose, stiff neck, pains in the chest and back, carbuncle, feverish sensation in the chest, general fever. Puncture: 1.5—3 cm obliquely (It is not advisable to puncture deep). Moxibustion: 3—5 moxa cones or 5—15 minutes with warming moxibustion.

Fengfei point 风痱穴 [fēng fèi xué] An extra point, one located 1.8 cm below Zhongwan (CV 12), the other two 1.8 cm bilateral to Zhongwan (CV 12), 3 in total. Moxibustion: 3—5 moxa cone or 5—10 minutes with warming moxibustion.

Fengmenrefu 风门热府 [fēng mén rè fú] I. e., Fengmen (BL 12).

Fengshi (GB 31) 风市 [fēng shì] A meridian point of Gallbladder Meridian of Foot-*shaoyang*. Originally an extra point, also termed Zuishou. Location: 2 dm above the horizontal line of the cubital transvers crease between the lateral side of the thigh. Stand erect, with the two arms put by side. It is where the tip of the middle finger touches. Regional anatomy: Passing through the iliotibial boundle, reaching musculus vatus lateralis. There are the muscular branches of the lateral femoral circumflex artery and vein. The lateral femoral cutaneous muscle and the muscular branch of the femoral nerve are distributed. Indications: Apoplexy, hemiplegia, atrophy of the lower limbs, itch of the whole body, foot *qi*. Puncture: 3—4.5 cm perpendi-cularly. Moxibustion: 3—5 moxa cones or 5—10 minutes with warming moxibustion.

Fengyan 风眼 [fēng yǎn] An extra point, located at the dorsopalmar boundary of the head of the transverse crease of the metacarpal bone, on the radial side of the thumb. Indications: Anxiety and fulllness of the chest and abdomen, vomiting, hiccup, pain and difficulty in the movement of the five fingers, night blindness, mature lens opacity. Puncture: 0. 3—0. 6 cm perpendicularly. Moxibustion: 3—5 moxa cones or 5—10 minutes with warming moxibustion.

Fengchi (GB 20) 风池 [fēng chí] A point of Gallbladder Meridian of Foot-*shaoyang*, the confluence of foot-*shaoyang* meridian and Connecting Vessel of Yang. Location: At the level with Fengfu (GV 16) between sternocleidoumastoidous muscle and trapezius muscle, posterior to the mastoid process. Regional anatomy: Passing through the splenus muscle of head, the semispinal muscle of head to reach the lateral aspect of the greater straight muscle of the posterior head. There are the branches of the occipital artery and vein. The branch of the lesser occipital nerve is distributed. Indications: Headache, vertigo, stiff neck, congestion and pain in the eye, epistaxis, rhinitis, deafness, apoplexy, deviated mouth and eyes, malaria, febrile diseases, common cold, goiter. Puncture:1. 5—3 cm with the tip of the needle slightly downward, obliquely toward the tip of the nose. Moxibustion: 3—7 moxa cones or 5—15 minutes with warming moxibustion.

feeling of pulse 脉诊 [mài zhěn] The diagnostic method that a physician touches and compresses the patient's radial pulse proximal to the carpal joints, so as to assess its changes.

Fengcitong 风齿痛 [fēng chǐ tòng] An extra point, Location: 3-7 cm above the transverse cease of wrist, similar to Neiguan (PC 6). (Fig 31)

Fengyan 风岩 [fēng yán] An extra point, located 1. 5 cm antrior to the midpoint of the line connecting the midpoint of the posterior hairline and the inferior edge of the lobre. Indications: Mania, hysteria, headache, neurasthenia. Puncture: 3—4 cm perpendi-

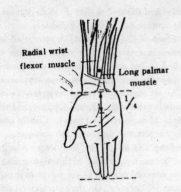

Radial wrist flexor muscle

Long palmar muscle

1/4

Fig 31

cularly.

Fenzhong 分中 [fēn zhōng] Referring to Huangtiao (GB 30).

Fenshui 分水 [fēn shuǐ] I. e., Shuifen (CV 9).

Fenrou 分肉 [fēn ròu] 1. Referring to sinew; 2. an alternate term for Yangfu (GB 38).

Feidi 肺底 [fèi dǐ] An alternate term for Lingtai. (GV 10).

Fegufu (GV 16) 风府 [fēng fǔ] A GV point of the confluence of GV and Connecting Vessel of Yang. Also termed Sheben and Caoxi. Location: 3 cm above the postrior hairline on the midline of the nape. Regional anatomy: Passing through the ligament of nape to reach the posterooccipital membrane. There is the branch of the occipital artery. The 3rd cervical nerve and the greater occipital nerve are distributed. The cerebromedullary cistern and the bulb are in the deeper. Indications: Mania, epilepsy, hysteria, apoplexy, hemiplegia, vertigo, stiffness and pain in the neck, sore throat, ocular pain, epistaxis. Puncture:1. 8—3 cm perpendicularly or downwardly obliquely. (Forward, upward and deep puncture is prohibited) Moxibustion is prohibited.

Feimu 肺募 [fèi mù] 1. One of anterior referred points of the viscera, i. e., Zhongfu (LU 1); 2. An extra point.

Feishu (BL 13) 肺俞 [fèi shū] A point of bladder Meridian of Foot-*taiyin*, the back *shu* point of the lungs. Location: 4. 5 cm lateral to Shenzhu (GV 12) between the spinal process of the 3rd and 4th thoracic vertebrae. Regional anatomy: Passing through the trapezius muscle and the rhomboid muscle. There is the medial branch of the posterior branch of the 3rd intercostal artery and vein. The medial cutaneous branch of the posterior branch of the 3rd thoracic nerve is distributed. The lateral branch of the posterior branch of the 3rd thoracic nerve is in the deeper. Indications: Cough, asthmatic breath, steaming of bones and tidal fever, night sweat, full chest, spitting blood, sore throat, pain in the lumbar spine. Puncture: 1. 5—2. 5 cm obliquely.

(it is not advisable to puncture deep). Moxibustion: 3—5 moxa cones or 5—15 minutes with warm needling.

fifteen collateral points 十五络穴 [shí wǔ luò xué] The points of the fifteen collateral meridians. See fifteen collateral meridians and their points.

fifteen collateral meridians 十五络 [shí wǔ luò] Also termed *shi wu bie luo*. In the four extremities, the twelve meridians branch a collateral meridian each; in the trunk, there is the collateral meridian of CV (at the anterior trunk), the collateral meridian of GV (at the posterior trunk) and the big collateral meridian of spleen (at the lateral trunk). Each collateral meridian has a point and its indications. They are tabuleted as follows. (Table)

Fifteen Collateral Meridians	Name of Point	Distribution	Excess Syndrome	Deficiency Syndrome
Hand-*taiyin*	Lieque (LU 7)	Running over Hand-*yangming*	Feverish sensation in the palms	Yawning, frequent urination
Hand-*shaoyin*	Tongli (HT 5)	Hand-*taiyang*		Aphasia
Hand-*jueyin*	Neiguan (PC 6)	Hand-*shaoyang*	Cardialgia	Anxiety
Hand-taiyang	Zhizheng (SI 7)	Hand-*shaoyin*		Wart
Hand-*yangming*	pianli (LI 6)	Hand-*taiyin*	Dental carrier deafness	Cold teeth
Hand-*shaoyang*	Waiguan (TE, SJ 5)	Hand-*jueyin*	Spasm of elbow	
Foot-*taiyang*	Feiyang (BL 58)	Foot-*shaoyin*	Nasal suffocation, pains in the head, back	Epistaxis
Foot-*shaoyang*	Guangming (GB 37)	Foot-*jueyin*	jue syndrome	
Foot-*yangming*	Fenglong (ST 40)	Foot-*taiyin*	Sore throat, sudden mutism, mania	
Foot-*taiyin*	Gongsun (SP 4)	Foot-*yangming*	Cholera, pain in abdomen	Tympanite
Foot-*shaoyin*	Dazhong(CV, RN 17)	Foot-*taiyang*	Anxiety, uioschesis	Lumbago
Foot-*jueyin*	Ligou (LR 5)	Foot-*shaoyang*	Swoleen testes, hernia	Sudden itch
CV	Jiuwei (CV 5)	Merging into the abdomen	Pain in the atdomenal shin	Skin itch
GV	Changqiang (GV 1)	Ascending along to the nape and merging into the head	Stiff spine	Heaviness of head
Big colleteral of spleen	Dabao (SP21)	Distributed over the chest and axilla	Pain in the whole lody	

fifteen collateral meridians 十五络脉 [shí wǔ luò mài] Also termed *shiwu bieluo*. At the four limbs, the twelve meridians branch a collateral each; at the trunk, there is the collaterat of Conception Vessel (anterior to the body), the collateral of Governor Vessel (posterior to the body and the big collateral of spleen (lateral to the body). Each collateral meridian has a connecting point and its indications.

fifty-nine points 五十九刺 [wǔ shí jiǔ cì] fifty-nine points used for treating febrile diseases in ancient China. They are as follows. Shaoze (SI 1), Guanchong (SJ 1), Shangyang (LI 1), Zhongchong (PC 9), Shaochong (HT 9), Houxi (SI 3), Zhongzhu (TE 3), Sanjian (LI 3), Shaofu (HT 8), Shugu (BL 65), Zulinqi (GB 41), Xiangu (ST 43), Taodao (SP 3), Wuchu (BL 5), Chengguang (BL 6), Tongtian (BL 7), Toulinqi (GB 15), Chengling (GB 18), Naokong (GB 19), Tinghui (GB 2), Wangu (GB 12), Chengjiang (CV 24), Yemen (GV 15), Baihui (GB 20), Xinhui (GB 22), Shenting (GV 24), Fengfu (GV 16), Lianquang (CV 23), Fengchi (GB 20) and Tianzhu (BL 10).

fifty-nine points for febrile diseases 热病五十九俞 [rè bìng wǔ shí jiǔ shū] The fifty-nine points for treating febrile diseases. According to Wang's Notes, they are Shangxing (GV 23), Xinhui (GV 22), Qianoling (GV 21), Baihui (GV 20), Houding (GV 19), Wuchu (BL 5) Chengguang (BL 6), Tongtian (BL 7), Luogue (BL 8), Yuzhen (BL 9), Linqi (BL 41), Muchuang (BL 18), Zhengying (GB 17), Chengling (GB 18), Zhengying (GB 17), Chengling (GB 18), Naokong (GB 19), Dazhu (BL 11), Zhongbu (LU 1), Quepen (ST 12), Fingunen (BL 12), Qichong (ST 30), Zusanli (ST 36) Shousanli (LI 10), Shangjuxu (ST 37), Xiajuxu (ST 39), Yunmen (LU 2) Jianyu (LI 15), Yaoshu (GV 2), Pohu (BL 42), Shentang (GV 24), Hunmen (BL 47), Yishe (BL 49), Zhishi (BL 52), Weizhong (BL

40).

fifty-seven lumbosacral points 肾俞五十七穴 [shèn shū wǔ shí qī xué] Referring to 57 points for treating water disease. According to Wang Bin's notes, they include 25 points at the lumbosacral region: Jizhong (GV 6), Xuanshu (GV 5), Mingmen (GV 4), Yaoshu (GV 2), Changqiang (GV 1), Dachangshu (BL 25), Pangguangshu (BL 56), Huangmen (BL 51), Zhishi (BL 52), Baomen (BL 53), Zhibian (BL 54); 20 points at the lower abdomen: Zhongzhu (KI 15), Siman (KI 14), Qixue (KI 13), Dahe (KI 12), Henggu (KI 11), Wailing (ST 16), Daju (ST 27), Shuidao (ST 28), Guilai (ST 29), Qichong (ST 30); 12 points below the knee: Dazhong (KI 4), Fuliu (KI 7), Yingu (KI 10), Zhaohai (KI 6), Jiaoxin (KI 8), Zhubin (KI 9). Those located in the centre are the single points but those at the bilateral side are double.

fitness moxibustion 保健灸 [bǎo jiàn jiǔ] A moxibustion technique to approach the strengthening of body resistance and preserving health by reinforcing the human body's anti-disease ability. I. e., to prevent from disease by continuous supprurative moxibustion. The commonly-used points are Zusanli (ST 36), Fuanyuan (CV 4), Qihai (CV 6), Gaohuang (BL 43), etc.

fixed quality of acupuncture anesthesia 针麻定量 [zhēn má dìng liàng] A term of acupuncture anesthesia. It refers that in the course of acupuncture anesthesia the manifestation and examination of the parameter of stimulation of acupuncture anesthesia. Refer parameter of stimulation of acupuncture anesthesia.

five points at back spine 脊背五穴 [jí bèi wǔ xué] An extra points. One is located at the higher spot of the spinal process of the 2nd thoracic vertebra; the 2nd is located at the end of coccyx; the 3rd is at the spinal bone of the line connecting the above-mentioned points. Then form an equilateral triangle with a rope (1/2 of the line connecting the previous to points). Indications: Mania, epilepsywith fright. Moxibustion: 3—5 moxa cones for each point. (Fig 32)

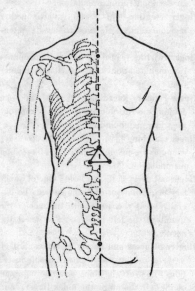

Fig 32

first lateral line of chest 胸第一侧线 [xiōng dì yī chè xiàn] A line for locating the meridian point, 6 cm to the line of chest, where Kidney Meridian of Foot-*shaoyin* passes through, Shufu (KI 27), Yuznong (KI 26), Shenque (CT), Lingxu (KI 23), and Bulang (KI 2৬) are distributed.

fifty-nine points for febrile diseases 热俞五十九穴 [rè shū wǔ shí jiǔ xué] I. e. , fifty-nine points for febrile diseases.

fine needle 微针 [wēi zhēn] Also termed small needle. Generally referring to the nine needles, contrary to *bian* (sharp) stone.

first lateral line of back 背第一侧线 [bèi dì yī chè xiàn] a line locating the meridian point. The aea 4. 8 cm distal to the midline of the back is where Bladder Meridian of Foot-*taiyang* passes through where the points such as Dazhu (GV 14), Fengmen (BL 12), Feishu (BL 13), Jueyinshu (BL

14), Xinshu (BL 15) Dushu (BL 16), Geshu (BL 17), Ganshu (SP 16), Danshu (BL 19), Pishu (BL 20), Weishu (BL 21), Sanjiaoshu (BL 22), Shenshu (BL 23), Qihaishu (BL 24), Dachangshu (BL 25), Guanyuanshu (BL 26), Xiaochangshu (BL 27), Pangguangshu (BL 28), Zhonglushu (BL 29) and Baihuanshu (BL 30) are distributed over.

finger needling 指针 [zhǐ zhēn] To replace the needle with the finger, e. g. press, pinch or knead, etc. (Fig 33)

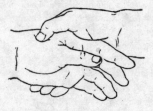

Fig 33

finger pulling 指拔 [zhǐ bá] I. e. , the technique of withdrawing the needle.

finger poking technique 指拨法 [zhǐ bá fǎ] An acupuncture manipulation. To hold the handle of needle with the thumb and index finger and to gently poke the body of needle with the middle finger, so as to strengthen needling sensation.

finger holding 指持 [zhǐ chí] An acupuncture manipulation. i. e. , needle-held method. (Fig 34)

finger-pushing manipulation 循法 [xún fǎ] An accessary acupuncture manipulation, i. e. , push the fingers to and fro along the meridian. (Fig 35)

fifteenth vertebra 第十五椎 [dì shí wǔ zhuī] Referring to the third lumbar vertebra.

filiform needle 毫针 [háo zhēn] One of the nine ancient needles, most commonly used for treating varieties of cold, heat, pain and blockage since it is thready and small in its body, antipathogenic *qi* of the human body in its body may not be injured.

finger-eyes 指目 [zhǐ mù] A physician feels

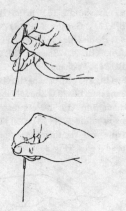

Fig 34

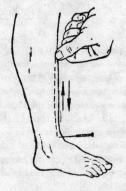

Fig 35

the patient's pulse with the most senstive touch of the lips of his or her fingers.

Finger 指 [zhǐ] An ear point at the lower edge of the helix at the upper end of the scaphoid fossa.

finger *cun* 指寸 [zhǐ cùn] The patient's hand is taken as the proportional *cun* for selecting the point. Its method is divided into middle finger *cun*, thumb *cun* and transverse finger *cun*.

fingernail-pressing manipulation 爪法 [zǎo fǎ] An auxiliary insertion of the needle during acupuncture.

fingernail pressing 爪摄 [zǎo shè] An auxiliary acupuncture manipulation.

finger retention 指留 [zhǐ liú] An acupuncture manipulation. Referring to needle retention.

finger twirling 指捻 [zhǐ niǎn] An acupuncture manipulation, i. e. , twirling manipulation.

finger rotatory kneading 指搓 [zhǐ cuō] An acupunctue manipulation, i. e. , rotatory kneading manipulation.

finger searching 指循 [zhǐ xún] An accessary acupuncture manipulation, i. e. , searching manipulation.

fingernail press 爪切 [zǎo qiè] One of auxiliary manipulations of acupuncture. To laterally press the point with the nail of the thumb of the left hand so as to insert the needle.

fingernail press and needle insertion 爪切进针 [zǎo qiè jìn zhēn] One of needle insertions. To press the point with the fingernail of the left thumb or the index finger, and swiftly insert the needle by the side of the fingernail with the right hand holding the needle. Suitable for insertion of the short needle. Fingernail press can fix the point and aid in inserting the needle and relieve pain and strengthen needling sensation.

five decisive actions 五决 [wǔ jué] The five decisive actions of the livver heart, spleen, lungs and kidneys on diagnosis of diseases. "The five decisive actions refer to inspecting the diseases of the five storing viscera to decide whether the patient will be alive or dead, which is the guideline of diagnosing diseases. " (Classified Classsic)

five constituents 五体 [wǔ tǐ] 1. Referring to the skin, muscle, vessel, tendons and bones. They correspond with the five storing viscera; 2. Referring to the two hands, two feet and head.

five-type persons 五态之人 [wǔ tài zhī rén] People were divided into the five types in ancient China. "The *taiyin* people, *shaoyin* people, *taiyang* people, *shaoyang* people, and peope with moderate yin-yang. They have different tendons, bones, *qi* and blood. " (One who is good at using acupuncure and moxibustion treats the patient according to the five types of people. Reduce if he is sthenic, reinforce if he is asthenic. " (Miraculous Pivot).

five-circle theory 五轮 [wǔ lún] A theory of ophthalmology in traditional Chinese medicine. It divides the eye from its periphery to the centre into five circles, namely, *rulun* (muscle circle), *xuelun* (blood circle) *qilun* (*qi* circle), *fenglun* (wind circle), and *shuilun* (water circle) to explain physiopathological changes of the eyes, a guidance of diagnosis and treatment. 1. *Rulun* refers to the upper and lower eyelids, belonging to the spleen and their disease are usually related to the pleen and stomach; 2. *Xuelun* refers to the external and internal canthi, belonging to the heart and their diseases are usually related to the heart and small intesting; 3. *Qilun* refers to the white part of the eye, belonging to the lung, its disease is usually related to the lung and large intestine; 4. *Fenglun* refers to the black part of the eye, belonging to the liver and its disease is usually related to the liver and gallbladder. *Shuilun* refers to the pupil, belonging to the kidney and its disease is usually related to the kidney.

five correspondences 五主 [wǔ zhǔ] It is called five correspondences that heart, liver and kidneys correspond with the skin, muscle and vessels. The lungs relate to the skin, the liver relates to the tendons, the spleen relates to the muscles and the kidneys relate to the bones.

five excesses 五过 [wǔ guò] Excess of acupuncture reinforcing-reducing. "Excess of reducing weakens anti-pathogenic qi. That is the five excesses. " (Classified Classic). "Since the five storing viscera externally correspand with the skin, vessels, muscles, tendons, bones and have their excess and deficient states, it is advisable to regulate them. If reinforcing and reducing are excessive, it is called five excesses. "

five exhaustions 五夺 [wǔ duó] The cases of five exhaustions of primordial *qi*, namely, excessive emaciation, severe hemorrhage, exhaustion of yang after severe perspiration, exhaustion of yin after severe diarrhea, metrorrhagia after delivery. When coming across the above conditions, reducing manipulation of acupuncture must be administered.

five emotions produce fire 五志化火 [wǔ zhì huà huǒ]Certain fire(tense heat)manifestations induced by patholoigc hyperfunction due to disorder of emotional reactions, such as joy, anger, anxiety, worry and apprehension.

five correspondences and ten variations 五门十变 [wǔ mén shí biàn] A term of midnight-noon ebb-flow needling. Five correspondances refer to the ten heavenly stems corresponding with one another.

five constituents 五大 [wǔ dà] The two hands, two feet and head, also called *wuti*.

five points of Tianyou 天牖五部 [tiān yōu wǔ bù] I. e. , Renying (ST 9), Futu (LI 18), Tianrong (TE, SJ 16), Tianzhu (BL 10), Tianfu (LU 3).

five critical cases 五逆 [wǔ nì] Five kinds of critical diseases or syndromes that the pulse does not accord with the syndrome. "It is termed five *ni* that the diseases do not accord with the syndrome. " "The 1st is that the pulse is quiet in febrile diseases, and then the pulse is full and rapid after perspiration; The 2nd is dirrhea, the pulse is full and large; The 3rd is fixed blockage, general fever, faint pulse; The 4th is emaciation, general fever, pale complexion; The 5th is chills and fever, firm pulse.

Chinese gall 五倍子[wǔ bèi zǐ]The drug used for applying it on the point. The excrescence produced by an insect on the leaf of Rhuschinensis, R. pungahensis, R. pungabensis sinta (Ancardiaceae).

five punctures 五刺 [wǔ cì] The five needlings that were formed in accordance with the correspodance between the five storing viscera and the five constituents (skin, vessel, tendon, muscle and bone), i. e. superficial puncture corresponds with the lungs (related to skin), leopard-spot puncture corresponds with the heart (related to vessels), joint puncture corresponds with the liver (related to tendons), *hegu* puncture correpsponds with the spleen and *shu* puncture corresponds with the kidneys. (related to bones)

five emotions 五志 [wǔ zhì] The five kinds of mental changes are joy, anger, anxiety, worry and fear.

five softenesses 五软 [wǔ ruǎn] A collective term for the five symptom complexes in infancy, namely, softness of the heal, softness of the neck, softness of the arm and legs, softness of the muscles, and softness of the mouth.

five storing viscera 五脏 [wǔ zàng] A collective term for the heart, liver, spleen, lungs, and kidneys. According to traditional Chinese medicine, this term may eihter refer to the acutual organs or chiefly to external reflections of their functioning and pathologic processes. Hence, each of them has its own intrinsic chracteristics. According to Internal Classic their functions are mainly "storing the refined principle but not emptying or excreting. "

five variations 五变 [wǔ biàn] The corresponding relationship between the five storing viscera and the five elements. The five storing viscera have the five variations, i. e. , five times, five elements, five sounds, five colors; The five variations correspond with five *shu* points. In each storing viscus, there are five *shu* points, i. e. , stream-like point prunctured in spring, *shu* points punctured in summer, sea-like point punctured in autumn, and well-like point punctured in winter. So there are actually 25 points,

which corrspond with five times.

five varied needlings 五变刺 [wǔ biàn cì] Selection of the five *shu* points for acupuncture according to five cases. "For the disease at the storing viscera, select the well-like point; For the disease of complexion and pulse select the spring-like point; For the disease that sometimes becomes mild but sometimes becomes severe, select the *shu* point; For the disease of abnormal voice, select the river-like point; For the disease at the stomach due to improper diet, select the sea-like point. (Miraculous Pivot)"

five merilans 五经 [wǔ jīng] The meridians of the liver, heart, spleen, lung and kidney.

five-evil needlings 五邪刺 [wǔ xié cì] The theory of needling techniques in Internal Classic. That is to use different needling techniques for treating different disease conditions. "For carbuncle, the sword-like needle is used to evacuate pus", "for pathogenic *qi* of *shi* (excess) type, the sharp prismatic needle is used to reduce its excess", "for pathogenioc *qi* of *xu* (deficiency) type, the sharp-round needle is used to supplement its insufficiency", "for cold pathogenic *qi*, the filiform needle is used to warm it. " (Miraculous Pivot)

five elements 五行 [wǔ xíng] Chinese ancestors thought that the five kinds of matterials—metal, wood, water, fire and earth—were the indispensible and most fundamental elements in constituting the Universe. There exist the promoting, inhibiting and restraining relationships among them. They are also in constant motion and change. In traditional Chinese medicine they are used to explain and expand a series of medical problems by comparing with and deducing from such properties and mutual relatoonships.'

five-element theory 五行学说 [wǔ xíng xué shuō] Originally it was a philosophical theory in ancient China. Later, it was adapted in medical practice, becoming an important part of the theories of traditional Chinese medicine. It relates the properties of five elements (metal, wood, water, fire and earth) to universally interdependent and mututally restraining relationsips of matters. It played a definitive role in development of traditional Chinese mediccine. In ancient Greece, there was the four-element theory, which was similar in its contents to the five-element theoy. This reflects that the thought of Chinese ancients and Greek ancients agreed without prior consultation.

fire cupping technique 火罐法 [huǒ guàn fǎ] A kind of cupping. That is to make use of ignited fire and burning to get rid of air in the cup to form negative pressure, so as to make the cup absorb the body surface. The commonly-used one is divided into the fire-thrown one and the fire-flushed one. The former is to throw a small piece of ignited paper into the cup, then immediately cover the absorbed part with it. The latter is to pinch a cotton ball rinsed with 95% of alcohol, ignite it and then put it in the cup for a moment and then withdraw it with forceps. And then swiftly cover the selected area with the cup. (Fig 36)

fire needling 火针 [huǒ zhēn] An acupuncture technique, also referring to the needling instrument. The large needle in the nine needles in ancient times was written as fire needle and also called *fanzhen* which is 1.2 dm in length, and is used for swelling and poisoning, relieving muscular spasm and drain poison. Later it was made of stainless steel, the body of the needle is comparatively long. It is mainly used for treating carbuncle, swelling and supputrative ulcer, scrofula, wart, nevus, etc. While using it, the puncture point must be accurate and the needle must not be inserted too deep.

first lateral line of head 头第一侧线 [tóu dì yī chè xiàn] The line to locate the meridian point, which connects Qucha (BL 4) and Tianzhu (BL 10) where Gallbladder Meridian of Foot-*taiyang* passes through. Qucha

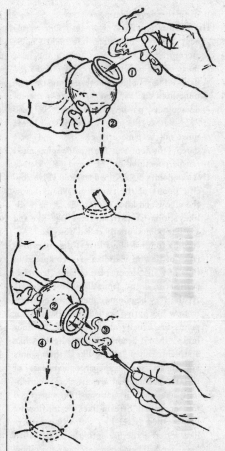

Fig 36

(BL 4), Wuchu (BL 5), Chengguang (BL 6), Tongtian (BL 7), Luoque (BL 8), Yuzhen (BL 9) and Tianhu (BL 10) are distributed over.

five movements and six climates 五运六气 [wǔ yùn liù qì] Chinese ancients combined six kinds of climate (wind, heat, warmth, dampness, dryness and chills) to deduce the relationship between the changes of weather and the occurrence of disease in humans. This theory is somewhat similar to the modern climatological medicine and worthy of further investigating.

five prohibitions 五禁 〔wǔ jìn〕One of the acupuncture prohibitions in ancient China. According to Miraculous Pivot, the head must not be punctured on '甲', and '乙' dates, the shoulder and throat must not be punctured on '丙' and '丁' dates, the abdomen must not be punctured on '戊' and '己' dates, the joints, the hip and knees must not be punctured on '庚' and '辛' dates, the foot and the tibial region must not be punctured on '壬' and '癸' dates.

five shu points 五腧穴〔wǔ shū xué〕Five specific points of the twelve meridians below the elbow and knee joints, viz., the well-like, spring-like, stream-like, river-like and sea-like points, briefly called"five-shu". According to Miraculous Pivot, the characteristics of flow of meridian qi is compared to flow of water, from small to large, from superficial to deep, from distal to proximal. At the very beginning, meridianal qi starts to flow like spring, called "well like," their points are usually at the ends of the flour limbs, then it becomes bigger slightly, like a stream, called "spring-like," their points are near the metacarpophlangeal or metatarspohalangeal areas; more flourishing, like water irrigationg from superficial to deep, called"Stream-like", water flowing long, called "river-like", finally it gathers like water gathering into the sea, called "sea-like". Their points are near the elbow and knee joints. As to application of five-shu points "select well like points for the diseases of the storing viscera; select spring-like points for the diseases of complexion; select the stream-like point for the diseases occurring sometimes mildly but sometimes severely; select the river-like points for the diseases of voice; select the river-like points for stomach trouble and disorder due to improper diet. "(Miraculous Pivot). "The well-like point is for fullness in the epigastric region, the spring-like point for general fever, the stream-like

point for asthmatic breath, cough, chills and fever, and the sea-like point for diarrhea due to adverse flow of qi. This explains that the indications of the five-shu points have their characteristics each, and they can be used not only to treat local pathological changes but also to treat disorders at the distal area and those of viscera concerned. (Fig 37)

fire wrapped by cold 寒包火〔hán bāo huǒ〕The body has accumulated heat internally and is then affected by cold externally, resulting in pathological manifestations of an external envelop of cold with an internal core of heat.

firm pulse 牢脉〔láo mài〕The pulse that can only be felt by deep palpation, and is firm, forceful, large, taut and long. It is frequently seen in the condition due to accumulation of yin cold.

first lateral line of abdomen 腹第一侧线〔fù dì yī chè xiàn〕The line for locating the meridan points, 1.5 cm to the abdominal midline, where Kidney Meridian of Foot-shaoyin passes through. Distributed are Youmen (KI 21), Futonggu (KI 20), Yindu (KI 19), Shiguan (KI 18), Shangqu, (KI 17), Gaohuang (KI 16), Zhongshu (KI 15), Siman (KI 14), Qixue (KI 13), Dahe (KI 12), Henggu (KI 11).

flying manipulation 飞法〔fēi fǎ〕An acupuncture manipulation. Hold the shaft of the needle with the thumb and index and middle fingers oppositely, twirl it and then take off them. While twirling, flex the index and middle fingers inwardly to make the needle rotate left; While taking off the fingers, extend the index and middle fingers outward as a flying bird extends its wings. (Fig 38)

flaming of hepatic fire 肝火上炎〔gān huǒ shàng yán〕The liver meridian becomes substantial and flaming, leading to obvious febrile symptoms in the upper part of the body. The main symptoms are the same as those of hepatic fire.

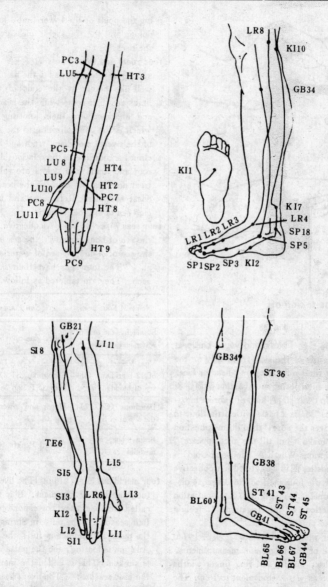

Fig 37

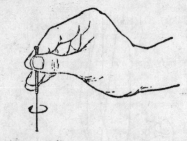

One twirling

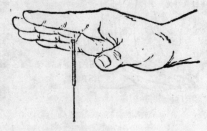

One taking off

Fig 38

flat wart 扁平疣〔biǎn píng yòu〕The pea-shaped grow of the skin frequently on the backs of the hands, fingers, head or face.

flour paste-interposing moxibustion 隔面饼灸〔gé miàn bǐng jiǔ〕A kind of indirect moxibustion. "Make a paste with little flour to use it cover the sore, then do moxibustion on it to make it hot till the juice appears." (Prescriptions Worth A Thousand Gold)

four diagnostics 四诊〔sì zhěng〕A collective term for the four methods to diagnose disease, namely, 1. inspection; 2. auscultation and olfaction; 3. interrogation; 4. feeling pulse and plpation.

four-finger-width measurement 一夫法〔yī fú fǎ〕One of the finger-*cun* measurements. The index, middle and ring finger widths are taken as *yi fu*, equivalent to 1 cm. The index, middle, ring and small fingers are held together. The widths at the middle segments are taken as *yi fu*. Frequently used for the vertical measurement of select-ing the point at the lower limb, lower abdomen and the transverse measurement of the back.

four roots and three knots 四根三结〔sì gēn sān jié〕It refers that as to the merdians the well-like points at the ends of the four limbs are their roots while the head, chest and abdomen are their knotting places, which is the generalization to the locations of the twelve meridians' root and knot. In clinic, accodrding to the relationship of this root and knot, the points are selected to treat diseases and pains of the head, face, chest abdomen. Refer root and knot and *biao-ben* of six meridians.

four seas 四海〔sì hǎi〕A collective term for the sea of bone marrow, the sea of blood, the sea of *qi* and the sea of water and cereal. "The four seas have their *shu* points each. They are tableted as follow.

Name of Four Seas	*Shu* Points
Stomach, the sea of water and cereals	Qijie; Zusanli (ST 36)
Vital Vessel, the sea of 12 meridians (the sea of blood)	Dazhui (GV, Du 14), Shangjuxu (ST 37), Xiajuxu (ST 39)
Danzhong (CV 17), the sea of *qi*	Upper and lower Renying (St 9)
Brain, the sea of medulla	Baihui; Fengfu (GV 16)

four meridians 四经〔sì jīng〕The liver, heart, lung and kidney meridians. It is therefore called because they correspond with the four seasons. "The pulse in Spring is wiry, the pulse in Summer is full, the puase in Autumn is foating, and the pulse in Winter is sunken. This is called the meridians of the four seasons." "The liver, heart, lungs and kidneys coresond with *qi* in the four seasons." "The liver (wood) corresponds with the Spring, the heart (fire) with the Summer, the lungs with the Autumn and the kidney (water) with the Winter. ”

four general points 四总穴 [sì zǒng xué] The four commonly-used points, namely, Zusanli (ST 36), Weizhong (BL 40), Lieque (LU 7) and Hegu (LI 4). The Song of Four General Points recorded in Conplete Book of Acupuncture generalises the ditail indications of these four points, which has been read out by acupuncture lerarners. For abdominal disorders Zusanli (ST 36) is retained, for waist and back disorders Weizhong (BL 40) is searched. For head and neck disorders Lique (LU 7) is persured, for face and mouth disorders Hegu (LI 4) can solve.

foot-*taiyang* meridian 足太阳脉 [zú tài yáng mài] The name of the meridian during early period. Same with foot-*taiyang* meridian.

foot-*taiyin* meridian 足太阴脉 [zú tài yīn mài] The name the of meridian during early period. Same as foot-*taiyin* meridian.

Four Books of Acupuncture 针灸四书 [zhēn jiǔ sì shū] A series of books compiled by Dou Guifang in Yuan Dynasty (1271 — 1368), including Acupuncture Classic of Mid-night-noon Ebb-flow, Huangdi's *Mintang* Acupuncture Classic, Keys to Acupuncture Classic and Moxibustion Technique on Gaohuangshu Points. It was first published in 1311. Besides the separate edition, its main contents were collected in Prescriptions of Universal Relief.

foot-*yangming* meridian 足阳明脉 [zú yáng míng mài] The name of the meridian during the early period. Same as foot-*yangming* meridian.

foot-jueyin meridian 足厥阴脉 [zú jué yīn mài] The name of the meridian during the early period, same as foot-*jueyin* meridian

foot ju yang meridian 足巨阳脉 [zú jù yáng mài] An alternate term for meridian at early period. Same as foot-*taiyang* meridian.

four yong-wei points 荣卫四穴 [róng wèi sì xué] According to Outline of Medicine, they are located at “5. 5 cm superior, inferior, left and right to the back spine, 9 cm below

Yaoyan (CX-B7), 12 cm lateral to the spine, 4 on the bilateral side. ” Approx. 6 cm lateral the posterior foramens of the 1st, 2nd, 3rd, and 4th sacrums repsectively.

four nutritional and defenvic points 营卫四穴 [yíng wèi sì xué] I. e. , *yong wei si sue.*

Forehead 额 [é] An ear point at the edge of the caritillege of the antitragus at the centre of the lower zone.

fourteen extra points for mania 过梁针 [guò liáng zhēn] Referring to the fourteen extra points for treating mental disorders such as mania, insanity, etc. They are: 1) Tianting: 1. 5 cm lateral (inward) and directly above the anterior edge of the axiliary fossa, select it by putting the hand by the body. Puncture: 15—18 cm slightly obliquely outward. 2) Yeting: located 1. 5 cm directly slightly below the anterior edge of the axilla, at the inferior edge of the muscle. puncture: 15—18 cm deep. 3) Quweiyong. located stlightly lateral to the end of the transverse crease of the flexed elbow; Puncture: 4—9 cm. 4) Chirao, located in the centre from the transverse crease of the extensor side of the forearm to the transverse crease of elbow, 19 cm above the wrist. Puncture: 4—9 cm. 5) Zhongrao located at the extensor side of the upper limb, 12 cm above the transvese crease of wrist. Puncture: 3—7 cm. 6) Cunrao located at the extensor side of the upper limb, 6 cm above the transverse crease of wrist. Puncture: 3—4 cm. 7) Naogen located in the depression between the lateral ankle and Achilles tendon, 3—6 cm between the tibia and fibula. Puncture: 6—9 cm. 8) Zhongping located 15 cm below the knee. Puncture: 3—6 cm between the tibia and fibula. Puncture: 6— 9 cm. 9) Yinwei, located on the lateral side of the thigh, 3 cm above the transverse crease of the cubital fossa, in the depression between the biceps muscle of thigh and the lateral muscle of thigh. Puncture: 9—15 cm. 10) Yinwei located 3 cm above Yinwei. Puncture: 9—15 cm. 11) Yinwei 3 cm above

Yinwei. Puncture; 9—15 cm. 12) Silian located 3 cm above Yinwei. Puncture; 9—15 cm. 13) Wuling located 6 cm above Yinwei. Puncture; 9—15 cm. In clinical application, the depth of puncture should accord with the patient's condition. (fat or thin, weak or sthenic), according to the above-mentioned puncture depth of the various points. It is not advisable to puncture too deep.

fourteen manipulations 十四法[shí sì fǎ]The fourteen manipulations applied in the course of acupuncture operation. Originally called "reinforcing and reducing manipulations by fingers. "I. e. , moving, withdrawing, kneading, inserting, spiralling, twirling, springing, rotating, searching, kneading and closing, pinching pressing, scratching, and fingernail pressing manipulations.

fourteen meridians 十四经 [shí sì jīng] The twelve meridians pulse Governor Vessel and Conception Vessel.

fragrant-flower garlic-interposing moxibustion 隔韭灸 [gé jiǔ jiǔ] A kind of indirect moxibustion. "After ulceration of sore, swelling and pain appear due to invasion of wind and cold. Use fragrant flower gaitn to make a paste after pounding it into small pieces and then put it on the affected area, and do moxibustion on it to make hot qi into it. " (Compendium of Sore Medicine).

fresh and rippened 生熟 [shēng shóu] A term used in moxibustion techique 'Sheng' refers to less moxibustioin and slower fire; 'shou' refers to much moxibustion and quicker fire, also divided into slightly quicker fire and greater quicker fire.

Frenulum of tongue 舌柱[shè zhù]Nemenclatured as the name of the extra point, and can be punctured by a triangular needle to cause its upper part bleeding slightly. (Fig 39)

frontal angle 耳角 [ěr jiǎo] The angles at the outer ends of the anterior hair lines.

fu 跗 [fù] The dorsum of the foot.

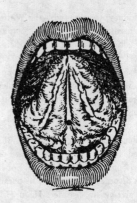

Fig 39

Fuqu腹屈 [fù qū] An alternate term for Fujie (SP 14).

Fuai 腹哀 [fù āi] A point of Spleen Meridian of Foot-*taiyin*.

Fuyang 付阳 [fù yáng] I. e. , 跗阳.

Futu (ST 32) 伏兔 [fú tù] A point of Stomach Meridian of Foot-*yangming*, also termed Waigou. Location; 18 cm above the knee-cap on the line connecting the anterosuperior spine of ilium and the lateral side of the knee-cap, on the anterolateral side of te thigh. Reginal anatomy; There are the branches of the lateral femoral circumflex artery and the lateral circumflex femoral vein at musculus femoris. The anterior cutaneous nerve of thigh and the lateral cutaneous nerve of thigh are distributed. Indications; Pains in the waist, cold and paralysis of knees and legs, foot *qi*, hernia, abdominal distension, cold and paralysisof knees and legs. Puncture; 4—4. 5 cm perpendicularly. Moxibustion; 3—5 moxa cones or 5—10 minutes with warming moxitustion.

Fuliu 复留 [fù liú] I. e. , Fuliu (KI 20).

Fufen（BL 41）附分[fù fēn]A point of Bladder Meridian of Foot-*taiyang*, the confluence of *taiyang* meridians of hand and foot. Location; 9 cm lateral to the interspace between the 2nd and 3rd thoracic vertebrae. Regional anatomy; Passing through the trapezius muscle and the rhomboic muscle, reaching at the iliocostal muscle. There is the descending branch of the transverse artery of neck, at the lateral branch of the posterior branch of the lst and 2nd thoracic nerve. The dorsal scapular nerve is in the deeper. Indications: contracture of the shoulder and back, stiffness and pain in the neck, numbness of the elbow and arm. Puncture: 1. 5— 2. 5 cm obliquely. (It is not advisable to puncture it deep). Moxibustion: 3—5 moxa cones or 5—15 minutes with warm needling.

Fuyang 附阳 [fù yáng] I. e., 跗阳 (BL59).

Fuzhongshu 府中俞 [fǔ zhōng shū] An alternate term for Zhongfu (LU 1).

Fuhui 府会 [fǔ huì] I. e., confluence of the emptying viscera.

Futonggu (KI 20) 腹通谷 [fù tōng gǔ] A point of Kidney Meridian of Foot-*shaoyin*, the confluence of Vital Vessel and foot-*shaoyin* meridian. Location: 15 cm above the umbilicus, 1. 5 cm lateral to Shangwan (CM, RN 13). Regional anatomy: At the medial edge of the straight muscle of abdomen. There is the branch of the epigastric superior artery and vein. The 8th intercostal nerve is distributed. Indications: abdominal pain, abdominal distension, vomiting, cadrdialgia, palpitaion. Puncture: 1. 5—3 cm perpendicularly. Moxibustion: 3—7 moxa cones or 5—10 minutes with moxa stick.

Fujie (SP 14) 腹结 [fù jié] A point of Spleen Meridian of Foot-*taiyin*, also termed Fuqu, Changku. Location: 12 cm lateral to the umbilicus, 4 cm below Daheng (SP 15) of 9 cm above Fushe (SP 13). Regional anatomy: Passing through the trapezius muscle of abdomen, and medial trapezius muscle of abdomen, reaching at the transverse muscle of abdomen. The 11th intercostal nerve is distributed. Indications: Pain in the surrounding umbilicus, hernia, cold abdomen and diarrhea. Puncture: 3—4. 5 cm perpendicularly. Moxibustion: 3—5 moxa cones or 5—10 minutes with warming moxibustion.

Fucheng 扶承 [fú chéng] I. e., Chengfu (BL 36).

Futu (LI 18) 扶突 [fú tū] A point of Large Intestine Meridian of Hand-*yangming*, also termed Shuixue. Location: At the level with Adam's Apple, at the posterior edge of sternocleidomastoidous musche, on the lateral side of the neck. Regional anatomy: Passing through the broadest muscle of neck, and the posterior edge of sternocleidomastoidous musche, reaching at the levator muscle of scapula, there is the deep cervical artery and vien in the deeper. The great auricular nerve, the cervical cutaneous nerve and lesser occipital nerve, and the accessary nerve are distributed. Indications: Cough, asthmatic breath, sore throat, sudden aphonia, goiter, scrofula. Puncture: 1. 5—2 cm perpendicularly. Moxibustion: 3—5 moxa cones or 5—10 minutes with warming moxibustion.

fugu 辅骨 [fǔ gǔ] 1. Referring to the protruding bone bilateral to the knee. The medial one is called inner *fu*, (the medial condyle of bibia) while the outer one outer *fu*, the head of fibula; 2. referring to radius of the upper limb.

Fubai (GB 10) 浮白 [fú bái] A point of Gallbladder Meridian of Foot-*shaoyang*, the confluence of foot-*taiyang* meridian and foot-*shaoyin* meridian. Location: Posterosuperior to the mastoid process of the temporal bone behind the ear. At the crossing point of the upper 1/3 and middle 1/3 of the line connecting Tianchong (GB 9) and Wangu (SI 4). Regional anatomy: There is the posterior aural artery and vein. The branch of the greater occipital nerve is distributed. Indications: Heachache, tinnitus, deafness, toothache, goiter, stiffness and pain in the neck, scrofula, pain in the arm, atrophy of feet. Puncture: 0. 6—1. 5 cm horizontally. Moxibustion: 1—3 moxa cones or 3—5 minutes with warming moxibustion.

Fushe (SP 13) 府舍 [fǔ shè] A point of Spleen

Meridian of Foot-*taiyin*, the confuence of foot-*taiyin* meridian, Connecting Vessel of Yin and *jueyin* meridians. Location: 21 cm above and 12 cm lateral to Qugu (CV, RN 2) at the midpoint of the suprior edge of symphysis pubis. Regional anatomy: Superolateral to the inguinal ligament. There is the superficial vein of the abdominal wall. The ilio-inguinal nerve is distributed. Indications: Abdominal pain, hernia, abdominal fullness, cholera and diarrhea. Puncture: 3—4.5 cm perpendicularly. Moxibustion: 3—5 moxa cones or 5—10 minutes with warm ming moxitustion.

fu-shu **points** 府俞 [fǔ shū] Referring to various points of well-like, spring-like, streamlike and sea-like points of the yang meridians of six emptying viscera. The meridians of six emptying viscera have 36 points unilaterally and bilaterally.

Fuxi (BL 38) 浮郄 [fú xī] A point of Bladder Meridian of Foot-*taiyang*. location: Laterosuperior to the cubital fossa. At the medial edge of the biceps muscle of thigh, 3 cm directly above Weiyang (BL 39). Select it when the knee is flexed. Regional anatomy: There is the lateral artery and vein of the knee. The posterior cutaneous nerve of thigh and the common peroneal nerve are distributed. Indications: Numbness of hip and thigh, spasm of the poplitial tendon. Puncture: 3—4.5 cm perendicularly. Moxibustion: 3—5 moxa cones or 5—10 minutes with warming moxibustion.

fuluzhimai 伏膂之脉 [fú lǚ zhī mài] See *fu chong zhi wai*.

Fuliu 伏溜 [fú liú] I.e., Fuliu (KI 7).

fumigating moxibustion 熏灸 [xūn jiǔ] A kind of moxibustion to fumigate the affected area with hot air of boiling moxa or other drugs with water, or fumigate the affected area with ignited moxa.

Fuliu (KI 17) 腹溜 [fù liū] A point of Kidney Meridian of Foot-*shaoyin*, the river-like point (metal) of the meridian, also termed Cangang, Fubai. Location: At the midpoint of the horizontal line connecting the posteromedial ankle and Achilles tendon, 6 cm directly above Taixi (KI 3d), at the lower end of the soleus muscle that transverses to the medial side of Achilles tendon. Regional anatomy: There is the posterior tibial artery and vein in the deeper. The medial cutaneous nerve of calf and that of leg are distributed. The tibial nerve is in the deeper. Indications: Abdominal distension, borborygmus, diarrhea, edema, swollen legs, atrophic feet, night sweat, faint, small pulse, general fever with no sweat, stiffness and pain in the lumbar spine. Puncture: 2—4 cm perpendicularly. Moxibustion: 3—5 moxa cones or 5—10 minutes with warming moxibustion.

full pulse 洪脉 [hóng mài] The pulse that comes on forcefully and fades away like surf. It usually indicates *shi* (excess) heat.

Fubai 伏白 [fú bái] Another name of Fuliu (KI 7).

G

gaohuang 膏肓 [gāo huāng] 1. Originally, they are below the heart and abover the diaphragm. Later on it is used to decribed a deeply seated and incurable disease so the disease has invaded *gaohuang*; 2. The name of the acupuncture point, Gaohuang (BL 43).

Ganshu (BL 18) 肝俞 [gān shū] A point of Bladder Meridian of Foot-*taiyang*, the back *shu* point of the liver. Location: 4. 5 cm lateral to Jinsuo (GV 8) between the spinal processes of the 9th and 10th thoracic vertebrae. Reginal anatomy: Passing through the broadest muscle of back, reaching between the longest muscle and iliocostal muscle. There is the medial branch of the dorsal branch of the 9th intercostal artery and vein. The medial cutaneous branch of the posterior branch of the 9th thoracic nerve is distributed. The lateral branch of the posterior branch of the 9th thoracic nerve is in the deeper. Indications: Jaundice, pains in the hypochonrium, spitting blood, epistaxis. congestive eyes, blurred vision, nebula, night blingness, mania, epilepsy, pain in the back spine. Puncture: 1. 5—2. 5 cm obliquely. Moxibustion: 3— 5 moxa cones or 5—15 minutes with warming moxibustion.

gallbladder concerned with judgement 胆主决断 [dǎn zhǔ jué duàn] In traditional Chinese medicine, one of the functions of the gallbladder is related to certain functional activities of the central nervous system. The gallbladder plays an important, role in preventing and eliminating some of the unplesant influences of emotional disturbances, e. g. , being suddenly startled.

gastric yang 胃阳 [wèi yáng] It refers to the functions of the stomach, and pathologically is related to the ebb and flow of the cold or the heat. If with hot symptoms, it is regarded as gastric yang in excess. If the stomach is hypofunctional in combination with cold, it is regarded as gastric yang in deficiency.

gastric yin 胃阴 [wèi yīn] The fluid in the stomach.

gastric connection 胃系 [wèi xì] Referring to the esopagus.

Gap-like point 郄穴 [xī xué] A kind of name of the classified meridian point. The twelve meridians and Motility Veessel of Yin, Motility Vessel of Yang, Connecting Vessel of Yin, and Connecting Vesel of Yang at the four limbs have a gap-like point each, collectively called sixteen gaplike points. They are usually used in treating acute disorders in clinic. e. g. , for spitting blood Kongzui (LU 6) is cooperated; for cardialgia Ximen (PC 4) is cooperated, for stomachache Liangqiu (ST 34) is cooperated.

Gallbladder Meridian of Foot-shaoyang (GB) 足少阳胆经 [zú shào yáng dǎn jīng] One of the twelve meridians. The course: It crosses and emerges behind hand-*shaoyang* meridian, enters into the supraclavicular fassea. Tbe branch enters into the ear from the posterior ear, emerges and runs in front of the ear. After reaching the outer canthus, another branch splits from the outer canthus, descends to Daying (ST 5), meets hand-*shaoyang* meridian and reaches at the inferior eye; its lower part runs over Jiache (ST 6) to the neck, meets at the supraclavicular fossa. It descends to the inner chest, passses through the diaphragem, connects with the liver, pertains to the gallbladder, Then it runs along the inner hypochondrium, emerges from the groove, winds the hair area of the pubic region, runs transversely to enter into the hip joint. The main stem descends from the supraclavicular fossa to the axilla, passes through the hypochondrium, runs down and neets at the hip joint. It descends along the lateral aspect of the thigh, emerges from the lateral side of the knee, descends to the head of the anterior fibula, again runs downward to the lower segement of fibula, emerges in front of the lateral ankle, enters into the end of the 4th toe along the dorsal foot, enters into the interspace of the great toe, then emerges from the end of the toe along the interspace between the 1st and 2nd metatarsal bones, and turns back to pass through the toenail and emerges from the hair area of the dorsal toe (to connect with Liver Meridian of Foot-*jueyin*).

gallbladder 胆 [dǎn] One of the six emptying viscera. Gallbladder Meridian of Foot-*shaoyang* pertains to the gallbladder and Liver Meridian of Foot-*jueyin* connects with the gallbladder. Its back-*shu* point is Danshu (BL 19), its anterior referred point is Riyue (GB 24) and its joining point is Yanglingquan (GB 34).

gallbladder meridian of foot-*shaoyang* 胆足少阳之脉 [dǎn zú shào yáng zhī mài] The original name of Gallbadder Meridian of Foot-*shaoyang*.

garlic 大蒜 [dà shuàn] One of drugs for dressing and moxibustion. Pound garlic into small pieces and dress it on the point, which can make the skin hot even blistering, cut it into pieces to be used for interposing. It is called garlic-interposing moxibustion if a moxa cone is used to administer moxibustion.

garlic-interposing moxibustion 隔蒜灸 [gé shuàn jiǔ] A kind of indirect moxibustion.

Gaogu 高骨 [gāo gǔ] An extra point located at the higer spot of the styloid process of radius. Indications: Pain in the wrist. Puncture: 1—1.5 cm horizontally. Moxibustion: 3—7 moxa cones or 5—10 minutes with warming moxibustion.

Gaohuang 膏肓 [gāo huāng] 1. The interspace above the diaphragm and below the heart;

2. Referring Gaohuangshu (BL 43).

Gaohuangshu (BL 43) 膏肓俞 [gāo huāng shū] A point of Bladder Meridian of Foot-*taiyang*. Location: 9 cm lateral to the spinal process of the 4th thoracic vertebra. Regioinal anatomy: Passing through the trapezius muscle and rhmoid muscle, reaching at the iliocostal muscle. There is the decending branch of the posterior branch of the 4th intercostal artery and the descending branch of the cervical transverse artery. The medial cutaneous branch of the posterior branches of the 2nd and 3rd thoracic nerves and the dorsal scapular nerve are in the deeper. Indications: Pulmonary tuberculosis, cough, asthmatic breath, spitting blood, night sweat, amnesia, spermatorrhea, indigestion, pains in the scapular region and back. Puncture: 1—1.5 cm obiquely. (It is not advisable to puncture deep) Mocibustion: 7—15 moxa cones or 20—30 minutes with warming moxibustion.

GB points 足少阳胆经穴 [zú shào yáng dǎn jīng xué] According to Systematic Classic of Acupuncture they are Tonziliao (GB 1), Tinghui (GB 2), Shangguan (GB 3), Hanyan (GB 4), Xuanlu (GB 5), Xunli (GB 6), Qubin (GB 7), Shuaigu (GB 8), Tianchong (GB 9), Fubai (GB 10), Touqiaoyin (GB 11), Wangu (GB 12), Benshen (GB 13), Yangbai (GB 14), Toulinqi (GB 15), Muchuang (GB 16), Zhengying (GB 17), Chengling (GB 18), Naokong (GB 19), Fengchi (GB 20), Jianjing (GB 21), Yuanye (GB 22), Zhejin (GB 23), Riyue (GB 24), Jingmen (GB 25), Daimai (GB 26), Wushu (GB 27), Weidao (GB 28), Juliao (GB 29), Huantiao (GB 30), Fenghshi (GB 31), Zhongdu (GB 32), Xiyanguan (GB 33), Yanglingquan (GB 34), Yangjiao (GB 35), Waiqiu (GB 36), Guangming (GB 37), Yangfu (GB 38), Xuanzhong (GB 39), Qiuxu (GB 40) (soure), Zulinqi (GB 41) (well-like), Diwuhui (GB 42), Xiaxi (GB 43), Zuqiaoyin (GB 44), 44 in total.

GB diseases 足少阳胆经病［zú shào yáng dǎn jīng bīng］ They are mainly unilateral headache, swelling and pain in the neck, swelling below the axilla, scrofula, chills and fever, malaria, bitter mouth, belching, pain in the epigastrium and below the hypochondrium, and pain in the area where the meridian runs over.

Gemen 阁门 ［gé mén］ A extra point, also called Lanmen. Located 9 cm lateral to the midpoint of the root of the penis at the infrerior edge of pubis. Puncture: 1. 5—3 cm perpendicularly. Moxibustion: 3—5 moxa cones or 5—10 minutes with waring moxibustion.

General Introduction to Miraculous Moxibustion 神灸经纶 ［shén jiǔ jīng lún］ A medical book written by Qu Yiding in Qing Dynasty (1644—1911), 4 volumes. In the book moxibustion techniques are introduced. It was characterized by special attention paid to pulse-feeling and syndrome differentiation. It is a special book dealing with moxibustion techniques, comparatively wholesided in its contents, completed in 1851.

General Line of Administering Acupuncture in Rhythm 行针总要歌 ［xíng zhēn zǒng yào gē］ It contains some key points of needling technqures. For instance, "While locating the point and administering acupuncture, the patient must be minutely differentiated. (thin or obese, tall or short) For the obese patient, the depth of the needle inserted is 1 cm, for the thin one, the depth is 0. 5 cm for the paitent being neither obese nor thin, the depth is between 0. 6—1 cm. In this way there will be no mistake but there will be successful. "

General Collection for Holy Relief 圣济总录 ［shèn jì zǒng lù］ The original name of the book is Zhonghe Shenji Zhonglu. The officially revised edition, 200 volumes in total, consisting of 69 categories, over 20,000 formuulas recorded, a great synthetic medical book. In this book the 191th—194th voumes are the acupuncture category in which general description of bone measurement, general description of the meridians were recorded and the twelve meridians, eight extrra meridians and points were respectively described; secondly general descripiton of the nine needles, puncture, the techniques of moxibustion and acupuncture for varieties of diseases as well as prohibitions of moxibustion and acupuncture were also recorded. It was completed in 1117.

gen, liu, zhu and ru 根溜注入 ［gēn liū zhù rù］ The classified names of points. 'Gen' (root) refers to the well-points at the ends of the four limbs, same as that of gen-jie; 'liu' means cirulating and refers to the source points; 'zhu' means irrigating and refers to the meridian points; 'ru' means being from superficial to deep and refers to the points of the meridians at the neck and the connecting points at the four limbs. Their names are as follows.

Geguan （BL 46） 膈关 ［gé guān］ A point of

Meridian	Points			
	gen	Liu	zhu	Ru
Foot-gaiyang	Zhiyin(BL 67)	Jinggu(BL 64)	Kunlun(BL 60)	Tian zhu(BL 10) Feiyang (13L 58)
Foot-shaoyang	Zugiaoyin(GB 44)	Biuxu(GB 40)	Yangfu(GB 38)	Tianrong(SI 17)Guangming(GB 37)
Foot-yanganing	Lidui(ST 45)	Chongyang(ST 42)	Zusanli(ST 36)	Renying(ST 9) Fenglong(ST 40)
Hand-taiyang	Shaoze(SI 1)	Yanggu(SI 5)	Xiaohai(SI 8)	Tianchuang(SI 16) Zhizheng(SI 7)
Hand-shaoyang	Guangchong(TE 1)	Yangchi(TE 4)	Zhigou(TE 6)	Tianrou(TE 16) Waiguan(TE 5)
Hand-yangming	Shangyang(LI 1)	Hegu(LI 4)	Yangxi(LI 5)	Futu(LI 18) Pianli(LI 6)

Bladder Meridian of Foot-*taiyang*. Location: Below the spinal process of the 7th thoracic vertebra, 9 cm lateral to Zhiyang (GV, OU 9). Regional anotomy: Passing Through the broadest muscle of back, reaching at the iliocostal muscle. There are the posterior branches of the 7th intercostal artery and vein. The medial cutaneous branch of the posterior branch of the 6th and the 7th thoracic nerves are distributed. The lateral branches of the posterior branches of the 6th and the 7th thoracic nerves are in the deeper. Indications: Anorexia, vomiting, betching, stiffness and pain in the back spine. Puncture: 1. 5—2. 5 cm obliquely. (It is not advisable to puncture deep.) Moxibustion: 3—5 moxa cones or 5—15 minutes with warming moxibustion.

Geshu(BL 17)膈俞[gé shū]A point of Bladder Meridian of Foot-*taiyang*, the blood confluence of the eight confluential points. Location: Below the spinal process of the 7th thoracic vertebra, 4. 5 cm lateral to Zhiyang(GV, DU 9). Regional anatomy: At the inferior edge of the trapezius muscle and the broadest muscle of back, reaching at the long muscle, there is the medial branch of the dorsal branch of the 7th intercostal artery and vein. The medial cutaneous branch of the posterior branch of the 7th thoraic vertebra is in the deeper. Indications: Distension and pain in the epigastrium, vomiting, hiccup, anorexia, cough, asthmatic breath, spitting blood, tidal fever, night sweat, pain in the back, stiff neck. Puncture: 1. 5—2. 5 cm obliquely. (It is not advisable to puncture deep.) Moxibustion: 3—5 moxa cones or 5—15 minutes with warming moxibustion.

gehuang 鬲肓[gé huāng]The adipose membrane located above the diaphragm and below the heart.

general principle 总纲[zhǒng gāng]Referring to the two guiding principles, yin and yang, among the eight guiding principles, which have the action to guide the other six. The exterior, heat and excess belong to the category of yang while the interior, cold and deficiency belong to yin.

Girdle Vessel 带脉[dài mài]One of the eight extra vessels. The course is to start from below the hypochodrium, winds the waist one circle. Then Foot-*shaoyin* meridian and that of foot-*taiyang* join it and to ascend to the branch of the kidneys, and then to emerge from the 2nd lumbar vertebra and pertain to Girdle Vessel. I. e. , Girdle Vessel is connected with GV, foot-*taiyang* and foot-*shaoyang* meridians at the waist and back. Its frontal part is connected with various meridians at the waist and abdomen. Its crossing point pertans to foot-*shaoyin* meridian.

glass model marked with meridians and points 经络经穴玻璃人[jīng luò jīng xué bō lí rén]An acupuncture teaching tool made of glass in Shanghai Medical Models Factory and Shanghai College of Traditional Chinese Medicine in 1958. Its appearance is a healthy man in a standing position. The bones and internal organs can be seen through the organic glass external shell, and the courses of the fourteen meridians and 361 points are distributed over its surface, of which 140 points and internal organs can give out light to manifest the relationship between the meridian points and internal organs. There is also the recording instruments. The lecture can be carried on along with the demonstrating sequence of the fourteen meridians.

glu for moxibustion sore 灸疮膏药[jiǔ chuāng gāo yào] The glu used for suppurative moxibustion. It can be applied on the local area directly after direct moxibustion, so as to promote moxibution and protect the surface of sore.

Golden Mirror of Medicine 医宗金鉴 [yī zōng jīn jiàn]A medical book written by Wu Qian in Qing Dynasty(1644—1911), 90 volumes. It contains 15 kinds of books dealing with the medical foundation and various clinical specialties, completed in 1742, of which Keys to Experiences of Acupuncture and Moxibustion, Key to Experiences of Bone Setting are the special books in the aspect of acupuncture and bone-setting.

Gold Neelde in Rhythm 金针赋[jīn zhēn fù] An acupuncture article in rhythm. First recorded in complete Book of Acupuncture by Xu Feng. In the book the needling techniques such as setting the mountain on fire, cool to a cear sky night, yin hiding in yang, yang hiding in yin, mid-night-noon, qi-insertion, qi retention, 'dark-green dragon sways its tail', 'white tiger shakes its head,' 'dark-green turtle explores the point', 'red phoenix extends its wings' have exerted a great influence upon latter generations.

gold needle 金针[jīn zhēn]1. Specially referring to the medial instrument made of met-

al. In 1968 the gold needle in Han Dynasty (206 B. C. —220 A. D.) was unearthed in Liu Shen's Tomb in Western Han Dynasty (206 B. C. —24A. D.); 2. Generally referring to the medial instruments made of metal.

Governor Vessel(GV)督脉[dū mài]1. One of the eight extra meridians. The course: Starting from the inner lower abdomen, running backward from the pubic region, running in the middle of the inner spine, ascendig to Fengfu (GV, DU 16), entering into the brain, ascending to the vertex, descending to the forehead, to the nose bridge and the upper teeth. The anterior and posterior part is communicated with CV, Vital Vessel, as well as foot-*taiyang* meridian and foot-*shaoyang* meridian, connecting with the heart, kidney and brain; 2. referring to Shenting (GV 24) or as the same of the extra point. (Fig 40)

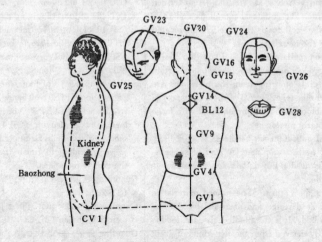

Fig 40

GV governing the sea of meridians 督领经脉 之海[dū lǐng jīng mài zhī hǎi]Referring to GV.

goiter 瘿气[yīng qì]An enlargement of the thyroid gland.

Gongsun (SP 4)公孙[gōng sūn]A point of Spleen Meridian of Foot-*taiyin*, the connecting point of the meridian. One of the eight crossing points, communicated with Vital Vessel. Location: On the medial side of the foot, at the dorsoventral boundary at the anteroinferior edge of the base of the 1st metatarsal bone or 3 cm posterior to Taibai(SP 3), the medial artery of the dorsal foot and that of the network of the dorsal vein. The branches of the porper nerve and the femoral superficial nerve are distributed. Indications: Stomachache, indigestion, borborygmus, abdominal distension, diarrhea, dysentery, vomiting, frequent drinking, cholera, edema, anxiety, insomnia, mania, foot *qi*. Puncture: 1. 5—3 cm perpendicularly. Moxibustion: 3—5 moxa cones or 5—15 minutes with warming moxibustion.

grouped points 组穴[zhǔ xué]Referring to the combination of over two points and application with the new name. e. g., "*siguang*" consists of Hegu(LI 4), Taichong(GB 9); "*Liu zhi jiu*" cosists of Geshu(BL 17), Ganshu(BL 18), pishu(BL 20).

grandson vessels 孙脉[sūn mài]Also termed *sun luo*. The collateral meridians and their smaller collaterals all are communicated with the meridians.

grandson collaterals 孙 络 [sūn luò] Also termed *sun mai* and *sun lue*, *zhimai*. Certain colaterals splitting from the meridians are approximately 365. All of them transport *qi* and blood and are communicated with large collateral meridians.

granual subcutaneous needle 颗粒式皮内针 [kē lì shì pí nèi zhēn]A kind of subcutaneous needle. For details, see subcutaneous needle.

grain qi 谷气[gǔ qì]The refined material in food as digested and absorbed by the human body. It is so called because the food is chiefly derived from the five kinds of grain (rice, two kinds of millet, wheat, and beans).

great reinforcing-reducing maniulations 大补大泻[dà bǔ dà xiè]Contrary to moderate reinforcing-reducing manipulation. The reinforcing-reducing manipulation with greater power and larger volume of stimu-

lus.

great meridian-connected method 大接经法 [dà jiē jīng fǎ]One of the point-combined methods, a special point for treating apoplexy and hemiplegia with atrophy and numbness. Including "from yang to yin" and "from yin to Yang", of which the well-like points of the twelve meridians are selected. The first one is selected from Zhiyin (BL 37), the well-like point of foot-*taiyang* meridian to Yongquan (KI 1) of foot-*shaoyin* meridian, Zhongchong (PC 9) of hand-*jueyin* meridian, Guanchong (TE 1) of hand-*shaoyin* meridian, Zuqiaoyin (GB 44) of foot-*shaoyang* meridian, Dadun (LR 1) of foot-*jueyin* meridian, Shaoshang (LU 11) of hand-*taiyin* meridian, Shaochong (HT 9) of hand-*shaoyin* meridian, Shaoze (SI 1) of hand-*taiyin* meridian, sequentially to finish the puncture of the twelve meridians. The 2nd one is to select from Shaoyang (LU 1) of hand-*yangming* meridian, Lidui (ST 45) of foot-*yangming* meridian, Yinbai (SP 1) of foot-*taiyin* meridian, Shaochong (HT 9) of hand-*shaoyin* meridian, Shaoze (SI 1) of hand-*taiyang* meridian, Zhiyin (BL 67) of foot-*taiyang* meridian, Yongquan(KI 1) of foot-*shaoyin* meridian, Zhongchong(PC 9) of hand-*jueyin* meridian, Guanchong(TE, SI 1) of hand-*shaoyang* meridian, Zuqiaoyin (GB 44) of foot-*shaoyang* meridian, Dadun (LR 1) of foot-*jueyin* meridian to finish the puncture of the twelve meridians.

Guanming 关明[guān míng]I. e., Guanmen (ST 22).

Guanliang 关梁 [guān liáng] An alternate term for Jinmen (BL 63).

Guanling 关陵[guān líng]An alternate term for Xiyangguan (GB 33).

Guanyi 关仪[guān yí]An extra point located 3 cm at the level with and 3 cm to the lateral side of the knee. Puncture: 1. 5—3 cm perpendicularly. Moxibustion: 3—7 moxa cones or 5—15 minutes with warming moxibustion.

guan zhe 关蛰[guān zhé]One of the cutaneousregions of six meridians, the portion of the body surface pertaining to *tayin* meridians of hand and foot. '*Guan zhe*' means the key point and hiding. It is so called because the yin meridians relate to internal syndromes and *taiyin* meridian is their key.

guan, he, shu 关阖枢[guān hé shū] '*Guan*' implies the door bolt, '*he*' the door plank, and '*shu*' the pivot. They were used to explain the function of the three yang meridians and three yin meridians, so as to expound characteristics of diseases or syndromes. the three yang meridians, *taiyang* is at the superficial of the yang aspect so that it is called *guan*, *yangming* is in the middle so that it is called *he*, the three meridians, *taiying* is at the superficial of the yin aspect so that it is called *guan*, *shaoying* is in the middle so that it is called *shu*, *jueyin* is in the deep so that it is called *he*. The cutaneous regions of the six meridians are also nomenclatured in combination with *guan*, *he*, and *shu*.

Guanchong (TE 1) 关冲[guān chōng] A point of Triple Energizer Meridian of Hand-*shaoyang*, the well-like (metal)point of the meridian. Location: Approx. 0. 3 cm lateral to the corner of the fingernail on the ulnar side of the ring finger. Regional anatomy: There is the arterial and venous network formed by the digital and palmar proper artery and vein. The digital and plamar proper nerve from the ulnar nerve is distributed. Indications: Headache, congestive eyes, deafness, sore throat, stiff tongue, febrile diseases, anxiety. Puncture: 0. 3—0. 6 cm obliquely or prick to cause little bleeding. Moxibustion: 1—3 moxa cones or 5—10 minutes with warming moxibustion.

Guanyang 关阳[guān yáng]I. e. , Xiguan (LR 7).

guanshu 关枢[guān shū]One of the cutaneous regions of the six meridians. The portion of the body surface pertaining to *taiyang* meridians of hand and foot. Guanshu means the key point or the pivot. It is therefore called because *taiyang* meridian relates to superficial syndrome.

Guanyuanshu(BL 26)关元俞[guān yuán shū] A point of Bladder Meridian of Foot-*taiyang*. Location: 4. 5 cm lateral to the interspace between the 5th lumbar vertebra. Regional anatomy: In the sacrospinal muscle. There is the posterior branch of the lowest artery of loin. The posterior branch of the 5th lumbar nerve is distributed. Indications: Abdominal pain, borborygmus, diarrnea, rest dysentery, emaciation-thirst disease, enuresis, frequent or difficult urination, etc. Puncture: 3—4. 5 cm perpendicularly. Moxibustion: 3—7 moxa cones or 5—15 minutes with warming moxibustion.

Gumen 谷门[gǔ mén]An alternate term for Tianshu(ST 25).

guiding qi 导气[dǎo qì]An acupuncture manipulation. A method to insert the needle slowly and withdraw it slowly after acquiring *qi*. It has the action of regulating *qi*. By using this method, pathogenic *qi* can not attack deeply and anti-pathogenic *qi* can be recovered. In modern times it has been called the *qi*-guided method that the manipulation of administering acupuncture can promote needling induction to propagate along the coure of meridian. For details, see *xin qi fa*.

Guimen 鬼门[guǐ mén]An extra point. Located 0. 6 cm below the nipple. Indications: Waggering of tongue, sudden epilepsy. (by moxibustion)

Guexin 鬼心[guǐ xīn]I. e. , Daling(PC 7).

Guishi 鬼市[guǐ shì]I. e. , Chengjiang (CV 24).

Guixue 鬼穴[guǐ xué]1. Referring to various points for treating mania, called the thirteen ghost points; 2. Referring to Fengfu (CV 16)

Guicheng 鬼臣[guǐ chéng]I. e. , Quchi (LI 11).

Guixie 鬼邪[guǐ xié]An alternate term for Zusanli(ST 36).

Guidang 鬼当[guǐ dāng]I. e. , Dazhijiahou. (At the end of the transverse crease of the 2nd point of the lateral thumb)

Guichuang 鬼床[guǐ chuáng]I. e. , Jiache(ST 6).

Guizhen 鬼枕[guǐ zhěn]I. e. ,Fengfu(GV 16)

Guishou 鬼受[guǐ shòu]Referring to Chize (LU 5).

Guiyu 鬼域[guǐ yù]An extra point. Same as Shixuan (EX-UE 11)in location. Located at the tips of the ten fingers, 0. 3 cm to the fingernail. Indications:Coma, syncope, high fever, sunstroke, epilepsy, triangular neuralgia.

Guifeng 鬼封[guǐ fēng]An extra point,same as Haiquan(EX-HN 11) in location.

Guixin 鬼信[guǐ xìn]I. e. , Shaoshang (LU 13).

Guigong 鬼宫[guǐ gōng]I. e. , Shuigou (GV 26).

Guiketing 鬼客厅[guǐ kè tīng] I. e. , Shuigou (GV 26).

Guilu 鬼垒[guǐ lěi]I. e. , Yinbai(SP 1).

Guguan 股关[gǔ guān]An ear point at the upper edge of the lower foot of the antihelix to form a triangle with Sciatic and Hip.

Guiku 鬼哭[guǐ kū] I. e. ,an extra point.

Guiying 鬼营[guǐ yíng]Referring to Jianshi (PC 5) or Laogong(PC 8).

Guitang 鬼堂[guǐ táng]1. I. e. , Shangxin (GV 23);2. Referring to Chize(LU 5).

Guilai (ST 29)归来[guǐ lái]1. A point of Stomach Meridian of Foot-*yangming*, also termed Xixue. Location:6 cm lateral to Zhongji (RN 3),1. 2 dm below the umbilicus. Regional anatomy:Passing through the lateral edge of the straight muscle of abdomen and the internal oblique muscle of abdomen to reach the transverse fascia. There are the hypogastric artery and vein at its lateral side. The inferior nerve of abdomen is distributed. Indications:Pain in the bilateral lower abdomen,amenorrhea, profuse uterine,leukorrhea,herna,pain in

the penis. Puncture:3—4 cm perpendicularly. Moxibustion:5—7 moxa cones or 10—20 minutes with warming moxibustion;2. An extra point located 6—7 cm bilateral to Zhongji(CL 3). Indication:Enuresis.

gu 谷[gǔ]The hollow soft area of the lateral chest wall below axilla.

Guanyuan (CV 4)关元[guān yuán]A CV point, the anteriorly referred point of the small intestine,the confluence of three yin meridians of foot and CV, also termed Cimen, Sanjiejiao, Xiaji, Dajizhong, Dazhongji. Location:9 cm below the umbilicus on the abdominal midline. Regional anatomy:On the white abdominal line. There are the branches of the superficial artery and vein of the abdominal wall and the branches of the inferior artery and vein of the abdominal wall. The medial branch of the anterior cutaneous branch of the 12th intercostal nerve is distributed. The small intestine and the bladder being full are in the deeper. Indications:Collapse due to apoplexy,consumptive disease, weakness and emaciation, pain in the bilateral abdomen,cholera and diarrhea and vomiting, dysentery, prolapse of anus, hernia, bloody stools, dysuria, frequent ruination, anuria, spermatorrhea,impotence,premature ejaculation,irregular menstruation,amenorrhea, dysmenorrhea,leukorrhea,prolapse of uterine,metrorrhagia,itch of external genitalia, retention of the placenta,emaciation-thirst disease, vertigo. Puncture:3—4. 5 cm perpendicularly. (Be cautious in the case of the pregnant woman.)Moxibustion:3—7 moxa cones or 5—15 minutes with warming moxibustion.

Guomen 过门[guò mén]The wrong form of Tongjian,another name of Sanyangluo(TE 8).

Guanmen(ST 22)关门[guān mén]A point of Kidney Meridian of Foot-*yangming*. Location:6 cm lateral to Jianli (RN 11). Regional anatomy:At the straight muscle of abdomen and its sheath. There are the branchesof the 8th intercostal artery and vein and the branches of the superior artery and vein of the abdominal wall. The branch of the 8th intercostal nerve is distributed. Indications:Abdominal pain,abdominal distension, borborygmus, diarrhea, poor appetite, edema, enuresis. Puncture: 3—4. 5 cm perpendicularly. Moxibustion: 3—5 moxa cones or 5—10 minutes with warming moxibustion.

Guangming (GB 37)光明[guāng míng]1. A point of Gallbladde Meridian of Foot-*shaoyang*, the connecting point of the meridian. Location:At the anterior edge of fibula, 15 cm directly above the tip of the lateral ankle. Regional anatomy: Between the long extensor muscle of the toe and the short muscle of fibula. There are the branches of the anterial tibial artery and vein. The superficial fibular nerve is distributed. Indications:Pain in the eyes,night blindness, flaccidity and blockage of the lower limb, swelling of the cheek, distension and pain in the breast,night blindness. Puncture: 3—4 cm perpendicularly. Moxibustion;3—5 moxa cones or 5—10 minutes with warming moxibustion; 2. I. e. , Mingguang,another name of Zanzhu;3. An extra point same in position with Yuyao(EX-HN 4). Indications:Conjuctivites,ptosis of eyelids, pain in the supraorbital bone, ametropia, supraorbital neuralgia. Puncture:1—1. 5 cm obliquely.

Guiyan 鬼眼[guǐ yǎn]1. An extra point located at the corner of the root of the raidal (tibia) side of the thumb (great toe). See it by taking the two fingers (toes) together. Indications: Epilepsy, mental trouble, syncope. Moxibustion: 3—7 moxa cones re-

spectively;2. An alternate term for Yaoyan (EX-B7);3. An alternate term for Xiyan (EX-LE 5).

Guilu 鬼路[guǐ lù]Referring Shenmai(Bl 62) or Jianshi(PC 5).

Guitui 鬼腿[guǐ tuǐ]Referring Quchi(LI 11).

Guiku 鬼窟[guǐ kū]Referring Laogong (PC 80).

Guilu 鬼禄[guǐ lù]An aternate term for Xuanming.

Guicang 鬼藏[guǐ cáng]Referring to Huiyin (CV 1) or Yumentou.

GV collateral 督脉络[dū mài luò]One of the fifteen collaterals. The name of Changqiang (GV 1). (Fig 41)

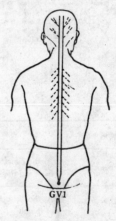

Fig 41

GV diseases 督脉病[dū mài bìng]As GV runs along the inner spine and its diseases and symptoms are stiff spine,opisthotonos, headache,stiff neck,mania,epilepsy due to fright,vertigo,pain in the lumbar spine.

GV points 督穴[dū xué]1. The points pertaining to GV;2. Referring to Houxi(SI 3).

H

hand needling 手针 [shǒu zhēn] An acupuncture technique of puncturing the patient at the hand, the point on the hand, associated with the meridian points and the extra points at the hand and the points used for massage can be used to treat diseases and symptoms at the various parts of the body. It is the application of selection of distal points. (Fig 42). For the points, see the following chart.

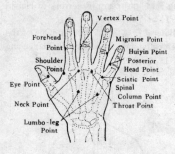 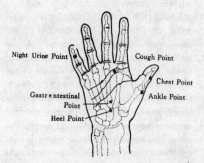

Fig 42

Name of point	Location
Waist-leg point	At the radial aspect of the extensor muscle of the 2nd index finger of the dorsal hand and the ulnar aspect of the extensor muscle of the ring finger, 2 in total
Ankle point	At the dorsopalmar boundary at the radial side of the metarcarpophalangeal joint of thumb
Chest point	At the dorsopalmar boundary at the radial aspect of the phalangeal joint of thumb
Eye point	At the dorsopalmar boundary at the radial aspect of the phalangeal joint of thumb
Shoulder point	At the dorsopalmar boundary at the radial side of the metacarpophalangeal joint of the index finger
Anterior Head point	At the dorsopalamr boundary, at the ulnar side of the phalangeal joint at the proximal end of the index finger
Vertex point	At the dorsopalmar boundary at the phalangeal joint, at the proximal end of the middle finger
Deviated point	At the dorsopalmar boundary at the ulnar side of the phalangeal joint at the proximal end of the ring finger

Continued

Name of point	Location
Huiyin point	At the dorsopalmar boundary at the radial side of the proximal end of the small finger
Spinal Column point	At the dorsopalmar boundary of the ulnar side of the metacarpophalangeal joint of the small finger
Sciatic point	Between the 4th and 5th metacarpophalangeal joints of the dorsal hand,proximal to the 4th metacarpophalangeal joint
Throat point	Between the 3rd and 4th metacarpophalangeal joints of the dorsal hand,proximal to the 2nd metacarpophalangeal joint
Gastrointestinal point	At the midpoint of the line connecting Laogong (PC 8) and Daling (PC 7)
Asthmatic Cough point	At the ulnar side of the metacarpophalangeal joint,distal to the palmar surface
Heel poont	At the midpoint of the line connecting Daling(PC 7) and Gastrointestinal point

hang 胻[háng] I. e. ,tibia.

hand-*yangming* meridian 臂阳明脉[bì yáng míng mài]An early name of the meridian, similar to Hand-*yangming* Meridian.

han 颔[hàn]Referring to the soft tissue superior to the neck and inferior to the mandible.

hand-supported position 托颐位[tuō yí wèi] The name of the body position in acupuncture. For details see sitting position.

Handbook of Acupuncture Science 针灸学手册[zhēn jiǔ xué shǒu chè]A book compiled by Wang Xuetai, published by People's Health Press in 1956. It was revised and reprinted in 1962. The reprinted edition contains six chapters,respectively introducing a brief history of acupuncture,needling techniques, moxibustion techniques, the courses of meridians and diseases and sympoms of meridians, points, treatment of dieases. Quite a few reference data were cited and more illustrations and charts were cooperated,the points used were differentiated into the major ones and minor ones, rich in contents. It offers reference for clinical research.

hand-*juyin* meridian 臂巨（钜）阴脉[bì jù yīn mài]An early name of the meridain,similar to hand-*taiyin* meridian.

hand-*shaoyang* meridain 臂少阳脉[bì shào yáng mài]An early name of the meridian, similar to hand-*shaoyang* meridian.

hand-*shaoyin* meridian 臂少阴脉[bì shào yīn mài]An early name of the meridian,similar to hand-*shaoyin* meridian.

Hanyan（GB 4）颔厌[hàn yàn]A point of Gallbladder Meridian of Foot-*shaoyang*,the confluence of hand-*shaoyang*, foot-*shaoyang* and foot-*yangming* meridians. Location: At the upper temporal corner. Make a connecting line from Touwei(at the corner of the hailine lateral to the forehead) to Qubin (in the temporal hair anterior to the root of ear),at the crossing point of upper 1/4 and lower 3/4, i. e. , between Touwei(ST 8) and Xuanlu(GB 6). Regional antomy:At the temporal muscle. There is the pariatal branch of the superficial temporal artery and vein. The temporal branch of the oculotemporal nerve is distributed. Indications: Headache, vertigo, tinnitus, pain in the outer canthus,epilepsy due to fright.

Puncture: 1—1.5 cm horizontally. Moxibustion: 1—3 moxa cones or 3—5 minutes with warming moxibustion.

Handbook of acupuncture classic 针经指南 [zhēn jīng zhǐ nán] A book written by Dou Hanqing during the Jin and Yuan dynasties (1115—1368). It records *Zhenjing Biao You Fu*, *Zhenjing Zhi Shuo*, *Liuzhu Baxue*, *Shou Zhi Bu Xie*, etc. Of them, *Zhenjing Biao You Fu* was widely popular; *Zhenjing Zhi Shuo* explains the meanings of some words in Miraculous Pivot; *Liuzhu Baxue* introduces the origin of the eight confluential points; *Shouzhi Buxie Fa* are the fourteen manipulations such as shaking, withdrawing, rotatorily inserting, spiraling, shaking, springing, twirling, touching, kneading and closing, pinching, pressing, finger pinching by fingernail etc. *Ye Zhe Gong Tu* deals with prohibitions of the "nine palaces", Dou Guigang in Yuan Dynasty (1271—1386) had got this handed-down book in 1276. In 1311 it was written in Four Books of Acupuncture that he had edited. Its contents were recorded in Prescriptions for Universal Relief.

Haidi 海底 [hǎi dǐ] An alternate term for Huiyin (CV 1).

Haiquan 海泉 [hǎi quán] An extra point, located at the midpoint of the frenulum of tongue. There is the lingual artery and vein, the lingual nerve and the tympanic cord of the facial nerve locally. Indications: Vomiting, hiccup, distending tongue, flaccidity of tongue, sore throat, diarrhea, emaciation-thirst disease. Puncture: 0.3—0.6 cm deep perpendicularly or to prick cause little bleeding with a triangular needle. (Fig 43)

haiguan 骸关 [hái guān] Referring to the knee joint.

hanggu 胻骨 [háng gú] Tibia.

Heart Meridian of Hand-*shaoyin* (HT) 手少阴心经 [shǒu shào yīn xīn jīng] One of the twelve meridians. The course: Starts from the heart, emerges and pertains to the car-

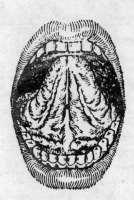

Fig 43

diac connection, passes through the diaphragm and disappears in the small intestine. One branch ascends from the cardiac connection and runs along the esophagus, connects with the cardiac connection, turns back and ascends to the lungs, descends and emerges from under the axilla, runs along the posterior aspect of the medial side of the upper arm, runds behind the hand-*taiyin* and hand-*jueyin* meridians, then reaches at the process of the styloid ulna posterior to the palm, and then enters in to the medioposterior aspect of the medial side of the palm, runs along the radial side of the small finger and emerges from its tip. (to connect with Small Intestine Meridian of Hand-*taiyang*)

harmony between heart and kidney 心肾相交 [xīn shèn xiāng jiāo] The heart is located in the upper energizer and pertains to the 'fire'. The kidney is in the lower energizer, and pertains to the 'water'. Under normal circumstances, the heart and kidney are mutually communicating and reuglating. Cardiac yang may descend to the kidney and nourish renal yang while renal yin may ascend to the heart and nourish cardiac yin. In this way, the dynamic equilibrium of yin and yang between the heart and kidney may be maintained.

hair border 毛际 [máo jì] The border of the pubic hair in the lowe abdomen. CV ascends to the hair border. Gallbladder Meridian of Foot-*shaoyang* "winds the hair border," and Liver Meridian of Foot-*Jueyin* "enters into the hair border."

half exterior and half interior 半表半里 [bàn biǎo bàn lǐ] The pathologic changes that are neither located in the exterior nor in the varieties of diseases.

hastening *qi* 催气 [cuī qì] To apply various acupuncture manipulations to obtain induction when *qi* is not acquired during acupuncture.

hairline 发际 [fà jì] 1. The border of the hair. The front one is called the anterior hairline, the posterior one the posteior hairline; 2. Referring to Shenting (GV, DU 24); 3. Faji, the extra point located on the midline of the forehead at the midpoint of the anterior hairline. Indications: Headache, dizziness, vertigo.

hand-*taiyang* meridian 臂太阳脉 [bì tài yáng mài] An early name of the meridian, similiar to Hand-*taiyang* meridian.

hai 骸 [hài] 1. Generally referring to the skeletion; 2. another name of the tibia.

Hanfu 寒府 [hán fǔ] An alternate term for Xiyangguan (GB 33).

hangsang 颃颡 [háng sāng] Referring to nasopharynx.

hejian 害肩 [hé jiān] The cuntaneous region of *juiyin* meridian, one of the six cutaneous meridians. Referring to the area of the body surface the *jueyin* meridians of hand and foot pertain to.

hefei 害蜚 [hé fēi] The cutaneous region of the *yangmings* meridian, one of the cutaneous regions of six meridians, referring to the area of the body surface the foot-*yangming* meridians of hand of foot pertain to.

heat blockage 热痹 [rè bì] A blockage syndrome caused by relative excess of pathologic heat, and characterized by redness, swelling, heat and pain of the joints often with generalized heat manifestations, such as fever, chills, thirst, yellowish coating of tongue, rapid pulse, etc.

heart 心 [xīn] One of the five storing viscera, located in the chest, the governor of the storing viscera. Its functiion is to store mind and controls blood vessels. Heart Meridian of Hand-*shaoyin* pertains to the cardiac connectioin. Small Intestine Meridian of Hand-*taiyang* connects with the heart, Pericadrdium Meridian of Hand-*jueyin* "internally connects with the heart and lungs." The branches of three yin meridians and of three yang meridians are all communicated with the heart. Its back-*shu* point is Xinshu (BL 15) and its anterior-referred point is Juque (CV 14).

heart meridian of hand-*shaoyin* 心手少阴之脉 [xīn shǒu shào yīn zhī mài] An original name of Headrt Meridian of Hand-*shaoyin* (HT).

Hemorrhoid point 痔疮穴 [zhì chuāng xué] An extra point. Indication: Hemorrhoids. Moxibustion can be done on it with 3—5 *zhuang* of moxa cone.

Heyang (BL 55) 合阳 [hé yáng] A point of Bladder Meridian of Fot-*taiyang*. Location: 6 cm directly below Weizhong (BL 40) at the midpoint of the transverse crease of the cubital fossa, between the heads of gastrochemius muscle. Indications: lumbovertebral pain referring to the abdomen, pains in the lower limbs, metrorrhagia, hernial pain and paralyss. Puncture: 3—4.5 cm perpendicularly. Moxibustion: 3—5 *zhuang* of moxa cone or 5—10 minutes with war-ming moxibustion.

Hegu (LI 4) 合谷 [hé gǔ] A point of Large Intestine Meridian of Hand-*yangming*, the source (fire) point of the meridian. Another name of Hukou. Location: At the midpoint of the radial side of the 2nd metacarpal bone, between the 1st and 2nd metacarpal bones of the dorsal hand, at the highest point of the protruding muscle when the thumb and index finger are held together. Regional anatomy: Passing through the 1st dorsal uterosseous muscle, reaching at the adductor muscle of thumb. There is the dorsal venous network and the branch of the radial artery at the proximal side, which penetrates through the dorsal hand from the palm. The superficial radial nerve is distributed. The digital palmar proper nerve of the central nerve is in the deeper. Indications: Headache, vertigo, congestive, swollen and painful eyes, epistaxis, rhinitis, toothache, deafness, puffy face, deep-rooted sore, spasm of fingers, sore throat, aphonia, closejaw, mumps, pain in the arms, hemiplegia, fever and aversion o cold, no sweat, hypohidrosis, cough, amenorrhea, stomachache, abdominal pain, constipation, dysentery, infantile convulsion, scaby, dysentery. Puncture: 1. 5—3 cm perpendicularly. Moxibustion: 3—5 moxa cones or 5—10 minutes with warming moxibustion.

hegu puncture 合谷刺 [hé gú cì] One of the five needling fechniques for treating pamful muscles. It is to directly puncture the muscles of the affected region, obliquely right and left just like the claws of a chicken.

Henggu 横骨 [héng gǔ] 1. Henggu (KI 11), a meridian point pertaining to Kidney Meridian of Foot-*shaoyin*, the confluence of Vital Vessel and foot-*shaoyin* meridian, also termed Xiaji, Xiaheng. Location: 1. 5 cm below the umbilicus, 1. 5 cm lateral to Qugu (CV 2). Regional anatomy: At the medial side of the straight muscle of abdomen. There is the epigastric artery, and the lateral artery of the external genitalia. The branch of the ilioepigastric nerve is distributed. Indications: Fullness and pain in the lower abdomen, difficulty in urination, pain in the pubic region, lumbago and impotentce, nocternal emission, enuresis, hernia, urethritis, sexual hypofunction. Puncture: 3—4. 5 cm perpendicularly. Moxibustion: 3—5 moxa cones or 5—10 minutes with warming moxibustion. 2. Referring to symphesis pubis.

heart transferring its fire to small intestine 心移热小肠 [xīn yí rè xiǎo cháng] Excessive cardiac fire affects small intestine. The main symptoms are dysphoria, ulcers of the mouth and the tongue, red tip of the tongue, scanty dark colored urine, or stabbing pain with urination cmaturia, etc.

heat stroke 中暑 [zhòng shǔ] The disease caused by prolonged exposure to hot environment in summer. It is manifested as fever, nausea and vomiting, restlessness, profuse sweating or no sweating at all, hypernea, pale complexion or fainting spells, loss of consciousness, convulsion and trismus, etc. The mild case: Dazhui (GV 14), Hegu (LI 4), Xiangu (ST 43), Neiguan (PC 6), Zusanli (ST 36); 2. The severe case: Baihui (GV 20), Shuigou (GV 26), Shixuan (KI 5), Quze (PC 3), Weizhong (BL 40), Quchi (LI 11).

Hepatic Yang₁ 肝阳₁ [gān yáng yī] An ear point at the upper edge of the helix condyle notch.

Hepatic Yang₂ 肝阳₂ [gān yáng èr] An ear point at the lower edge of the helix condyle notch.

Helix 1,2,3,4,5,6 轮 1, 2, 3, 4, 5, 6 [lún yī èr sān sì wǔ liù] Ear points. Helix₁ is located inferior to the helix notch, Helix₆ is located at the lower edge of Tonsil on the lobre. The distance from Helix₁ to Helix₆ is divided into the four equivalent parts. They are Helixz, Helix₃, Helix₄ and Helix₅ from upper to lower.

hegu 核骨 [hé gǔ] The sesamoid bone behind the first metatarsophalangeal joint.

hemorrhage 出血 [chū xuè] It is generally termed hemorrhage that the blood does not circulate normally but exudes from the mouth and nose or exudes into the muscle and skin. Hemoptysis: 1. Hemoptysis caused by invasion of the lungs by hepatic fire: Feishu (BL 13), Yuji (LU 10), Laogong (PC 8), Xingjian (LR 2); 2. Excess fire due to deficiency of yin.

heavenly stratum 天部 [tiān bù] Referring to

the superficial stratum of the point at the subcutaneous arera, also called *tiancai*.

heat sensation measured examining method 知热感度测定法 [zhī rè gǎn dù chè dìng fǎ] To measure the degree of heat sensation of the well-like or back *shu* points of the twelve meridians and compare the different numerical values of the left and right side. It is generally carried on with an incence burnees or a heat sensation measured apparatus. If incence burners are taken as heat source, they should be moved by appointing to the well-like point once every other 1/2 second till the patient feels scorching and the times are recorded as the degree of heat sensation of the meridian the point is located. Or the heat source is appointed to the point at a fixed position to measue the time the patient needs to be feel scorching. After the examination, the deficiency and excess of various meridians and the condition of imbalance are analysed from the numerical value of heat sensation of the twelve well-like points or back *shu* points examined or the different number of thé left and right sides. In the well-like points examined, some points' positions are changed due to the need of examination.

heavenly stems 天干[tiān gān]Also called ten stems, i. e. , 甲, 乙, 丙, 丁, 戊, 己, 庚, 辛, 壬, 癸, which were originally the names of recording the dates and hours. Combined with twelve branches, it is called stem-branch, respectively called heavenly tems and earthly branches. Used in point combination according to time.

heaven-pole bone 天柱骨 [tiān zhù gǔ] Referring to cervical vertebrae.

Hepatomegaly Zone 肝肿大区 [gān zhǒng dà qū] An ear point at the area where the crus of the helix disappears and the area superoinfesior to Lateral Stomach.

heat enters into the pericardium 热入心包 [rè rù xīn bāo] Pathogenic heat invades the inside of the body and affects the mind, giving rise to such symptoms as high fever, coma, delirium lethargy, etc.

heart being coupled with small intestine 心合小肠 [xīn hé xiǎo cháng] Referring to the mutual relationship and influence between the heart and the small intestine. It is recognized through the relationship between the heart meridian and the small intestine meridian and some of their physiopathologic reflections.

held fingers and holding hand 骈指 押手 [bǐng zhǐ yá shǒu] One of holding hands during acupuncture, also termed *bing zhi jia shou*. To hold the four fingers together, press the point with the surface of the palm, and hold the needle with another hand and to make the tip of the needle penetrate through the intérspace between the two fingers into the point. (Fig 44)

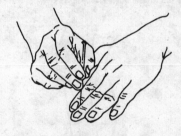

Fig 44

heat moxibustion 热灸[rè jiǔ]Contrary to cold moxibustion by applying drugs to cause blistering. It generally refers to carrying on moxibustion treatment by making use of heat energy. E. g. , moxibustion with mugwort, lampwick moxibustion with rush, moxibustion with buclerry, moxibustion with congenge, moxibustion with electroheat, etc.

hernia *qi* 疝气 [shàn qì] Generally referring to enlargement and pain of the testicles, scrotum and the bilateral lower abdomen.

headache 头痛[tóu tòng]A symptom complex commonly seen in clinic, frequently occuring in varieties of chronic diseases, and being extremely complicated in its etiology.

Henu 合颅 [hé nú] An alternate term for Nao-hu (GV 17).

Heel 跟 [gēn] An ear point slightly lateral to the end of the upper foot of the antihelix.

heat syndrome 热证 [rè zhèng] The symptoms and signs caused by an invasion of pathogenic heat or hyperactivity of yang *qi*, for example, fever, dampness in the chest, chiefly manifested as upper back pain, feeling of suffocation in the chest, shortness of breath, cough with copious phlegm, etc.

Heding 鹤顶 [hé dǐng] 1. An extra point, located in the depession slightly above the midpoint of the patella, at the superior edge of the patella. Indications: Pain in the knee, weakness of foot, paralysis of the lower limbs, beriberi; 2. "located 10.5 cm into the hairline, directly above the nose from at the vertex. (Fig 45)

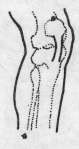

Fig 45

henggu 横骨 [héng gǔ] 1. The pubic bone; 2. the name of the acupuncture point, Henggu (KI 11), located on the upper border of symphysis pubis, about 2 cm lateral to the midpoint, bilaterally.

heart governing the mind 心主神明 [xīn zhǔ shén míng] In traditional Chinese medicine the heart is supposed to govern mental, intelligent and emotional activities. Some of activities of the cerebrum are assigned to the heart. It is the Chief of the internal organs and comparable to the commander-in-chief.

Heyu 合颠 [hé yǔ] 1. Referring the xiphoid

process of stern; 2. An alternate term for Jiuwei (CV 15).

Huantiao 环跳 [huán tiào] I.e., Huantiao (GB 30).

Henghu 横户 [héng hù] An alternate term for Yinjiao (CV 7).

Hengshe 横舍 [héng shè] I.e., Sheheng, an alternate term for Yamen (GV 15).

hepatic blockage 肝闭 [gān bì] I.e., a blockage syndrome of muscles and tendons, which is refractory to prolonged treatment. progresses to affect the liver, and thus, includes the symptoms of headache, dreaminess, thirst, freqent urination, abdominal distention, lumbago, hypochondriac pain, etc.

Heat point 热穴 [rè xué] An ear point between Sacral Vertebra and Lumbar point, approx. at the level with Hip point.

Hepatitis point 肝炎点 [gān yán diǎn] An ear point in the middle of Asthma point and Shenmen.

Heart point 心脏点 [xīn zàng diǎn] An ear point in the depression at the tip of the tragus.

Hemorroidal nucleus point 痔核点 [zhì hé diǎn] An ear point at the medial side of the tip of ear, superior to Blood-pressure Lowering Spot.

he 颌 [hé] The part of the manidible bone below the ear.

hip joint 髀枢 [bì shū] Also termed *biyan*, referring to the hip joint.

hidden pulse 伏脉 [fú mài] The pulse that is deeply situated and can be felt by pressing the bone. It may be seen in the conditions such as fainting, excruciating pain, and sequestration of pathogenic *qi*.

Hip joint 髋关节 [kuān guān jié] An ear point in the middle between Scaral Vertebra and Toe.

high fever 高热 [gāo rè] It is called high fever that the body temperature exceeds 39℃. It is a common symptom in clinic, and can be seen in many a disease, and 1. Invasion of the lungs by wind-heat: Dazhui (GV 14),

Quchi (LI 11), Hegu (LI 4), Yuji (LU 10), Waiguan (TE 5); 2. *Jue* symptom-complex.

hiccup 呃逆 [è nì] Repeatedly reflux of air, producing a sharp quick sound in the throat.

Hip 臀 [tún] An ear point at the edge of the starting point of the lower foot of the antihelix.

horizontal puncutre 沿皮刺 [yán pí cì] Also termed *heng ci* (transverse puncture). Referring to puncturing along the subcutaneous region with the body of needle and the sking surface of the point formed a 10°—20° angle. It suits the points at the head, face, chest, etc. Where the muscles are thin or just at the bone surface.

hovering moxibustion 悬起灸 [xuán qǐ jiǔ] A kind of moxibustion with a moxa stick, contrary to touching moxibustion. To do moxibustion with a moxa stick hanging over the point lest the skin should be injured. (Fig 46)

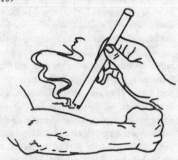

Fig 46

holding open *couli* (the junctlure between muscle and skin) 扦皮开腠理 [hàn pí kāi zhòu lǐ] Referring to the way to insert the needle. It means to hold open *couli* with the left hand along the interspace between the tendons and the muscle, insert the needle gently and slowly with the right hand to make the patient not feel fright but the disease cured.

Houding (CV19) 后顶 [hòu dǐng] A GV point, another name of Jiaochong. Location: 20 cm to the anterior hairline, on the midline of the head, i. e 4 cm posterior to Baihui (GV DU 20). Regional anatomy: At galera aponeurotica. There are the branches of the left and right occipital artery and vein. The cervical nerve is distributed. Indications: Headache, vertigo, stiff neck, mania, epilepsy, anxiety, insomnia. Puncture: Headache, vertigo, stiff neck, mania, epilepsy, anxiety, insomnia, Puncture: 1—1.5 cm horizontally. Moxibustion: 3—5 moxa cones or 5—10 minutes with warming moxibustion.

Houshencong 后神聪 [hòu shén cōng] One of Shencong. Located 3 cm posterior to Baihui (GV 20).

Houye 后腋 [hòu yè] I. e., Houyexia point.

Houyexia point 后腋下穴 [hòu yè xià xué] An extra point, located at the end of the plica of the posterior axilla. Indications: Spasm of the shoulder and back, cervical scrofula, sore throat, wind blockage. Puncture: 1.5—3 cm perpendicularly. Moxibustion: 3—6 moxa cones or 5—15 minutes with warming moxibustion.

Houxi (SI 3) 后溪 [hòu xī] A point of Small Intestine Meridian of Hand-*taiyang*, the stream-like (wood) point of the meridian, one of the eight confluential points, communicated with GV. Location: Posterior to the small head of the 5th metacarpal bone, on the ulnar side of the hand. When a fist is formed, it is located at the end of the transverse crease of the palm at the dorsopalmar border. Regional anatomy: At the abductor muscle of the little finger and the opposing muscle of the little finger. There is the dorsal digital artery and vein and the venous network of the distal hand. The branch of the ulnar nerve is distributed. Indications: Stiffness and pain in the head and neck, deafness, nebula, spasm of the elbow and finger, febrile diseases, malaria, mania, epilepsy, night sweat, vertigo, scabies.

Puncture: 1.5—3 cm perpendicularly. Moxibustion: 3—5 moxa cones or 5—10 minutes with warming moxibustion.

hollow pulse 芤脉 [kōu mài] The pulse that is superficial, large and hollow, giving the feeling of that of scallion. It is usually seen after severe hemorrhages.

houhe 喉核 [hóu hé] Tonsils.

holistic concept 整体观念 [zhěng tǐ guān liàn] It is an important idea of traditional Chinese medicine in preventing and treating diseases. It has two main components. 1. A human body is regarded as an integral, with special emphasis on the harmonic and integral interrelationship between the viscera and the superficial structures in the close phsyiologic connections and their mutual pathologic influence. Thereby, in traditional Chinese medicine, the local pathologic changes are always considered in conjunction with other tissues and organs of the entire body, instead of considered alone; 2. Special attention is paid to the integration of the human body with the external environment. The onset, the evolution and the changes of the disease are considered in conjunction with the climatic, geopgraphic, social and other environmental factors, rather than considering the disease as an isolated incident.

host and guest 主客 [zhǔ kè] In composing the points in acupuncture the major ones are called the 'host', the cooperative one the 'guest'. The composition of one major point and one auxiliary point is called "The host corresponds with the guest. E. g., in eight confluence points, Neiguan (PC 6) and Gongsun (SP 4), Houxi (SI 3) and Shenmai (BL 62), Waiguan (TE 5) and Linqi, Lieque (LU 7) and Zhaohai (KI 6) are cooperatively applied. If they are composed and applied together with source points and connecting points, it is called host-guest and source-connecting points composition.

hottest summer 三伏 [sān fú] A seasonal term, the hottest summer in a lunar calendra, about the middle of July to the middle of August. It is divided into early, middle and later 'fu'. It is called fu acupuncture or fu moxibustion that chronic diseases are often treated in hottest summer in acupuncture clinic.

hou 喉 [hóu] Larynx.

houguan 喉关 [hóu guān] The part of oropharynx formed the tonsil, uvula, and the root of the tongue.

house of primordial mind 元神之府 [yuán shén zhī fǔ] Referring to cerebral medulla.

Houqu 后曲 [hòu qū] An alternate term for Tongziliao (GB 1).

Houguan 后关 [hòu guān] An alternate term for Tinggong (SI 19)

HT points 手少阴心经穴 [shǒu shào yīn xīn jīng xué] According to Systematic Classic of Acupuncture they are Jiquan (HT 1), Qingling (HT 2), Shaohai (HT 3) (sealike), Lingdao (HT 4) (river-like), Tongli (connection) (HT 5), Yinxi (HT 6) (gaplike), Shenmen (HT 7) (stream-like source), Shaofu (HT 8) (spring-like), Shaochong (HT 9) (well-like), 9 in total. There are also Xinshu (BL 15) pertaining to foot-*taiyang* meridian; Juquan (CV 14) pertaining to CV. (Fig 47)

HT diseases 手少阴心经病 [shǒu shào yīn xīn jīng bìng] They are mainly cardialgia, pains in the chest and hyrochondrium, anxiety, short breath, restlessness, vertigo, yellow eyes, dry throat, thirst, clammy cold, and pain in the posterior part of the medial side of the upper limb, feverish sensation in the palm.

Huantiao (GB 30) 环跳 [huán tiào] A point of Gallbladder Meridian of Foot-*shaoyang*, the confluence of foot-*shaoyang* and foot-*taiyang* meridians, also termed Bingu, Fenzhong, Piyan, Kuangu. Location: Posterior to the great trochanter of femurus, at the crossing point of the lateral 1/3 and medial 2/3 of the line connecting the great trochanter and the hiatus of the sacral tube. Select it in the side position and the

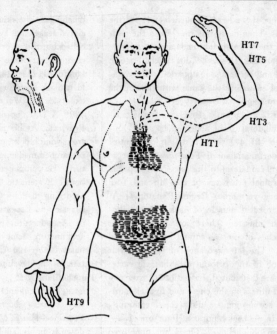

Fig 47

flexed thigh. Regional anatomy: There is the greatest gluteal muscle. Passing through the inferior edge of the piriformis. There is the inferior gluteal artery and vein at its medial side. The inferior gluteal cutaneous nerve and the inferior gluteal nerve are distributed. The sciatic nerve is in the deeper. Indications: Lumbago, hemipligia, atrophy of the lower limbs, general rash, lumbago due to strain, swollen and painful knees and ankles. Puncture: 6—9 cm perpendicularly. Moxibustion: 5—10 moxa cones or 15—30 minutes with warm needling.

Huantiao 环铫 [huán tiào] I. e., 环跳 (GB 30).

Huiyang (BL 35) 会阳 [huì yáng] A point of Bladder Meridian of Foot-taiyang, also termed Liji. Location: At the lower end of the coccyx. 1.5 cm lateral to it. Regional anatomy: At the medial side of the greatest gluteal muscle. There are the branches of the artery and vein. The coccygeal nerve is distributed. Indications: Abdomial pain, diarrhea, dysentery, impotence, leukorrhea, pain in the leg. Puncture: 3—4.5 cm perpendicularly. Moxibustion: 3—7 moxa cones or 5—15 minutes with warming moxibustion.

Huiqi 回气 [huí qì] An extra point, i. e., the tip of the sacrum. Moxibustion: 3—5 moxa cones or 5—10 minutes with warming moxibustion.

Huifawuchu 回发五处 [huí fā wǔ chù] An extra point located at the centre of the spiraling hair at the vertex and its anterior, posterior, left and right areas. First measure the patient's mouth, then measure the length between the two lateral edges of the two nostrils. Put the midpoint of the whole length on the centre of the spiraling hair and its anterior and posterior parts of the hairline of the head. The two ends are the points. Then make this rope cross the midline, the left and right ends are the points. Indications: Headache due to pathogenic wind and vertigo. Moxibustion: The number of *zhuang* is the same with that of the patient's age, twice per year.

huanjin 缓筋 [huǎn jīn] Referring to the muscles bilateral to the abdomen.

Hunmen (BL 47) 魂门 [hún mén] A point of Bladder meridian of Foot-*taiyang*. Location: 9 cm lateral to Jinsuo (GV8) between the spinal processes of the 9th and 10th thoracic vertebrae. Regional anatomy: At the broadest muscle of back and the iliocostal muscle. There are the posterior branches of the 9th intercostal artery and vein. The lateral branch of the posterior branch of the 7th and 8th thoracic vertebrae are distributed. Indications: Distension and fullness in the chest and hypochondrium, borborugmus and diarrhea, vomiting, pain in the back, anorexia. Puncture: 1.5—2.5cm obliquely. (It is not punctured deep). Moxibustion: 3—5 moxa cones or 5—15 minutes with warming moxibustion.

Hunhu 魂户 [hún hù] The wrong form of Pohu (BL 42).

Hunshe 魂舍 [hún shè] An extra point located 3 cm bilateral to the umbilicus. Puncture: 1.5—3 cm perpendicularly. Moxibustion: 3—5 moxa cones or 5—10 minutes with warming moxibustion.

Huigu 回骨 [huí gǔ] The wrong form of Qugu (CV 2).

Houfaji point 后发际穴 [hòu fà jì xué] An extra point. According to Medical Talk, "It is located in the centre of the hair line posterior to the nape," I. e., Yamen (GV, DU 15), According to Systematic Classic of Acupuncture, Yamen is "at the hairline." Accoding to 'Bronge Figure,' "It is 1.5 cm into the hairline."

horizonal puncture 直针刺 [zhí zhēn cì] One of twelve needling techniques. It refers to puncture along the subcutaneous region by pinching up the skin, so as to treat superficial disease and syndrome. It is usually called horizontal or transverse puncture in contemporary times.

Huangfu Mi (215—282 A. D.) 皇甫谧 [huáng fǔ mì] A literary man and acupuncture expert during Wei and Jin Periods (220—420 A. D.) born at Lingtai, Gansu Province. At his middle age, he suffered from wind blockage but he still learned and researched medicine, particularly acupuncture. He completed the compilation of the book, Systematic Classic of Acupuncture according to Plain Question, Acupuncture Classic and Essentials of Mingtang Points of Acupuncture, which summarized the acupuncture achievements before Jin Dynasty (265—420 A. D.) and laid a foundation for the development of acupuncture.

Hu Zhuiliang 胡最良 (1853—1923) [hú zuì liáng] An acupuncture expert in contemporary times, born at Wuxi, Jianshu Proivince. His TCM knowledge was handed down from his family and he was very good at applying midnight-noon ebb-flow, etc. He usually treated infantile diseases with finger needling and got very favourable effects. He was respected by the people at that time because he treated the poor and gave them drugs.

huai 踝 [huái] Malleoli, same as in Western medicine.

huoni 火逆 [huǒ nì] The varied symptom due to misuse of moxibustioin. The varied symptom-complex due to wrong use of moxibustioin.

huiyin vessel 会阴之脉 [huì yīn zhī mài] A branch of foot-*taiyang* meridian passing through the waist to the sacral region.

Huizong (TE 7) 会宗 [huì zōng] A point of Triple Energizer Meridian of Hand-*shaoyang*, the gap-like point of the meridian. Location: 9 cm above the transerse crease of the dorsal wrist, at the radial side of the ulna. Select it at 1 transverse finger-width at the ulnar side of Zhigong (TE 6).

Regional anatomy: Running between the ulnarextensor muscle of wrist and the proper extensor muscle of the small finger, reaching at the proper extensor muscle of the index finger. There is the dorsal interosseous artery and vein of the forearm. The dorsal cutaneous nerve of forearm and medial cutaneous nerve of forearm are distributed. The dorsal interosseous cutaneous nerve of forearm and the palmar interosseous nerve are in the deeper. Indications: Deafness, epilepsy, pain in the skin of the upper limbs. Puncture: 1.5—3 cm perpendicularly. Moxibustion: 3—5 moxa cones or 5—10 minutes with warming moxibustion.

Huiyuan 会原 [huì yuán] An alternate term for Chongyang (ST 42).

Huiwei 会维 [huì wéi] An alternate term for Dicang (ST 4).

Huie 会额 [huì è] An alternate term for Naohu (GV 17).

Huanzhong 环中 [huán zhōng] An extra point located at the hip, at the midpoint of the line connecting Huangtiao (GB 30) and Yaoshu (GV 2). Indications: Sciatica, lumbago, pain in the leg. Puncture: 3—6 cm perpendicularly. Moxibustion: 10 moxa cones or 15 minutes with warm moxibustion.

Huangang 环冈 [huán gāng] I. e., Tuangang. Huangang, the two points are located between the transverse crease 6 cm below Xiaochangshu (BL 27). Its indication is anurrhea.

Huang Zhuzai (1886—1960) 黄竹斋 [huáng zhú zāi] A contemporary acupuncture expert, born at Xi'an, Shanxi Province. He once compiled Illustrative Study on Meridian Points of Acupuncture, 8 volumes, and had a systematic texual study on the meridian points. He also revised Illustrative Classic of Bronze Figure Marked with *Shu* Points of Acupuncture, and also wrote Notes to Treatise on Cold Injury and Notes to Synopsis of the Golden Chamber, etc.

hungry horse shakes the bell 饿马摇铃 [è mǎ yáo líng] An acupunctre manipulation, symetrical to the phoenix extends its wings. It implies that while twirling the needle the thumb is mainly used to twirl the needle forward, and the needle is slowly rotated just like the hungry horse.

Huangmen (BL 51) 肓门 [huāng mén] A point of Bladder Meridian of Foot-*taiyang*. Location: 9 cm lateral to Xuanshu (GV 5) between the spinal processes of the 1st and 2nd lumbar vertebrae. Regional anatomy: Passing through the broadest muscle of back, reaching at the iliocostal muscle. There is the posterior branch of the 1st lumbar artery and vein. The lateral branch of the posterior branch of the 12th thoracic nerve is distributed. Indications: Pain in the upper abdomen, abdominal mass, constipation, breast trouble. Puncture: 1.5—2.5 cm obliquely. (It is not advisable to puncture deep.) Moxibustion: 5—7 moxa cones or 5—15 minutes with warming moxibustion.

Huang Shu (KI 16) 肓俞 [huāng shū] A point of Kidney Meridian of Foot-*shaoyin*. The confluence of Vital Vessel and foot-*shaoyin* meridian. Location: 1.5 cm lateral to shenque (CV 8) in the umbilicus. Regional anatomy: Passing through the fascia of the medial and lateral oblique muscle of abdomen and the straight muscle of abdomen, reaching at the transverse muscle of abdomen. There is the muscular branch of the inferior epigastric artery and vein. The 10th interostal nerve is distributed. Indications: Abdominal pain, abdominal distension. Puncture: 3—4.5 cm perpendicularly. Moxibustion: 5—7 moxa cones or 10—15 minutes with warming moxibustion.

Huangmu 肓募 [huāng mù] An extra point. Located at the midpoint between the nipple and the umbilicus. Indications: Pain caused by abdominal mass, jaundice, postpartum asthenia. Moxibustion: 3—7 moxa cones or 5—15 minutes with warming moxibustion.

Huatuojiaji 华佗夹脊 [huá tuó jiá jǐ] I. e., Jiaji points. It is therefore called because it was created by Huatuo.

Huagai (**CV 20**) 华盖 [huá gài] A CV point located at the level with the 1st intercostal space on the midline of chest. Regional anatomy: Cough, asthmatic breath, thoracalgia, pains in the hypochondrium, sore throat, swelling of cheek. Puncture: 0. 9—1. 5 cm horizontally. Moxibustion: 3—5 moxa cones of 5—10 minutes with warming moxibustion.

humen 户门 [hù mén] Referring to teeth. One of seven vital portals.

Huaroumen (**ST 24**) 滑肉门 [huá ròu mén] A point of Stomach Meridian of Foot-*yangming*. Location: 6 cm lateral to Shuifen (CV 9) 3 cm above the umbilicus. Regional anatomy: At the straight muscle of abdomen. There are the branches of the 9th intercostal artery and vein and the branches of the artery and vein of the hypogastric wall. The branch of the 9th intercostal nerve is distributed. Indications: Stomachache, hiccup, vomiting, borborygmus, diarrhea, mania, acute/chronic gastroenteritis, adhesion of intestine, schyzophrenia. Puncture: 3—4. 5 cm perpendiccularly. Moxibustion: 3—5 moxa cones or 5—10 minutes with warming moxibustion.

Hua Shou (1304—1386) 滑寿 [huá shòu] A medical expert in Yuan Dynasty (1271—1368). First he learned medicine from Wan Juzhong. Later he learned needling techniques from Gao Tongyang. The books he wrote are Original Meaning of Difficult Classic, Essentials of Diagnostics, Expounding of Fourteen Meridians. He has exerted a great influence upon academy of acupuncture.

Huanmen 患门 [huàn mén] An extra point, located 4. 5 cm lateral to the spinal process of the 5th thoracic vertebra. Indications: streaming of bones, and tidal fever, yellow face and emaciation, poor appetite, lassitude, rough and asthmatic breath with sputum, anxiety, fever and night sweat, nocturnal emission, cardialgia, pain referring to

the chest and back, Moxibustion: 3—7 moxa cones or 5—15 minutes with warming moxibustion. (Fig 48)

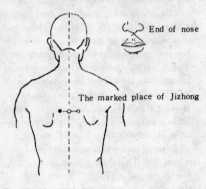

End of nose

The marked place of Jizhong

Fig 48

huantiao **needle** 环跳针 [huán tiào zhēn] I. e., a long needle.

Hua Tuo 华佗 [huá tuó] (208 B. C.) A famous medical expert at the end of Eastern Han Dynasty (208 B. C. —220 A. D.) born at Hao County, Anhui Province. He was very special in formulary and drugs. The prescriptions he prescribed and the points he punctured were only a few, but the therapeutic effects he got were very remarkable. He created *mafu* powder for general anesthesia to perform the operation on the abdominal cavity. Thus, he was the pioneer in performing surgical operation. He paid special attention to induction of *qi* while administering acupuncture. According to the record of *Sui* Book, he wrote one volume of Moxibustion and Acupuncture Classic in the Occiput, which had not been handed down. In Prescription for Emergency, Prescriptions Worth a Thousand Gold and Prescriptions of Medical Experiences part of his articles on acupuncture and moxibustion were remained. His disciple, Fan Ah was also very good at acupuncture and moxibustion.

Hukou 虎口 [hǔ kǒu] 1. An alternate term for

Hegu (LI 4); 2. An extra point, located at the dorso-palmar boundary, anterior to Hegu (LI 4). Indications: Headache, anxiety, fever, vertigo, insomnia, night sweat, cardialgia, toothache, infantile closed mouth. Puncture: 1—1.5 cm obliquely. Moxibustion: 5—7 moxa cones.

Huiyin (CV 1) 会阴 [huì yīn] A GV point, the confluence of CV, GV and Vital Vessel, also termed Pingi, Xiaji, Haidi. Location: In the center of perineum between the male anus and the root of scrotum of the male or between the female anus and the posterior symphysis. Indication: Drawning, suffocation, coma, maina, epilepsy, dysuria, pain in the pubic region, itch of external gentialia, sweat-dampness in the public region, external prolapse of uterine, prolapse of anus, hernia, hemorrhoids, irregular menstruation. Puncture: 1.5—3 cm perpendicularly. (Be cautious in the case of the pregnant woman.) Moxibustion: 5—10 minutes with warming moxibustion. (Fig 49)

huozhong 或中 [huò zhōng] I.e., Yuzhong (KI 26).

Huaijian 踝尖 [huái jiān] An alternate term for Neihuaijian.

hypochondrium 胁 [xié] A collective term for the lateral aspect of the chest from the axilla to the 12th rib.

Hyoscyamus niger L. 莨菪根 [làng dàng gēn] A kind of interposing thing for moxibustion used for treating scrofula.

hypoactivity of yang in the middle energizer 中阳不振 [zhōng yáng bú zhèn] Pathologic manifestations due to the decreased digestive and absorptive functions of the spleen and stomach. The main symptoms are anorexia, preference for hot foods and drinks, cold clammy limbs, nausea and vomiting, diarrhea, sallow complexion, pale lips, whitish coating of the tongue, slow pulse, etc.

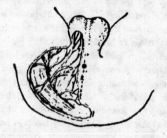

Fig 49

hypochondriac pain 胁痛 [xié tòng] One of the commonly seen symptoms in clinic. It generally refers to pain in the bilateral hypochondriac region.

Illustration of Selecting Points along the Meridans 金兰循经取穴图解 [jīn lán xuán jīng qǔ xué tú jiě] A book written by Hutaibinie in Yuan Dynasty (1271—1368). It first drew the anterior and posterior illurtrations of storing-emptying viscera, then described the course of three yin meridians and three yang meridians, finally recorded the course of the fourteen meridians with the notes and illutrations appended. Expounding of Fourteen Meridians is on the basis of it. The original has been lost.

Illustrations of Meridians 经络分图 [jīng luò fēn tú] A medical book, written by Luo Shaoju, four volumes. The sequence is arranged according to three yang and three yin meridians of hand and foot, different from that according to the sequence of flow of *qi* and blood. I. e., hand-*taiyang*, hand-*yangming*, hand-*shaoyang*, hand-*taiyin*. hand-*shaoyin*, hand-*jueyin*, foot-*taiyang*, foot-*yangming*, foot-*shaoyang*, foot-*tayin*, foot-*shaoyin*, and foot-*jueyin*. Then the eight extra vessels; GV, CV, Vital Vessel, Girdle Vessel, Motility Vessel of Yang, Motility Vessel of yin, Connecting Vessel of Yang, Connecting Vessel of Yin. And it also had a textual study and explanation of the meridians and points. It was completed in 1900.

Illustrated Manual of Points of the Bronze Figure 铜人腧穴针灸图经 [tóng rén shū xué zhēn jiǔ tú jīng] A book compiled by Wang Weiyi in Song Dynasty (960—1279A. D.), completed in 1026. Next year, two bronze models were remoulded in association with the book. Therefore its complete name is Illustrated Classic of Newly-Remoulded Bronze Model Marked with *Shu* Points of Acupuncture. In the book, there are the illustrations of the front, back, left and right sides of the figure and the indica-tions of the points, which had been also carved on the stones for popularization. The five rest stones were unearthed in Beijing during 1965—1971.

Illustrated Meridians 绘图经络图说 [huì tú jīng luò tú shuō] A book written by Zhang Ming in Ming Dynasty (1368—1644). It contains 14 colored pictures of meridians and *shu* points and one picture of the viscera. In each picture the meridians and *shu* points were explained and the bone-measurements and general introduction to the viscera are appeneed. It was written by 1630.

illness due to unacclimatization 水土不服 [shuǐ tǔ bù fú] When a person just arrives at a new place, as a result of the changes of the natural environment and living customs unacclimatization symptom may occur temporarily, such as anorexia, nausea, and vomiting, abdominal distension and pain, diarrhea, or irregularity of menstruation, etc.

impotence 阳萎 [yáng wěi] A failure of the penis to erect, resulting in inability to perform sexual act.

impairrment of the liver and the kidney 肝肾亏损 [gān shèn kuī sǔn] Also termed *gan shen yin xu*. The pathologic changes in which yin fluids of both the liver and the kidney are simultaneously impaired. The main symptoms are dizziness, feeling of distension of the head, blurred vision, tinnitus, fever, bitter taste, hot palms and soles, insomnia, soreness of the waist and knees, spermatorrhea, stringy, faint and rapid pulse, or faint and weak pulse, etc.

injecting-like needle insertion 注射式进针 [zhù shè shì jìn zhēn] One of needle insertion methods, also termed swift insertion of needle. (*kuai cha zhen*) To pinch the lower segment of the body of needle with the thumb and index finger, Let the tip of needle (about 0.6 cm) expose, then swiftly insert the needle. It suits perpendicular puncture. (fig 50)

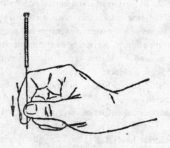

Fig 50

injury of the lungs by dry *qi* 燥气伤肺[zào qì shāng fèi] The pathologic manifestations due to pulmonary injuries by dry *qi*. The main symptoms are dry cough, dry nose, itchness and pains in the throat, pains in the chest and hypochondrium, even occasional bloody sputum, etc.

inspection 望神 [wàng shén] The diagnostic technique to evaluate the facial expression, complexion, general appearance, characteristics of the tongue, except the distribution of superficial venules of the infant's fingers, etc.

inspection of the body state and movement 望形态[wàng xíng tài] The diagnostic technique to evaluate the patient's body status and movements (including muscles, skin and skeleton posture, motility and strength, etc.)

intestinal blockage 肠闭[cháng bì] A blockage syndrome affecting large and small intestines with symptoms of abdomal distension, diarrhea, dysuria, etc.

intermingling of cold and heat 寒热错杂[hán rè cuò zá] The pathologic changes produced by the intemingling of the cold syndrome and heat syndrome.

invasion of the spleen by hepatic *qi* 肝气犯脾 [gān qì fàn pí] When the dispersing function of the liver is disturbed and affects the

spleen, there may appear simultaneous pathologic manifestations of the liver and th spleen. The main symptoms are vertigo, chest distress, hypochondriac pain, irritability and excitability, distension of the abdomen, loose stools, anorexia, stringy pulse, etc.

invasion of the stomach by hepatic *qi* 肝气犯胃[gān qì fàn wèi]Also termed *gan wei bu he*, when the dispersing function of the liver is disturbed and affects the stomach, there may appear simultaneous pathologic manifestations of both the liver and the stomach. The main symptoms are vertigo, chest distress, hypochondriac pain, irritability and irrascibility, epigastric distension and pain, anorexia, nausea and vomiting, regurgitation, stringy pulse, etc.

inevitable tansmutation of superposed yin into yang 重阴必阳 [chóng yīn bì yáng] A disease may be characterized by an excess of yin *qi* when the excess of its yin *qi* reaches a certain limit, it may exhibit yang characters or metamorphose toward yang. E. g., when a syndrome of chills develops to its climax, fever manifestations may appear.

insufficiency of *qi* in the middle energizer 中气不足 [zhōng qì bù zú] Pathologic manifestations due to weakness of the spleen and stomach in the middle energizer. The main symptoms are anorexia, abdominal distension after eating, dizziness, lassitude, chronic diarrhea, apathy, etc.

inability of renal *qi* 肾气不固 [shèn qì bú gù] The pathologic manifestations of incontinence of urine and spermatorrhea due to decreased renal function. The main symptoms are spermatorrhea, premature ejaculation, enuresis, frequent nocturia, incontinence of urine, persistent leukorrhea, lumbago, etc.

intestinal carbuncle 肠痈[cháng yōng]Acute suppurative inflammation of the intestine.

inward-outward rotation 内外转 [nèi wài zhuān]It is called the left outward rotation while twirling the needle; It is called the right inward rotation while withdrawing the thumb inward.

internal movement of hepatic wind 肝风内动 [gān fēng nèi dòng] All the symptoms which appear as moving, changing and sudden as wind are classified as the manifestations of liver disorders in traditional Chinese medicine.

insuffiiency of lactation 乳少 [rǔ shǎo] Very little lactation is secreted after delivey, which can not meet the neonate's need.

infantile malnutrition 疳积 [gān jī] Infantile malniutrition characterized by emaciation, abdominal distension, and nutritional disorder with chronic indigestion.

interior cold 里寒 [lǐ hán] It generally refers to the cold symptom complexes of the internal organs. It is chiefly manifested by chills, cold limbs, pale complexion, soreness and coldness of the waist and the knees, loose stools, copious clear urine, deep slow or small faint pulse, pale tongue with whitish moist coating, etc.

infantile needle 小儿针 [xiǎo ér zhēn] I. e., plum needle. It is therefore called because it is suitable for infants.

infantile enuresis 小儿遗尿 [xiǎo ér yí niào] A symptom that the young children at the age about 3 constantly feel that urine is spontaneously discharged in sleep and find it after being awaked.

indirect moxibustion 间接灸 [jiàn jiē jiǔ] A kind of moxibustion with moxa cone, also called ge wu jiu. Referring to administering moxibustion by putting a layer of an interposing thing between the moxa cone on the point. The moxa cone used is larger than that used for direct moxibustion. Along with different interposing things, it is respectively called jinger-interposing moxibustion (a piece of fresh jinger), garlic-interposing moxibustion (a piece of barlic), salt-interposing moxibustion, drug-paste-interposing moxibustion (prepared with ground drug), etc.

indirect moxibustion 间隔灸 [jiàn gé jiǔ] I.

e., jian jie jiu.

interior excess 里实 [lǐ shí] 1. Generally referring to the excess syndrome of the viscera. 2. Referring to a stagnation of formed qi in the intestinal truct with such manifestations as abdominal distension and pain, constipation. 3. Referring to the manifestations caused by accumulation of various pathologic products in the body, such as phlegm, sludging of blood, heliminthiasis, indigestion, etc.

indivuidual palpation 单按 [dān àn] To feel the pulse with one finger at one location.

interior heat 里热 [lǐ rè] Usually referring to the febrile disease manifested by higher fever, no chills, aversion to heat, thirst with polydipsia, restlessness, or uneasiness and bitter taste, scanty dark-colored urine, reddish tongue with yellowish coating, full and rapid or taut and forceful pulse, etc.

inevitable transmutation of superposed yang into yin 重阳必阴 [chóng yáng bì yīn] A disease may be characterized by an excess of yang qi. When the excess of yang qi reaches a certain limit, it may exhibit yin characters or metamorphose toward yin. For instance, when a heat synddrome reaches its climax, manifestations of chills may appear.

insomnia 失眠 [shí mián] The slight one is being hard to fall asleep, or being easily waken. The severe one is being unable to fall asleep all the night.

inserting techique 进法 [jìn fǎ] A method of waiting for qi adopted after the needle is inserted into a certain depth of the cutaneous region. For the thin patient, the needle is inserted superficially; For the fat one deeply and the needle js properly twisted so as to make qi arrive.

interior deficiency 里虚 [lǐ xū] Usually referring to the deficiency syndrome due to insufficiency of qi and blood, and impairment of the functions of the viscera.

interspace of the two eyebrows 两衡 [liǎng héng] The main location for color diagnosis. "The *qi* state of the five storing and six emptying viscera can be seen from *Mingtang* and the interspace between two eyebrows. " (Yong's Notes)

infantile diarrhea 小儿泄泻 [xiǎo ér xié xiè] It is characteriezed by increased times of passing motion, watery and thin stools or acqueous stools and caused by infant's weak spleen and stomach, abnormal sleep and irregular diet.

infrared radiation of point 红外线穴位照射法 [hóng wài xiàn xué wèi zhào sè fǎ] To treat diseases by using the infrared ray to radiate the point. That is to cover other parts of the body with a piece of white cloth, let the point expose, then radiate it with a generator of the infrared till the patient feels comfortable warming heat and the reddish color appears on the patient's skin. It can be used in treating asthma, chronic bronchitis, rheumatic arthritis, tenosynovitis, postpartum insufficiency of lactation, etc. It is not advisable to use it for the patient with high fever, the incomplete cardiovascular function and tendency of hemorrhage, and local obstruction of warm sensation.

insanity 癫狂 [diān kuáng] A general term for maniac-depressive pschosis.

interosseous space 骨空 [gǔ kōng] The interosseous space where the point is located.

inducing period of acupuncture anesthsia 针麻诱导期 [zhēn má yòu dǎo qī] A term of acupuncture anesthesia. It refers to the period of time during which from the bigining of inserting the needle into the point gaining needling sensation and administering a certain stimulating way till reaching the analgesic affect and that the operation can be performed. The duration of the continuous time and characteristic of the point applied are related to the method of stimulation. In general, 15—30 minutes is proper. If the point punctured is on the nerve stem of the nerve branch, the continuous time of the inducing period can be somewhat shorter. If the point punctured is distal to the operation area, it can be longer. The continuous time of the inducing period of acupuncture stimulation by manipulative needling is generally longer than that of electroacupuncture stimulation.

internal wind 内风 [nèi fēng] The syndrome characterized by 'movement', 'changes' and 'abruptness', similating the wind. However, it results from disturbance of visceral functions inside the body, instead of being affected by pathogenic wind from the exterior.

internal cold 内寒 [nèi hán] The syndrome which resulted from the impairment of the visceral functions and weakness of yang *qi*. It is originated from the interior of the body, instead of a direct invasion by pathogenic wind from the exterior.

internal dampness 内湿 [nèi shī] The syndrome due to retention of water and moiture from disturbance of visceral functions.

internal dryness 内燥 [nèi zào] The dryness due to deficiency of body fluids and aqueous essence.

inferior cubital fossa 郄下 [xī xià] Referring to the area directly below Weizhong (BL 40).

internal moxibustioin 内灸 [nèi jiǔ] The therapeutic method by swallowing fresh garlic.

injury by wind 伤风 [shāng fēng] 1. Diseases due to the invasion of pathogenic wind. 2. Common cold, flu. According to traditional Chinese medicine common cold can be divided into three types, namely, commom cold of wind-cold type, common cold of wind-heat type and common cold of summer-dampness type. Prescription: 1. The wind-cold type: Lieque (LU 7), Yingxiang (LU 20), Zhizheng (SI 7), Fengmen (BL 12), Fengchi (GB 20), Hegu (LI 4); 2. The wind-heat type, Chize (LU 5), Yuji (LU 10), Quchi (LI 11), Dazhui (GV 14), Waiguan (TE 5); 3. The summer-heat dampness type: Kongzui (LU 6), Hegu

(LI 4), Zhongwan (CV 12), Zusanli (ST 36), Zhigou (TE 6).

inner canthus 目内眦 [mù nèi zì] Referring to the inner corner of the eye.

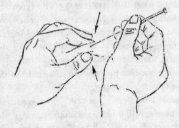

Fig 51

insertion of the needle by pinching the skin up 捏起进针 [niē qǐ jìn zhēn] One of needle insertions, also called *jia chi yia shou*. The two hands are in cooperation, then to pinch up the skin where the point is located with the thumb and the index finger of the left hand, and the right hand holds the needle and inserts it along the subcutaneous region. It suits the region where the skin and muscle are thin and superficial that can not be punctured deep. E. g., Dicang (ST 4) at the corner of mouth, Yingtang (EX-HN 3) between the two eyebrows. (Fig 51)

indications of *shu* points 孔穴主对 [kǒng xué zhǔ duì] Referring to the indications of the *shu* points.

index finger and 2nd toe 大指次指 [dà zhǐ cì zhǐ] In ancient times *zhi* (toe) and *zhi* (finger) were the same in meaning.

Internal Classic 内经 [nèi jīng] 1. A brief term for Yellow Emperor's Internal Classic; 2. the meridian internally running at the storing viscera, contrary to those running in the limbs.

irregular menstruation 月经不调 [yuè jīng bù tiáo] Referring to abnormalities in the cycle, amount, color and quality of the menstrual flow.

irregular pulse 涩脉 [sè mài] The pulse which is rirregular in rhythm, faint and slow, like scraping lightly with a knife. It usualy indicates deficiency of blood with impairment of yin or stagnation of *qi* and sludging of blood.

iron needle 铁针 [tiě zhēn] A acupuncture instrument, one of the nine needles in ancient China, also called *jian zhen* in latter generations.

J

Jade Key to the Secluded Chamber 重楼玉钥 [chóng lóu yù yào] A medical book written by Zhen Meijian 2 volumes. The lst volume describes the anatomy, physiology and pathology of throat, then diagnosis and treatment of the laryngology, appended with Meijian's description of the symptoms, which is somewhat unique in viewing differential treatment of diphteria. The 2nd volume describes acupuncture treatment on laryngological diseases. It was published in 1838.

jade house 玉房 [yù fáng] The region where primordial principle is stored.

jaundice 黄疸 [huáng dǎn] The name of the disease in traditional Chinese medicine, clinically characterized by yellow-brown pigmentation of the skin and sclera and yellow colored urine. It may be classified into two types, yang jaundice and yin jaundice.

jiao 角 [jiǎo] 1. The corner of the forehead, referring to the node of the timple; 2. An abrreviation of *jiao fa* (cupping technique).

Jiaoxin (KI 8) 交信 [jiāo xìn] A point of Kidney Meridian of Foot-*shaoyin*, the gap-like point of Motility Vessel of Yin. Location: 3 cm below Sanyinjiao (BL 22), about 1.5 cm anterior to Fuliu (KI 7), 6 cm above the tip of the medial ankle, at the medial side of the leg. Regional anatomy: At the posterior tibia and the long flexor muscle of toe. There is the tibial artery and vein in the deeper stratum. The medial cutaneous nerve of leg is distributed. The tibial nerve is in the deeper. Puncture: 3—4 cm perpencularly. Moxibustion: 3—5 moxa cones or 5—10 minutes with warming moxibustion.

ji **sitting position** 箕坐位 [jī zhuò wèi] A kind of body position. See body position.

Jiagen 甲根 [jiǎ gēn] An extra point located at the root of the inner and outer corners of the thumbnail, 4 in total.

Jiaochong 交冲 [jiāo chōng] An alternate term for Houding (GV 19).

Jiaji points 夹脊 [jiá jí] Orginally it refers to the meridian points bilateral to the spine. Later it was taken as the name of the extra point located 1.5 cm bilateral to and from the various inferior spinal processes from the 1st thoracic vertebra to the 5th lumbar vertebra. For their application refer back-*shu* point.

Jianwaishu (SI 14) 肩外俞 [jiān wài shū] A point of Small Intestine Meridian of Hand-*taiyang*. Location: 9 cm lateral to Taodao (GV, DU 13) below the spinal process of the 1st thoracic vertebra. Regional anatomy: At the trapezius muscle and the ramboid muscle. There is the transverse cervical artery and vein. The medial cutaneous branch and the accessary nerve of the posterior branch of the lst and 2nd thoracic nerves are distributed. The dorsal nerve of scapula is in the deeper. Indications: Soreness and pain in the shoulder and back, stiff neck, cold and pain in the upper limbs. Puncture: 1.5—2.5 cm obliquely. Moxibustion: 3—5 moxa cones or 5—10 minutes with warming moxibustion.

Jianshi (PC 5) 间使 [jiān shǐ] A point of Percardium Meridian of Hand-*jueyin*, the river-like (metal) point of the meridian. Location: At the palmar side of the forearm, 9 cm above the transverse crease of wrist, between the long palmar muscle and the radial flexor muscle of wrist. Select it by making the hand supine. Regional anatomy: Reaching at the superficial digital muscle and the deep digital muscle. There is the central artery and vein of the forearm. The palmar interosseous artery and vein of the forearm in the deeper. The medial cutaneous nerve of forearm, the lateral cutaneous nerve of forearm, and the palmar cutaneous branch of the central nerve are distributed. The palmar interosseous nerve of the forearm is in the deeper. Indications: Palpitation, cardialgia, stomachache, malaria, mania, epilepsy, anxiety, vomiting, febrile diseases, swollen axilla, spasmodic elbows, pain in the arm. Puncture: 1.5—3 cm perpendicularly. Moxibustion: 3—5 moxa cones or 5—10 minutes with warming moxibustion.

Jiangu 间谷 [jiān gǔ] An alternate term for Erjian (LI 2).

Jianchen 剑巨 [jiàn jù] An extra point located at the flexor side of the forearm; 10 cm above the transverse crease of the wrist, between the long palmar muscle and the radial flexor muscle of wrist. Indication: lymphadenilitis, scrofulosa in the neck and axilla. Puncture: 1.5—3 cm perpendicularly. Moxibuston: 3—5 moxa cones or 5—10 minutes with warm moxibustion.

jia 胛 [jiǎ] The scapular region.

jiangu 楗骨 [jiàn gǔ] Referring to tibia.

Jianneishu 肩内俞 [jiān nèi shū] An extra point located 3 cm directly below Jianyu (LI 15) of the midpoint of the line connecting Jianyu (LI 15) and Yunmen (LU 2). Indications: Pains in the shoulder and arm. Puncture: 1.5—3 cm perpendicularly. Moxibustion: 3—5 moxa cones or 5—10 minutes with warming moxibustion. (Fig 52)

Jiafeng 胛缝 [jiǎ fèng] An extra point located at the back, the upper and lower ends of the medial edge of the scapular bone, 4 in total. There are the posterior banches of the cervical transverse artery and of the intercostal artery, and the posterior branches of the dorsal scapular nerve of the pectoral nerve. Indications: Scapular neuralgia, scapular rheumatism. Puncture: 3 cm outward and horizontally. Moxibustion: 3—5 moxa cones or 5—10 minutes with warming moxibustion.

Jiache (ST 6) 颊车 [jiá chē] A point of Stomach Meridian of Foot-*yangming*, also

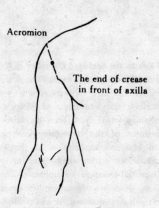

Acromion

The end of crease in front of axilla

Fig 52

termed Quya, Jiguan. Location: In the depression one finger-width anterosuperior to the corner of the mandible. At the protruding part of the masseter when the teeth is clenched. Regional anantomy: There is the masseter artery and vein. The greater aural nerve, the facial nerve and the masseter nerve are distributed. The masseter is below. Indications: Deviated mouth and eyes, toothache, swollen cheek, closejaw, stiffness and pain in the neck, aphonia. Puncture: 1—1.5 cm perpendicularly or 1.5—3 cm horizontally. Moxibustion: 5—10 minutes with warming moxibustion.

Jiaoyi 交仪 [jiāo yí] An alternate term for Ligou (LR 5).

Jixie 季胁 [jì xié] Also called *jilei*, referring to the lowerest ribs, i. e., the 11th and 12th ribs.

Jiaosun (TE 20) 角孙 [jiǎo sūn] A point of Triple Energizer Meridian of Hand-*shaoyang*, the confluence of *shaoyang* meridians of hand and foot and hand-*yangming* miridian. Location: In the hairline above the tip of ear when the auricle is folded. Reginal anatomy: At the temporal muscle. There are the branches of the superficial temporal artery and vein. The auriculotemporal nerve is distributed. Indications: Congestioin and swelling of the ocular region, congestive, swollen and painful eyes, nebula, toothache, dry lips, stiff neck, headache. Puncture: 1—1. 5 cm horizontally. Moxibustion: 1—3 moxa cones or 3—5 minutes with warming moxibustion.

Jinbi 颈臂 [jǐn bì] An extra point, located 3 cm abovre the crossing point of the medial 1/3 and lateral 1/3 of the clavicular bone at the posterior edge of the clavicular bone of sternocleidomastoidous muscle. The anterior branch of the supraclavicular nerve and the brachial plexus pass through locally. Indications: Numbness of the upper limb, paralysis, rheumatoid pain in the shoulder and arm. Puncture: 1. 5—3 cm perpendicuarly along the horizontal level. Do not puncture downward lest the tip of lung should be injured. (Fig 53)

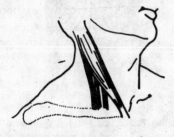

Fig 53

Jiali Point 颊里穴 [jiá lǐ xué] An extra point. located above the medial membrane of the medial cheek of the mouth, 3 cm at the level with the corner of mouth. Indications: Jaundice, pestilence, ulceration of gums. Puncture: 0. 3—0. 6 cm obliquely or to cause little bleeding with a triangular needle. (Fig 54)

jinger-interposing moxibustion 隔姜灸 [gé jiāng jiǔ] A kind of indirect moxibustion. To do moxibustion on the point interposed by a piece of jinger by moxa cone. The jinger is about 0. 3 cm in thickness and penetrated with holes by the small needle. If the patient feels scorching pain, the jinger

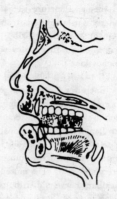

Fig 54

can be lifted for a while, then change it with another piece to continue moxibustion. In general, 3—5 moxa cones are used. Usually for treating epigastric pain, diarrhea due to cold affection, rheumatic cold blockage, etc. (Fig 55)

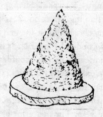

Fig 55

Jinhui 筋会 [jīn huì] One of eight confleuntial points.

Jinsu 筋束 [jīn sù] I. e., Jinsu (GV8).

jimao 聚毛 [jù máo] See *cong mao.*

Jianli (VC 11) 建里 [jiàn lǐ] A CV point. Location: At the abdominal midline, 9 cm above the umbilicus. Regional anatomy: At the white abdominal line. There is the banches of the superior and inferior epigastric artery and vein. The anterior cutaneous branch of the 8th intercostal nerve is distributed. Indications: Eipastric pain, distension of abdomon, vomiting, anoxexia, pain in the intestine, edema. Puncture: 3—4.5 cm perpendicularly. (It is cautious to be used for the pregnant woman.) Moxibustion: 3—7 moxa cones or 5—15 minutes with warming moxibustion.

Jianliao (TE 14) 肩髎 [jiān liáo] A point of Triple Energizer Meridian of Hand-*shaoyang*. Location: Posteroinferior to the acromion in the depression about 3 cm posterior to Jianyu (LI 15). Regional anatomy: At the deltoid muscle. There is the muscular branch of the posterior humeral circumflex artery and vein. The muscular branch of the axillary nerve is distributed. Indications: Heaviness of the shoulder, pain in the arm. Puncture: 3—4.5 perpendicularly. Moxibustion: 3—7 moxa cones or 5—15 minutes with warm needling.

Jianyu (LI 15) 肩髃 [jiān yú] A point of Large Intestine Meridian of Hand-*yangming*, the confluence of hand-*yangming* meridian and Motility Vessel of *Yang*, also termed Jianjing, Shangu, Pianjian, Shanggu, Piangu, Jianjian, Jianjing. Location: At the suprior deltoid muscle, between the end of aromion and the big node of humerus. It is in the depression anterior to the shoulder when the upper arm extends to the level position. Regional anatomy: On the deltoid muscle. There is the posterior humeral circumflex artery and vein. The posterior branch of the supraclavicular nerve and the axilary nerve is distributed. Indications: Pain in the shoulder and back, hemiplegia, spasm of the arms, feverish sensation in the shoulder, hemiplegia, urticaria due to wind-heat, scrofula. Puncture: 2.5—4.5 cm perpendicularly. Moxibustion: 3—5 moxa cones or 5—10 minutes with warming moxibustion.

Jinchong 颈冲 [jǐn chōng] An alternate term for Binao (LI 14).

Jin Zhitian 金治田 [jīn zhì tián] An acupuncutre expert in Qing Dynasty (1644—1911). He had a very deep study on moxibustion techniques. Inherited from Lei Shaoyi he wrote Secret Inheritage of Moxibustion Techniques.

Jin jing 金津 [Jīn jīng] See Jinjinyuye.

Jinjing-yuye 金津玉液 [Jīn jīn yù yè] An extra point. Jinjin (left) and Yuye (right) are located below the tongue proper on the vein bilateral to the frenulem of tongue. Select them by rolling the tongue. The glossal nerve and the hypoglossal nerve are at the local place. Indications: Heaviness, swelling and pain in the tongue, sore throat, aphasia, vomiting, diarrhea, jaundice, waisting-thirst disease. Prick to cause little bleeding with a triangular needle. (Fig 56)

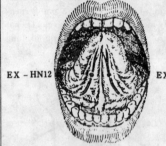

EX — HN12   EX — HN13

Fig 56

Jingling 精灵 [jīng líng] A point used for massage. Located at the dorsal hand, at the posterior edge of the interspace between the 4th and 5th metacarpal bones, in the depression at the midpoint of the line connecting the dorsal transverse crease of wrist and the small head of the metarcapal bone. Profuse sputum, hesitated qi and *qi* attack can be treated by pinching it. In modern times, it can be punctured.

Jinggong 精宫 [jīng gōng] 1. An alternate term for Zhishi (BL 52); 2. An alternate term for Mingmen (GV 4).

Jing lou 精露 [jīng lù] An alternate term for Shimen (CV 5).

***jiang*-interposing moxibustion** 隔酱灸 [gé jiàng jiǔ] A kind of indirect moxibustion. Used for treating prolapse of anus.

(*'jiang'* is a thick sauce made from soy beans, etc.)

Jianliao 肩聊 [jiān liáo] I. e., Jianliao (TE 14).

Jianjie 肩解 [jiān liě] 1. Referring to the scapular joint; 2. Referring to the upper portion of the spine of scapula.

Jianzhongshu (SI 15) 肩中俞 [jiān zhōng shū] A point of Small Intestine Meridian of Hand-*taiyang*. Location: 6 cm below Dazhui (GV 14) below the spinal process of the 7th cervial vertebra. Regional anatomy: At the trapezius muscle and the levator muscle of scapula. There is the transverse cervical artery and vein. The medial cutaneous branch and the accessary nerve of the posterior branch of the 1st and 2nd thoracic nerve are distributed. The dorsal nerve of scapula is in the deeper. Indications: Cough, asthmatic breast, pains in the shoulder and back, hemoptysis, chills and fever, blurred vision. Puncture: 1.5—2.5 cm obliquely. Moxibustion: 3—5 moxa cones or 5—10 minutes with warming moxibustion.

Jingmen (GB 25) 京门 [jīng mén] A point of Gallbladder Meridian of Foot-*shaoyang*, the anterior referred point of the kidney, also termed Qifu, Qishu. Location: At the lateral waist, approx. below the free end of the 12th rib. Regional anatomy: There is the external oblique muscle of abdomen, the transverse muscle of abdomen, and the 11th intercostal artery and vein. The 11th intercostal nerve is distributed. Indications: Borborygmus, diarrhea, abdominal distension, pains in the waist and hypochondrium. Puncture: 1.5—3 cm perpendicularly. Moxibustion with 3—5 moxa cones or 5—10 minutes with warming moxihustion.

Jinggu (BL 64) 京骨 [jīng gǔ] 1. A point of Bladder Meridian of Foot-*taiyang*, the source point of the meridian. Location: At the lateral edge of foot, below the protruding part of the tuberosity of the metatarsal bone, at the dorso-planter boundary. Regional anatomy: Below the abductor muucle

of the small toe. There is the lateral artery and vein of sole. The lateral cutaneous nerve of the dorsal foot is distributed. The lateral nerve of sole is in the deeper. Indications: Epilepsy, headache, nebula, stiff neck, pains in the waist and eyes, pain in the knee, spasm of feet. Puncture: 1—1.5 cm perpendicularly. Moxibustion: 3—5 moxa cones or 5—10 minutes with warming moxihustion; 2. Referring to the big bone protruding at the lateral side foot, i. e., the tuberosity of the 5th metatarsal bone.

Jiantou 肩头 [jiān tóu] An extra point, located in the depression of the scapular supraclavicular joint. I. e., mediosuperior to Jianyu (LI 15).

Jiulao 灸痨 [jiǔ láo] An extra point, located at the tip of the 3rd thoracic vertebra. Indications: Comsumptive disease with night sweat, cough, spitting suppurative blood, yellow face and emaciation, mental fatigue. Moxibustion: 3—7 moxa cones or 5—15 minutes with warming moxibustion.

Jiudianfeng 灸癫风 [jiǔ diàn fēng] An extra point. Located at the palmar side of the middle finger, slightly anterior to the midpoint at the transverse crease of the distal finger segment.

Jiuxiao 灸哮 [jiǔ xiào] An extra point, located at the back. Wind the neck with a rope and let it fall down to the tip of the xiphoid process of stern, and then turn it round to the back and make the midpoint of it be at the level with Adam's Apple. The place where the end of it touching the spine is the point. Indications: Asthma, cough, bronchitis. Moxibustion: 3—7 moxa cones or 5—15 minutes with warming moxibustion. (Fig 57)

Jianjing (GB 21) 肩井 [jiān jǐng] 1. A point of Gallbladder Meridian of Hand-*shaoyang*, the confluence of hand-*shaoyang* meridian and Connecting Vessel of Yang, also termed Bojing. Location: Above the spine of scapula, at the midpoint of the line connecting Dazhui (GV 14) and the acromion. Regional anatomy: Between the trapezius muscle, the levator muscle of scapula, and the supraspinal muscle. There is the cervical transverse artery and vein. The posterior branch of the suprascapular nerve and the accessary nerve are distributed. Indica-

tions: Pains in the shoulder and back, inability to raise the hand. Indications: Tinea, toothache, pains in the shoulder and back. Puncture: 1.5—3 cm perpendicularly. Moxibustion: 3—7 moxa cones or 5—15 minutes with warming moxibustion.

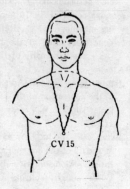 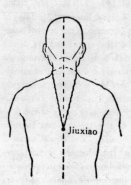

CV 15

Jiuxiao

Fig 57

Jianzhugu 肩柱骨 [jiān zhù gǔ] An extra point. Located at the highest point of the acromion of the scapula. Indications: Scrofula, pain in the shoulder and arm, inability of the hand to raise, toothache. Moxibustion: 3—7 moxa cones or 5—15 minutes with warming moxibustion.

Jianshu 肩俞 [jiān shū] An extra point, located at the midpoint of the line connecting Jianyu (LI 15) and Yuanmen (LU 2). Indications: Pains in the shoulder and arm. Puncture: 1.5—3 cm perpendicularly. Moxibustion: 3—5 moxa cones or 5—10 minutes with warming moxibustion.

Jingming 精明 [jīng míng] I.e., Jingming (BL 1).

Jingling-Weiling 精灵、威灵 [jīng líng wēi líng] A point used for massage, located at the dorsal hand, at the posterior edge of the interspace between the 4th and 5th and the 2nd and 3rd netarcarpal bones in the depression at the midpoint of the line connecting the transverse crease of the dorsal

wrist and the small head of the metacarpal bone. The anterior one is Jingling and the posterior, Weiling. To pinch and shake it to treat sudden death, first aid of sudden death, phlematic asthma and hasty breath. In modern times it can be punctured to treat headache, vertigo, tinnitus, convulsion, congestion and swelling of the dorsal hand, lumbar pain, inflamation of the wrist joint.

Jiexi (**ST 41**) 解溪 [jiě xī] A point of Stomach Meridian of Foot-*yangming*, the river-like (fire) point of the meridian. Location: At the centre of the transverse crease of the dorsal foot and ankle joint, between the long extensor muscle of thumb and the long extensor muscle of toe. Regional anatomy: Between the long extensor muscle of thumb and the extensor muscle of toe. There is the tibial anterior artery and vein. The fibular superficial and deep fibular nerves are distributed. Indications: Swelling in the head and face, flushed face, congestive eyes, headache, vertigo, abdominal distension, constipation, atrophy of the lower limbs, mania, feverish sensation in the stomach and abdomen. Puncture: 1.5—2.5 cm perpendicularly. Moxibustion: 3—5 minutes with warming moxibustion.

jilei 季肋 [jì lèi] The lateral thoracic region corresponding to that of the 11th and 12th costal cartilleges.

Jingzhong 睛中 [jīng zhōng] An extra point.

Jianzhen (SI 9) 肩贞 [jiān zhēn] A point of Small Intestine Meridian of Hand-*taiyang*. Location: 3 cm directly above the plica of the posterior axilla. Select it when the shoulder is put down and artery of scapula. The posterior cutaneous nerve of arm and the branch of the axillary nerve are distributed. The needle passes through the posterior fibre of the deltoid muscle to reach the quadrilateral foramen. Indications: pain in the scapular region, pain and numbness of the arms, supraclavicular pain, scrofula, tinnitus, deafness, toothache, scrofula, chills and fever. Puncture: 3—4.5 cm perpendicularly. Moxibustion: 3—7 moxa cones or 5—15 minutes with warming moxihustion.

Jianjian 肩尖 [jiān jiān] 1. An alternate term for Jainyu (LI 15); 2. An extra point.

Jinsuo (GV 8) 筋缩 [jīn suǒ] A GV point. Location: At the midline of the back, between the spinal processes of the 9th and 10 thoracic vertebrae. Regional anatomy: There is the posterior branch of the 9th intercostal space. The medial branch of the posterior branch of the 9th thoraic nerve is distributed. The spinal cord is in the deeper. Indications: Mania, contricture, stiff spine, pain in the back, stomachche, jaundice, looseness of the four limbs, contricture and spasm of the tendons. Puncture: 1.5—3 cm obliquely. Moxibustion: 3—5 moxa cones or 5—10 minutes with warming moxibustion.

Jielue 截疟 [jié luè] An extra point, located 12 cm directly below the nipple. Indica-

tions: Malaria, pains in the chest and hypochondrium. Moxibustion: 3—5 moxa cones or 5—10 minutes with warming moxibustion.

jiquan 极泉 [jí quán] An extra point, on the centre of the tongue surface. There is the lingual artery, the 2nd branch of the triangular nerve, the sublinqual nerve and the tympanic cord of the facial nerve locally. Indications: Asthma, cough, emaciationthirst disease, stiff tongue, paralysis of the lingual muscle. While puncturing it, tract the tongue outward with gauz. Puncture: 0.3—0.6 cm perpendicularly or prick to cause little bleeding with a triangular needle. (Fig 58)

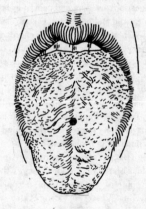

Fig 58

Jimen (SP 11) 箕门 [jī mén] A point of Spleen Meridian of Foot-*taiyin*. Location: At the medial side of thigh, 1.8 dm directly above Xuehai (SP 10). Regional anatomy: At the sartorius muscle. There is the greater proper vein. There is the femoral artery and vein at the lateral side in the deeper. The anterior cutaneous nerve of thigh is distributed. The proper nerve is in the deeper. Indications: Anuria, dribbling of urine or uroschesis, distension and pain in the groove. Puncture: 3—4.5 cm perpendicularly. Moxibustion: 5—10 minutes with moxa stick.

Jingming （**BL 1**）睛明 ［jīng míng］ A point
of Bladder Mieridian of Foot -*taiyang*, the
confluence of hand-*taiyang*, foot-*taiyang*
and foot-*yangming* meridians, also termed
Leikong. Location: At the infraorbital
edge, 0. 3 cm lateral to the inner canthus.
Regional antomy: Passing through the medial palpebral ligament, reaching at the internal straight muscle of eye. There is the
angular artery and vein. At the upper part
of the deep stratum. There is the basic stem
of the ocular artery and vein. The supra-
trochear and the infratrochear nerves are
distributed. The oculomotor nerve and the
ocular nerve are in the deeper. Indications:
Congestion, swelling and pain of eyes, aversion to cold and headache, vertigo, lacrimation, itch of the inner canthi, encroachment
of pterygium to the cornea, nebula, blurred
vision, myopia, night blindness, color blindness. Puncture: Advise the patient to close
his or her eyes. The doctor slightly pushes
the patient's bulbar eyeball outwardly and
then fixes it. Puncture 1. 5—3 cm perpendicularly along the edge of the orbital edge.
Moxibustion is prohibited.

Jinmen （**BL 63**）金门 ［jīn mén］ A point of
Bladder Meridian of Foot-*taiyang*, the gap-
like point of the meridian, pertaining to
Conecting Vessel of Yang, also termed
Guanliang. Location: Anteroinferior to the
anterolateral ankle, in the depression lateral
to the cuboid bone. Regional anatomy:
There is the short fibular muscle, the abductor muscle of the small toe, and the lateral artery and vein of the sole. The lateral
cutaneous nerve of the doral foot is distributed. The lateral cutaneous nerve of the
dorsal foot is in the deeper. Indications:
Epilepsy, infantile canvulsion, lumbago,
pain in the lateral ankle, pain in the lower
limbs. Puncture: 1—1. 5 cm perdicularly.
Moxibustion: 3—5 moxa cones or 5—10
minutes with warm needling; 2. Referring
to Huiyin(CV 1); 3. An extra point located

at the flexor side of the forearm, 9—15 cm
above the transverse crease of wrist, between the long palmar muscle and the radial flexor muscle of wrist, proximal to Jianshi
(PC 5). Indication: Scrofula. Puncture:
1. 5—3 cm perpendicularly. Moxibustion:
3—5 moxa cones or 5—10 minutes with
warm needling.

jiegu 接骨 ［jiē gǔ］ I. e., 接脊. Located in
the depression below the 12th vertebra.

Jingqu（**LU 8**）经渠 ［jīng qú］A point of Lung
Meridian of Hand-*taiyin*, the stream-like
(metal) point of the meridian. Location: on
the palmer side of forearm, 3 cm above the
transverse crease of wrist, at the pulsation
of the radial artery. Regional anatomy: Between the radial muscle of arm and the radial flexor muscle of wrist. There is the radial artery and vein. The lateral cutaneous
branch of the forearm and the radial superficial branch of the radial nerve are distributed. Indications: Cough, asthmatic
breath, sore throat, distension and fullness
in the chest, pains in the chest and back,
feverish sensation in the palms. Puncture:
1—1. 5 cm perpendieularly (avoiding the
artery). Moxibustion: 3—5 minutes with
warming moxibustion.

Jingzhong 经中 ［jīng zhōng］ An extra point,
located 9 cm lateral to Qihai (CV 6). Indications: Obstruction of defecation and micturition, leukorrhea, irregular menstruation, diarrhea. Puncture: 3—4 cm perpendicularly. Moxibustion: 3—5 moxa cones or
5—15 minutes with warm needling.

Jingmensihua 经门四花［jīng mén sì huā］An
extra point. See Sihua.

Jizhong （**GV 6**）脊中 ［jǐ zhōng］A GV point,
also termed Shenzong, Jishu. Location: At
the midline of the back, between the spinal
processes of the 11th and 12th thoracic vertebrae. Regional anatomy: There is the posterior branch of the 11th intercostal artery.
The medial branch of the posterior branch
of the 11th thoracic nerve is distributed.
The needle passes through the myofascia of

the waist and the back and reaches at the superior spinal ligament and the interspinal ligament. The spinal cord is in the deeper. Indication: Stiffness and pain in the waist, jaundice, diarrhea, dysentery, hemorrhoids, hematuria, prolapse of anus, epilpsy. Puncture: 1.5—3 cm obliquely. Moxibustion: 3—5 moxa cones or 5—10 minutes with warming moxibustion.

Jineishu 脊内俞 [jǐ nèi shū] An alternate term for Zhonglushu (BL 29).

Jisan qoints 脊三穴 [jǐ sān xué] An extra point, located at the posterior midline. One is located 3 cm below Yamen (GV 15), the other two are located below the spinal process of the 5th lumbar vertebra (Taodao) and in the depression below the 5th lumbar vertebra, three in total. Indications: Covulsive disease, pains in the waist and back, inflammation of the membrane of the spinal cord. Puncture: 1.4—3 cm obliquely. Moxibustion: 3—5 moxa cones or 5—15 minutes with warming moxibustion. (Fig 59)

Jibeiwu points 脊背五穴 [jǐ bèi wǔ xué] The 1st one is located at the highest point of the spinal process of the 2nd thoracic vertebra; the 2nd is located at the end of coccyx; the third one is located at the spinal bone on wich the midpoint of the line connecting the first two points is located. Then make an equilateral triangle with 1/2 of the connecting line folded as the three sides, with the base side at the level, the upper angle is at the middle point and the lower two angles are the last two points, 5 in total. Indications: Insanity, epilepsy. Moxibustion: 3—5 moxa cones for each point. (Fig 60)

Jingshi 经始 [jīng shǐ] An alternate term for Shaochong (HT 9).

Jieji 接脊 [jiē jǐ] An extra point, located at the posterior midline, in the depression below the spinal process of the 2nd thoracic vertebra. Indications: Indigestion, pains in the back spine, lumbago, enteritis, epilepsy. Puncture: 1.5—3 cm upwardly and obliquely. Moxibustion: 3—5 moxa cones or

5—10 minutes with warming moxibustion.

Jiquan (HT 1) 极泉 [jí quán] A point of Heart Meridian of Hand-*shaoyin*. Location: In the center of the axilla at the axillary artery. Select it with the arm raised and the axilla unfolded. Regional anatomy: There is the axillary artery at the lateral side. The ulnar nerve, central nerve and medial cutaneous nerve of arm are distributed. Indications: Cardialgia, depressed chest, palpitation, short breath, dry vomiting, pains in the hypochondrium and intercostal region, dry throat, anxiety and thirst, yellow eyes, scrofula, cold and pain in the elbow and arm, inability of the lower limbs to raise. Puncture: 1.5—3 cm perpendicularly upwardly to the axillary fossa. Moxibustion: 1—3 moxa cones or 3—5 minutes with moxibustion.

Jijupikuai point 积聚 (痞块穴) [jī jù pǐ kuài xué] An extra point located 12 cm lateral to the inferior of the spinal process of the 2nd lumbar vertebra. Indications: Accumulation and mass, stomachache, borborygmus, indigestion, amenorrhea, nocturnal emission. Puncture: 1.5—3 cm perpendicularly. Moxibustion: 3—5 moxa cones or 5—15 minutes with warming moxibustion.

Jimai (LR 12) 急脉 [jí mài] A point of Liver Meridian of Foot-*jueyin*. Location: 7.5 cm lateral to the midpoint of the inferior edge of symphysis pubis at the medial side of thigh. Regional anatomy: The public muscle is in below. There are the branches of the lateral cartery and vein in the public region and the public branch of the inferior epigastric artery and vein. There is the femoral vein externally. The ilioinguinal nerve is distributed. The anterior branch of the obductor nerve is in the deeper. Indications: Hernia, prolapse of uterus, pain in the penis, pain in the bilateral lower abdomen, pain in the medial aspect of thigh. Punctrue: 1.5—2 cm perpendicularly. Moxibustion: 3—5 moxa cones or 5—10 minutes with warming moxibustion.

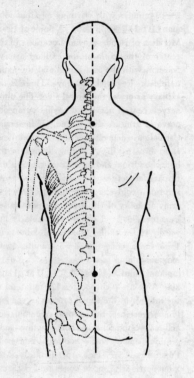

Fig 59

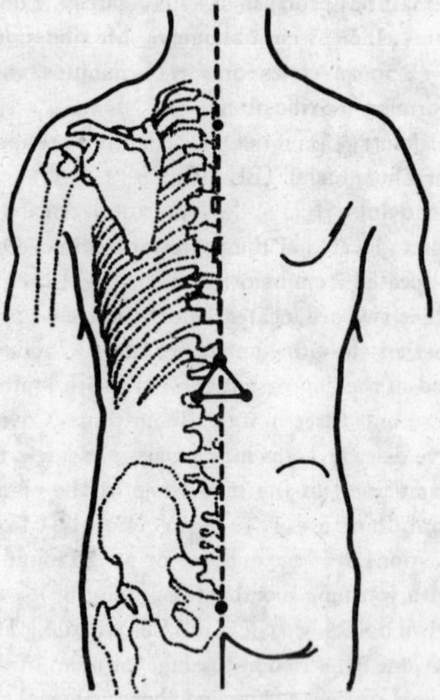

Fig 60

Jigujiezhong 脊骨解中 [jǐ gǔ jiě zhōng] An extra point located at the posterior midline on the spinal bone at the elevel with the nipple. Indication: Cough. Moxibustion: 3—5 moxa cones or 5—10 minutes with warming moxibustion.

Jishu 脊俞 [jǐ shū] An alternate term for Jizhong (GV 6).

Jiliangzhongyang 脊梁中央 [jǐ liáng zhōng yāng] An extra point, same with the extra point Duji in location.

Jipang 脊旁 [jǐ páng] I. e., Jiaji Point.

Jiuwei (CV 15) 鸠尾 [jiū wěi] 1. A meridian point, the connecting point of the vessel, the point of *gao*, also termed Weiyi. Location: Below the xiphoid process of the abdominal midline, 21 cm above the umbili-

cus. Reginal anatomy: At the starting area of the straight muscle of abdomen. There is the supperior epigastric artery and vein. The anterior cutaneous branch of the 7th intercostal nerve is distributed. Indications: cardialgia, palpitation, anxiety, epilepsy, mania, fullness and pain in the chest, cough and asthmatic breath, vomiting, hiccup, regurgitation, stomachache. Puncture: 1—1. 5 cm obliquely downwardly. (It is not advisable to puncture deep.) Moxibustion: 3—5 moxa cones or 5—10 minutes with warming moxibustion; 2. The xiphoid process of stern.

Jiuweiguduan 鸠尾骨端 [jiū wěi gǔ duān] An extra point. It is located at the lower edge of the xiphoid process of stern. Indication:

infantile sunken fontanell by puncturing it 1.5 cm.

Jiuxuebing 灸血病〔jiǔ xuě bìng〕An extra point located at the highest spot of the 3rd sacral spinal process of the 3rd sacral vertebra. Indicatioins: Spitting blood, expistaxis, hemafecia, metrorrhagia and other hemorrhagic symptoms. Moxibustion: 5—7 moxa cones or 10—15 minutes with warming moxibustion.

Jiuchitong 灸齿痛〔jiǔ chǐ tòng〕I. e. , Fengchitong.

Jiuliao 九窌〔jiǔ liào〕According to Yang Shangshan's Notes, it refers to Baliao plus Yaoshu. In Plain Questions, it was regarded as Baliao.

Jiuqu 九曲〔jiǔ qū〕A Brief term for *Jiuquzhongfu*.

Jiuquzhongfu 九曲中府〔jiǔ qū zhōng fǔ〕An extra point, located 9 cm below Zhushi Located directly below the middle axilla 9 cm below the 7th intercostal place. Indications: Pleuritis, disorders of the stomach, spleen and liver. Puncture: 1.5 cm obliquely. Moxibustion: 3—5 moxa cones or 5 minutes with warming moxibustion.

join points 合穴〔hé xué〕One of the five *shu* points, located near the elbow and knees. According to Difficult Classic, they are mainly suitable for treating disorders of six emptying viscera, of which those of six emptying viscera are the main. At the lower limbs, the large and small intestines and triple energizer have a joining poin each. With those of the stomach, bladder and gallbladder, they are collectively called the joining points of six emptying viscera.

joint puncture 关刺〔guān cì〕One of the five needling techniques for treating painful tendons. To directly puncture the muscles and ligments around the joints of the four limbs but to avoid hemorrhage. It is an ancient way to treat hepatic diseases.

Juchu 巨处〔jù chù〕I. e. , Wuchu (BL 5).

Juyang 巨阳〔jù yáng〕1. An alternate term for *taiyang* meridian; 2. Referring to Shenmai (BL 62).

Jugu (LI 16) 巨骨〔jù gú〕1. A point of Large Intestine Meridian of Hand-*yangming*, the confluence of hand-*yangming* meridian and Motility Vessel of Yang. Location: In the depression between the end of the clavicular acromion and the spine of scapula at the scapular region. Regional anatomy: Passing through trapezius and spinator muscles. There are the supraclavicular artery and vein. The postrerior branch of the supraclavicular nerve and the branch of the accesssary nerve are distributed. The supraclavicular nerve is in the deeepr. Indications: Pains in the shoulder and arm, epilepsy induced by terror, spitting blood, scrofula, lymphatic tuberculosis, goiter, inflammation of supraclavicular muscle, disorder of the shoulder and joint and its surrounding soft tissues; 2. *Jugu*, the clavicular bone.

Jueren point 绝孕穴〔jué yùn xué〕An extra point, according to Presciptions for Universal Relief, "If a woman wants to stop delivering the baby, she would be accept moxibustion at the interspace between 6 cm and 3 cm interspace below the umbilicus. It is called Jueren in Introduction to Accupuncture Points.

Jujue 巨觉〔jù jué〕I. e. , Chengjue.

Juliao (GB 29) 居髎〔jū liáo〕A point of Gallbladder Meridian of Foot-*shaoyang*, the confluence of foot-*shaoyang* meridian and Motility Vessel of Yang. Location: In the depression at the midpoint of the line connecting the superior spinal process of the anterior ilium and the greater trochanter of thigh. Regional anatomy: In the middle gluteal muscle and the least gluteal muscle. There is the superficial iliac circumflex artery and vein. The branches of the cutanous nerve of the superior cutaneous nerve of hip and the superior gluteal nerve are distributed. Indications: Pain in the waist and legs, paralysis, atrophic feet, hernia. Puncture: 3—4.5 cm perpendicularly.

Moxibustion: 3—5 moxa cones or 5—10 minutes with warming moxibustion.

juegu 撅骨 [jué gǔ] 1. Referring to coccyx; 2. Referring to Changqiang (GV 1).

Juxuxialian 巨虚下廉[jù xū xià lián]I. e. , Xiajuxu (ST 39).

Juxushanglian 巨虚上廉 [jù xū shàng lián] I. e. , Shangjuxu (ST 37).

Jueyang 厥阳[jué yáng]1. An alternate term for Feiyang (GB 58); 2. The name of symptom.

jueyinshu (BL 14) 厥阴俞 [jué yīn shū] A point of Bladder Meridian of Foot-*taiyang*, the back *shu* point of the Pericardium, also termed Jueshu. Location: 4. 5 cm lateral to the spinal process between the 4th and 5th thoracic vertebrae. Regional anatomy: At the trapezius muscle and the rhomboid muscle. There is the medial cutaneous branch of the doral lateral branch of the posterior branch of the 4th thoracic nerve is distributed. The lateral branch of the posterior branch of the thoracic nerve is in the deeper. Indications: Cardialgia, palpitation, depressed chest, cough, vomiting. Puncture: 1. 5—2. 5 cm obliquely. (It is not advisable to puncture deep) Moxibustion: 3—5 moxa cones or 5—15 minutes with warming moxibustion.

Juliao (ST 3) 巨髎 [jù liáo] A point of Stomach Meridian of Foot-*yangming*, the confluence of Motility Vessel and foot-*yangming* meridian. Location: With the eyes look forward, directly below the pupil, at the level with the inferior edge of ana nasi. Regional anatomy: Deviated mouth and eyes, tremor of the eyelids, congestion and pain in the eyes, nebula, epistaxis, toothache, swelling lips and chest, nebula. Puncture: 1—2 cm obliquely. Moxibustion: 3—5 moxa cones with warming moxibustion.

Juxu 巨虚 [jù xū] Referring to Shangjuxu (ST 33) and Xiajuxu (ST 39). The depression between the tendon and bone on the lateral side of tibia of the leg can be called *juxu*.

Juliao 巨窌 [jù liáo] 1. Same with Juliao (GB 29); 2. The wrong form of Muchuang (GB 16), another name of Sizukong (TE 23).

Juqueshu 巨阙俞[jù què shū]An extra point, located between the spinal processes of the 4th and 5th thoracic vertebra, on the posterior midline. Indications: Cough, asthmatic breath, bronchitis, neurasthenia. Moxibustion: 3—7 moxa cones or 5—15 minutes with warming moxibustion.

Juque (CV 14) 巨阙 [jù què] A CV point, the anterior referred point of the heart. Location: 18 cm above the umbilicus, on the abdominal midline. Regional antomy: In the white abdominal line. There are the hypergastric artery and vein. The anterior cutaneous branch of the 7th intercostal nerve is distributed. Indications: Thoracalgia, cardialgia, anxiety, palpitation with fright, mania, epilepsy, amnesia, full chest and short breath, cough, distension and sudden pain in the abdomen, vomiting, hiccup, acid regurgitation, jaundice, diarrhea. Puncture: 1. 5—3 cm perpendicularly (It is not advisable to puncture deep). Moxibustion: 3—5 moxa cones or 5—10 minutes with warming moxibustion.

Jue gu 绝骨[jué gǔ]1. Referring to the upper part of the lateral ankle in the depression between the long and short muscles of calf; 2. An alternate term for Xuanzhong (GB 39); 3. An alternate term for Yangfu (GB 38).

Jue **syndrome** 厥证 [jué zhèng] Sudden fainting with unconsciousness, cold.

K

kao 尻 [kāo] Referring to the sacrum and coccyx.

kan 顑 [kǎn] Approx. at the two temporal regions.

Kaoshan 靠山 [kào shān] A point used for massage, located at the end of the radial side of the transverse crease of radius. To pinch and knead it locally can treat malaria and profuse sputum.

Keliao 颏髎 [kē liáo] An alternate term for Chengjiang (CV 24).

Keshou Point 咳嗽穴 [kè sòu xué] See ji gu jie zhong.

Kezhu 客主 [kè zhǔ] I. e., Kezhuren, an alternate term for Shangguan (GB 3).

Kezhuren 客主人 [kè zhǔ rén] I. e., Shangguan (GB 3).

Key to Administering Acupuncture in Rythm 行针指要歌 [xíng zhēn zhǐ yào gē] In this rhythmic article some points used for common syndromes and symptoms were enumerated, which was recorded in Compendium of Acupuncture. The whole article is as follow: "For wind trouble, first puncture Fengfu (GV, DU 16) and Baihui (GV, DU 20). For stasis trouble, puncture the point of large intestine to reduce water. For consumptive disease, puncture Gaohuang (BL 43) and Bailao. For asthenic disorder puncture Qihai (CV 6), Dantian and Weizhong (BL 40). For *qi* trouble, puncture Danzhong (CV 17) only. For cough, do moxibustion on Feishu (BL 13), Fengmen (BL 12). For phlegm, first puncture Zhongwan (CV, RN 12) and Sanli (ST 36). For vomiting, puncture Zhongwan (CV 12), Qihai (CV 6) and Danzhong (CV 17) by reinforcing manipulation. For regurgitation and vomiting up indigested food use common therapy. There are very few people who know the secret of acupuncture."

kidney, the motive force of *qi* 肾间动气 [shèn jiān dòng qì] The kidney is the primary motive force to produce yang *qi* of the body.

Kidney Meridian of Foot-*shaoyin* (KI) 足少阴肾经 [zú shào yīn shèn jīng] One of the twelve meridians. The course: It starts from the inferior aspect of the small toe, runs obliquely to the sole, emerges from the tuberosity (Rangu) of the navicular bone, runs behind the medial ankle. Its branch enters into the heel, ascends to the inner leg, emerges from the medial side of the cubital fossa, ascends to the posteromedial side of the thigh, passes through the spinal column, pertains to the kidneys, and connects with the bladder. The vertical one, ascends from the kidney and passes through the liver and diaphragm. One branch emerges from the lungs, along the throat, by the root of tongue. The other branch emerges from the lungs, connects with the heart, disappears in the chest. (connects with Pericardium Meridian of Hand-*jueyin*).

KI *points* 足少阴肾经穴 [zú shào jīn shèn jīng xué] They are Yongquan (KI 1) (well), Rangu (KI 2) (spring), Taixi (KI 3) (stream, source), Dazhong (KI 4) (connecting), Shqiquan (KI 5) (gap), Zhaohai (KI 6), Fuliu (KI 7) (river), Jiaoxin (KI 8), Zubin (KI 9), Yingu (KI 10), Henggu (KI 11), Dahe (KI 12), Qixue (KI 13), Siman (KI 14), Zhongzhu (KI 15), Huangshu (KI 16), Shangqu (KI 17), Shiguan (KI 18), Yinxi (KI 19), Tonggu (KI 20), Youmen (KI 21), Bulang (KI 22), Shenfeng (KI 23), Lingxu (KI 24), Shenzang (KI 25), Yuzhong (KI 26), Shufu (KI 27), 27 in total. The points where Kidney Meridian crosses other meridians are Snyinjiao (BL 22) (foot-*taiyin* meridian), Changqiang (GV 1), Guanyuan (CV 14)) and Zhongji (CV 3). There is also Shenshu (BL 23) pertaining to foot-*taiyang* meridian, the anterior referred point Jingmen (BL 1) pertaining to foot-*shaoyang* meridian.

KI diseases 足少阴肾经病 [zú shào yīn shèn jīng bìng]The chief diseases and symptoms are dull complexion, short breath, spitting blood, blurred vision, palpitation, jaundice, diarrhea, feverish sensation in mouth, dry tongue, sore throat, dryness and pain in the throat, pains in the lumbar spine and the medial thigh, atrophy, clammny cold, lethargy, feverish sensation in the sole.

kidney meridian of foot-*shaoyin* 肾足少阴之脉 [shèn zú shào yīn zhī mài] The original name of *zu shao yin shen jing.*

kidney aborbs gases 肾主纳气 [shèn zhǔ nà qì]In traditional Chinese medicine, the respiratory activity is considered not only related directly to the lungs but indirectly to the kidey. The kidney may receive and absorb gases from the lungs. Clinically weakness of the kidney may arouse dyspnea, and it should be treated with the technique of strengthening the kidney. This is tonifying the kidney to accept pulmonary gases.

kidney 肾 [shèn] One of the five storing viscera, located at the waist, related to storing of primordial principle, the foundation of the whole body, specially related to bone marrow, will and aqueous liquids. Kidney Meridian of Foot-*jueyin* pertains to kidneys, Bladderr Meridian of Foot-*taiyang* cnnects with the kidneys and is communicated with GV, Vital Vessel and CV. Its back *shu* point is Shenshu(BL 23)and anterior referred point is Jingmen (GB 25).

kidney stores the essence 肾藏精 [shèn cáng jīng] The kindey stores the congenital essence (the essence of reporduction) and the acquired essence (from the grain and liquid in the five storing and six emptying viscera).

kidney as the congenital foundation 肾为先天之本 [shèn wéi xiān tiān zhī běn]The kidney is the foundation for a human's growth

and development and reproducing the next generation.

kidney concerned with water metabolism 肾主水 [shèn zhǔ shuǐ] The kidney plays an extraordinarily important role in regulating water metabolism of the human body.

kidney is concerned with repro duction 肾主生殖 [shèn zhú shēng zhí] The kidney concerned with the production, storage and excretion of the spleen and pays an important role in the growth, development and reproduction of the body.

kidney has the ears as its opening 肾开窍于耳 [shèn kāi qiào yú ěr] Some of the physiopathologic conditions of the kindey may generally be reflected as the changes of auditory acuity.

kidney opens into two yin 肾开窍于二阴 [shèn kāi qiào yú ěr yīn] Some physiopathological conditions of the kindey may be reflected by the change of urination, ejaculation, and defecation. The two yin refers to the anterior yin, the orifice of urethra and spermatic duct, and the posterior one, the anus.

Knee 膝[xī]An ear point at the starting point of the upper foot of the antihelix, laterosuperior to sacrococcygeal vertebra.

Kongzui (LU 6) 孔最 [kǒng zuì] A point of Lung Meridian of Hand-*taiyin*, the gap-like point of the meridian. Location: 2. 1 dm to Taiyuan (LU 9) on the line connecting Taiyuan (LU 9) and Chize (LU 5), on the palmar side of the forearm. Regional anatomy: Passing through the radial muscle of arm to reach the interspace between the round pronator muscle and long and short radial extensor muscles of wrist. There is the cephalic vein and the radial artery and vein. The lateral cutaneous nerves of forearm and the superifical branch of te radial nerve are distributed. Indicatioins: Headache, febrile diseases with no sweat, cough, asthmatic breath, aphonia, swelling and sore throat, pains in the shoulder, elbow and arm, hemorrhoids. Puncture:

1. 5—3 cm perpendicularly. Moxibustion: 3—7 moxa cones or 5—15 minutes with warming moxibustion.

Kouheliao (LI 19) 口禾髎 [kǒu hé liáo] A point of Large Intestine Meridian of Hand-*yangming*, also termed Changping, Changliao, Changjia. Location: 1. 5 cm at the level with Shuigou (DU 26) directly below the lateral edge of the nostril. Regional anatomy: At the end of the quadric muscle of the upper lip. There are the superior labial branches of the facial artery and vein. The anastomotic branch of the facial nerve and the infraorbital nerve are distributed. Indications: Nasal polyp, deviated mouth, closjaw, stuffy nose, epistaxis. Puncture: 1. 2 cm perpendicularly or obliquely. Moxibustion: 3—5 moxa cones.

Kufang (ST 14) 库房 [kù fáng] A point of Stomach Meridian of Foot-*yangming*. Location: At the 1st intercostal space, 12 cm lateral to Huagai (CV 20) at the midline of the chest. Regional anatomy: At the greater pectoral muscle and the lesser pectoral muscle. There is the acromial artery and vein and the lateral pectoral artery and vein. The branch of anterior pectoral nerve is distributed. Indications: Cough, adverse flow of *qi*, coughing purulent blood, distension and pain in the chest and hypochondrium. Puncture: 1—1. 5 cm obliquely. Moxibustion: 3—5 moxa cones or 5—10 minutes with warming moxibustion.

L

lacking seasonal variations of the pulse 脉逆四时 [mài nì sì shí] When the body cannot adapt to seasonal weather changes and the pulse fails to follow, pathogenic manifestations would appear, for example, in spring the pulse should be wiry, but it is floating in summer the pulse should be full, but it is deep in autumn the pulse should be floating, but it is wiry, in winter the pulse should be deep, but it is full.

Large intestine 大肠 [dà cháng] An ear point at the upper edge of the crus of helix, opposite to Mouth.

large pulse 大脉 [dà mài] The large pulse that fills the finger tip. If it is large and forceful, it indicates the excess syndrome and heat syndrome. If it is large and weak, it indicates the deficiency syndrome.

Lama point 喇嘛穴 [lǎ má xué] An extra point, located at the scapular region, on the line connecting Tianzong (SI 11) and the end of the posterior axillary plica. Indication: Lanrygitis. Puncture: 1.5—3 cm perpendicularly.

large intestine meridian of hand-*yangming* 大肠手阳明之脉 [dà cháng shǒu yáng míng zhī mài] The original name of Large Intestine Meridian of Hand-*yangming*.

laser needling 光针 [guāng zhēn] I. e., laser point radiation technique.

lateral ocular connection 目外维 [mù wài wéi] The connective tissue at the lateral side of the eyeball.

Laoshang 老商 [lǎo shāng] One of three *shang*. See Sanshang.

lateral thigh 髀阳 [bì yáng] Referring to the lateral side of thigh.

Lanwei Point 阑尾穴 [lán wěi xué] An extra point, located anterolaterior to the leg, 3—6 cm directly below Zusanli (ST 36) at the place where tenderness is most obvious, at the anterior muscle of the tibia. There is

the lateral cutaneous gascnemius nerve. There is the deep gascnemius nerve and the antrior tibial artery and vein in the deeper. Indications: Acute/chronic appendicitis, acute/chronic entritis, numbness or paralysis of the lower limb, puffy leg. Puncture: 3—4 cm perpendicularly.

lacking water with blazing fire 水亏火旺 [shuǐ kuī huǒ wàng] 1. Here water refers to renal water (renal yin) while fire to cardiac fire. An insuffciency of renal water with induce cardiac fire to flare up, and symptoms such as anxiety and insomnia will occur; 2. Water refers to renal water (renal yin), fire, vital fire (renal yang). An insufficiency of renal water will lead to an axcess of vital sexual desire and spermatorrhea will appear.

Lanmen 阑门 [lán mén] 1. Referring to the joining place of the large and small intestines, one of the seven vital portals; 2. An extra points, located 9 cm bilateral to Qugu (CV 2). Indications: Hernia, swollen pubic region. Puncture: 1.5—3 cm perpendicularly. Moxibustion: 3—5 moxa cones or 5—10 minutes with warming moxibustion; 3. An extra point, 4.5 cm above the umbilicus, used for unobstructing *qi* in the upper and lower parts of the body.

labial puncture 唇针 [chún zhēn] Referring to the needling technique of puncturing shuigou (CV 26) and Chengjiang (CV 24) at the lip. It can be applied for acupuncture anesthesia.

lacrimation 迎风流泪 [yíng fēng liú lèi] A syndrome that can be divided into cold tear and warm tear. In general, cold tear is usually severe in winter, but if it is prolonged for many years, it is severe in all seasons. Warm tear is usually the accompanying symptom of cateract.

large needle 巨针 [jù zhēn] Originally referring to the large needle in nine needles. In modern times there appears the large needle made of stainless steel, its diameter being 0.5—1 mm, its length being 9 cm, 15 cm, 3.3 dm, etc., used for transverse puncture along the subcutaneous region and puncture of muscle for treating paralysis and muscular spasm.

lamp-fire moxibustion 灯火灸 [dēng huǒ jiǔ] A kind of moxibustion, also called *deng cao jiu*. To scorch the point with the ignited rush rinsed with plantoil (sesame oil). In general it is advisable to do moxibustion swiftly by making the rush transversely or obliquely appoint the point. The oil rinsed is proper in amount lest the scald should occur due to dripping of hot oil. When the rush scorches the point the sound, 'pa', may appear and the rush fire may immediately go out. This is called one '*jiao*'. In general for each point one *jiao* of moxibustion is used, the slight red area may appear at the local area. Keep it clean lest infection should result. According to Outline of Materia Medica it is used for infantile convulsion, coma, ache and distension of the head due to pathogenic wind. In clinic it is also used for treating mumps, hiccup, vomiting, infantile indigestion, dysfunctional bleeding of uterus, clammy cold of hand and foot, etc. In recent years, a match stick has been used instead of the rush.

Large Intestine Meridian of Hand-*Yangming* (LI) 手阳明大肠经 [shǒu yáng míng dà cháng jīng] One of the twelve meridians. The course: Starts from the end of the index finger, runs along the radial side of the index finger, emerges between the lst and 2nd metacarpal bones, enters into the interspace of the two tendons (the long extensor muscle and short extensor muscle of tyumb), then enters into the lateral aspect of the elbow along the forearm, runs over the frontal side of the lateral aspect of the upper arm, ascends to the shoulder, emerges from the anterior acromion, ascends

again to meet Dazhui (GV 14), passes through the diaphragm, disappears at the large intestine. One branch ascends from the supraclavicular fossa to the lateral neck, passes through the cheek, enters into the teeth, emerges to wind the mouth, crosses at Shuigou (GV 26)—the left one runs right and the right one runs left—ascends by the nostril (to connect with Stomach Meridian of Foot-*yangming*).

large intestine 大肠 [dà cháng] One of six emptying viscera. Its actioin is to transport the residue of digested food. Large Intestine Meridian of Hand-*yangming* pertains to the large intestine while Lung Meridian of Hand-*taiyin* connects with the large intestine and foot-*taiyin* collateral and "connects with the intestine and stomach". Its back-*shu* point is Dachangshu (BL 25). Its anterior referred point is Tianshu (ST 25). Its lower-joining point is Shangjuxu (ST 37).

left-right twirling and flow of meridian *qi* 龙虎升腾 [lóng hǔ shēng téng] 1. *longhu* refers to the action of left and right spiral of the needle but *shenteng* refers to the flow of meridian *qi*. After inserting the needle, make the needle spiral left at the superficial stratum and press it downward, then make it spiral right and press it downward, and then press the body of the needle with the middle finger. Do like this repeatedly 9 times, then insert the needle into the deeper stratum, make the needle spiral right and thrust it one circle and then lift it, and press the body of the needle with the middle finger, repeat it 6 times. It can also be combined with finger press to make meridianal *qi* flow. It pertains to *feijing zhougi* and can be used for treating symptoms of stasis of *qi* and blood; 2. I. e. *longhu sheng jiang*. (Fig 61)

lesser occipital nerve 枕小神经 [zhěn xiǎo shén jīng] An ear point located at the medical aspect, 0.2 mm to the upper edge of the helix notch.

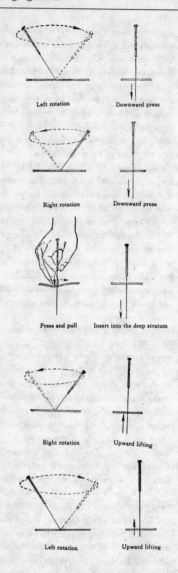

Fig 61

Laogong (PC 8) 劳宫 [láo gōng] A point of Pericardium Meridian of Hand-*jueyin*, the spring-like (fire point of the meridian, also termed Wuli, Zhangzhong. Location: Between the 2nd and 3rd metacarpal bones of the transverse crease of the palm, below the tip of the middle finger when a fist is formed, or between the 3rd and 4th metacarpal bones. Select it when the hand is in supine position. Regional anatomy: Passing through the interspace between the 2nd and 3rd superfical and deep flexor muscles of fingers, the 2nd lumbrical muscle and the starting point of the transverse head of the adductor muscle of thumb, reaching at the interosseous muscle. There is the common palmar digital artery. The 2nd common palmar digital nerve of the central nerve is distributed. Indications: Apoplexy and coma, sunstroke, cardialgia, mania, epilepsy, foul mouth tinea on the palm of the hand. Puncture: 1—1.5 cm perpendicularly. Moxibustion: 1—3 moxa cones or 3—5 minutes with warming moxibustion.

large joints 大节 [dà jié] 1. The large joints in the human body; 2. The 1st joint of a finger or a toe.

large needle 大针 [dà zhēn] An acupuncture instrument. One of nine needles in ancient times. "The nineth one is the big needle, 1.2 dm in length…as sharp as a small piece of bamboo. Its tip is somewhat rough, used to treat edema in the joint." (Miraculous Pivot), In ancient times, it was used to treat edema in the joint. (Miraculous Pivot), The successors use it to puncture after burning it red, called fire needle.

laser-radiating point technique 激光穴位照射法 [jī guāng xué wèi zhào shè fǎ] Also called laser needling, light needling. A therapeutic method to radiate the point with the radiating light yielded by the laser apparatus. The angle of the laser is narrow. It is good in direction and its energy is highly concentrated and powerful. A small amount of laser that can penetrate through the skin and acts on the deeper region can yield the light, heat, mechanic and electromagnetic effects, playing a role in treating diseases.

The lasers used for point radiation are He-Nelaser, hydrgen-ion laser, He-Cd laser, etc.

Lateral puncture 恢刺 [huī cì] One of twelve needling techniques. As for the diseases and symptoms such as contracture of tendon and muscle, anterior or posterior oblique puncture and lifting the body of needle are adopted, so as to unobstruct merdianal *qi*. This is a technique by using one needle for multiple purposes. It is similar to penetrating puncture in multiple directions applied in modern clinic.

Leitou 肋头 [lèi tóu] An extra point, located at the superior edge of the 2nd and 3rd ribs, at the bilateral edge of the stern, Indications: Cough, asthma, hiccup, intercostal neuralgia, bronchitis. Puncture: 1—1. 5 cm obliquely. Moxibustion: 3—5 moxa cones or 5—10 minutes with warming moxibustion.

Leixia 肋髀 [lèi xià] An extra point located in the intercostal space, 12 cm lateral to the nipple. Indications: Abdominal pain, hypochondriac and intercostal pain. Moxibustion: 3—5 moxa cones or 5—10 minutes with warming moxibustion.

Leihuo zhenfa 雷火针法 [lèi huǒ zhēn fǎ] 1. A kind of moxibustion with moxa stick, i. e., *lei huo zhen zhen*; 2. A book compiled by Liu Guoguang.

leihuo shenzhen (moxibustion with moxa stick) 雷火神针 [lèi huǒ shén zhēn] According to Outline of Materia Medica, the drugs used for preparing the moxa stick are: moxa powder 509, frankin cense, myrrh, pangolin scales, sulphur, realgar, wildaconite head, Sichua aconite head, bark of peach tree 2. 5 g (ground into powder mixed with moxa floss) each. Distribute the above-mentioned medicinal mugwort, then roll them in a stick with its diameter being as large as a transverse finger width and 9—12 cm in length, and then store it in the bottle and lie hidden in the earth 49 days, and finally take it out. Before using it, ignite it, blow out it, and puncture the affected area where ten layers of paper are interposed so that hot *qi* directly enters into the affected area.

leukorrhea 带下 [dài xià] Referring to the thready mucoid discharges of the vagina.

left-right twirling 左右转 [zuǒ yòu zhuàn] Referring to the direction of needle rotation. It is called left twirling or outward twirling that the needle is generally held by the right hand and the thumb moves foreward but the index finger withdraws; it is called right twirling or inward twirling that the thumb withdraws but the index finger moves forward. In latter generations, varieties of reinforcing-reducing manipulations were brought out in combination with rotation of the needle. (Fig 62)

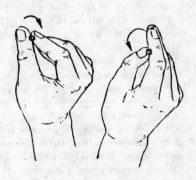

left twirling   right twirling
Fig 62

length of meridian 脉度 [mài dù] Referring to the length of the meridian. Three yang meridians of hand run from head to toot. their lengths are respectively 16 dm; three yin meridians of hand run from hand to chest, their lengths are respectively 10 dm; three yang meridians of foot from foot to head, their lengths are respectively 24 dm; three yin meridians of foot run from foot to chest, their lengths from foot to eye, are respectively 22 dm, GV and CV are respectively 13 dm. The lengths of meridians are accounted by taking the length of the body as 22 dm, i. e., on the base of the unit of bone.

left-right twirling and ascent-descent of *qi* 龙虎升降 [lóng hǔ shēn jiàng] An acupuncture manipulation. *Longhu* refers to left and right tiwirling of the needle but *shenjiang* refors to ascent and descent of *qi*. First twirl the needle forward with the thumb of the right hand. After the needle is inserted into the point, twirl the needle forward with the thumb of the left hand. After acquiring *qi*, twirl the needle left and right and lift and thrust it so as to make *qi* flow. If *qi* has not been flourishing, it can be used repeatedly. Also termed *longhu shenteng*.

left-right point-combined method 左右配穴法 [zuǒ yòu pèi xué fǎ] One of the point-combined methods, the application of the opposite points on the left and right sides. The twelve meridinas are of the same origin. Their points all are symetrical. In clinic the diseases of the internal organs are generally treated by selecting the points on the bilateral side, for stomach trouble Weishu (BL 21) of the bilateral side or Zuasnli (ST 36) of the bilateral side is selected.

left-right twirling and flow of meridian *qi* 龙虎交腾 [lóng hǔ jiāo téng] The acupuncture manipulation. *Longhu* refers to left-right rotation; *jiaoteng* refers to flow of meridian *qi*. It is to twirl the needle left and right 27 times, and twirl lit forward after acquiring *qi*, then push and tiwrl it into the deeper part, and then spring the tail of the needle to promote flow of *qi* and press down and thrust it to activate *qi*. It is used for treating febrile diseases such as red eyes (conjunctivitis), carbuncle at initial stage. (Fig 63)

Leikong 泪孔 [lèi kǒng] An alternate term for Jingming (BL 1).

leopard-spot puncture 豹文刺 [bào wén cì] Referring to the method to cause bleeding by puncturing the collateral meridian with a triangular needle for the purpose of puncturing small vessels. As the bleeding spots are many, it is called leopard-spot punc-

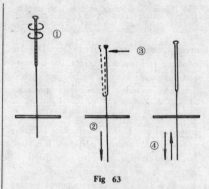

Fig 63

ture. Together with collateral puncture in nine needling techniques and related shallow puncture in twelve needling techniques it pertains to the method of puncturing collateral meridian to cause little bleeding.

Lianquan (CV 23) 廉泉 [lián quán] 1. A CV point, the confluence of connecting Vessel of Yin and CV, also termed Benchi, Sheben. Location: Above the Adam's Apple of the midline of neck, at the midpoint of the superior edge of the hyoid bone proper. Regional anatomy: Passing through the hyoid muscle reaching at the hyoid muscle, there is the anterior cervical vein. The cutaneous nerve of neck, the branches of the infrohyoid nerve and the glossopharyngeal nerve are distributed. Indications: Swelling and pain below the tongue, withdrawal of the root of the tongue, stiff tongue, appoplexy and aphasia, dry tongue and mouth, sores on the mouth and tongue, sudden aphonia, sore throat, deaf-mutism, cough, emaciation, thirst disease, anorexia. Puncture: 1. 5 cm obliquely toward the root of tongue. Moxibustion: 2—5 mmoxa cones or 5—10 minutes with warming moxibustion; 2. An extra poiont; 3. Refering to the sublingual gland which can secret mucoid liquid.

Liangqiu (ST 34) 梁丘 [liáng qiū] A point of Stomach Meridian of Foot-*yangming*, the gap-like point of the meridian. Location: At the anterolateral thigh, on the line connecting the anterosuperior iliospinal process of ilium and the lateral end of the patella base, 6 cm above the base of patella. Regional anatomy: Between the straight muscle of abdomen and the lateral muscle of thigh. There is the descending branch of the lateral circumsflex femoral artery. The muscular branch of the anterior cutaneous nerve of thigh, the lateral femoral cutaneouos nerve of thigh and the femoral nerve are distributed. Indications: Stomachache, swollen knees, paralysis. Puncture: 1. 5—3 cm perpendicularly. Mo-xibustion: 3—5 moxa cones or 5—10 minutes with warming moxibustion.

Liangmen (ST 21) 梁门 [liáng mén] A point of Stomach Meridian of Foot-*yangming*. Location: 6 cm lateral to Zhongwan (CV 12), 12 cm above the umbilicus. Regional anatomy: At the straight muscle of abdomen. There are the branches of the 8th intercostal nerve of the artery and vein and the branches of the superior epigastric artery and vein. The branch of the 8th intercostal nerve is distributed. Indications: Stomache, vomiting, anorexia, loose stool. Puncture: 3—4. 5 cm perpendicularly. Moxibustion: 3—5 moxa cones or 5—10 minutes with warming moxibustion.

lian 廉 [lián] An ancient Chinese anatomical term meaning 'side' or 'aspect'. For example, *shanglian* refers to the superior surface and *wailian*, the lateral aspect or side.

Liaoliao 髎髎 [liáo liáo] An extra point, located at the medial aspect of the knee, joint, 9 cm directly below Yinlingquan (SP 9). Indications: Metrorrhagia, irregular menstruation, wind sores, itch and pain in the medial aspect of the leg. Puncture: 1. 5—3 cm perpendicularly. Moxibustion: 2—5 moxa cones or 5—10 minutes with warming moxibustion.

Lidui (ST 45) 厉兑 [lì duì] A point of Stomach Meridian of Foot-*yangming*, the well-like (metal) point of the meridian. Location: 0. 3 cm lateral to the corner of the root of the toenail. Regional anatomy: There is the network of the artery and vein formed by the dorsal artery and vein of toe. The dorsal nerve of toe of the superficial femoral nerve is distributed. Indications: Swollen face, deviated mouth, toothache, epistaxis, yellow nasal discharge, distension and fullness in the chest and abdomen, cold feet, febrile disease, nightmare, manaia. Puncture: 0. 3—0. 6 cm obliquely. Moxibustion: 1—3 moxa cones or 3—5 minutes with warming moxibustion.

Liver Meridian of Foot-*Jueyin*(LR) 足厥阴肝经 [zú jué yīn gān jīng] One of the twelve meridians. The course: It starts from the hair region at the dorsum of the toe, ascends along the medial side of the dorsal foot, 3 cm to the medial ankle, ascends to the medial side of the leg, 24 cm to the medial ankle, crosses and emerges behind foot-*taiyin* meridian, ascends to the medial side of the cubital fossa, enters into the pubic region, along the medial side of the thigh, winds the pubic region, arrives at the lower abdomen, runs by the stomach, pertains to the liver, connects with the gallbladder; ascends to pass through the diaphragm, distributes itself over the hypochondriac region, runs along the posterior throat (esophagus), ascends to enter into the Adam's Apple and the nose, connects with the 'ocular connetion' (the connective itssue posterior to the eye), ascends to emerge from the forehead, crosses GV at the vertex. One branch descends from the 'ocular connection' to the internal mouth and cheek, winds the inner lips. The other splits from the liver, passes through the diaphragm, ascends to flow into the lungs. (connects with the Lung Meridian of Hand-*taiyin*)

lift, press and search 举、按、寻 [jǔ àn xún] The technique of pulse diagnosis by varying the digital pressure and maneuver. 'Lift' is to touch gently to asceratin the supericifial sensation; 'Press' is to press harder to obtain the deeper sensation; and 'Search' is to vary the pressure or the location of the fingers to get the better feeling of the pulse.

Liver 肝[gān]An ear point located posterosuperior to Stomach.

Lieque (LU 7) 列缺 [liè quē] A point of Lung Meridian of Hand-*taiyin*. The connecting point of the meridian, one of the eight confluential meridians, communicating with CV. Also called Tongxuan. Location: At the radial edge of the forearm, above the styloid process of radius, 4. 5 cm above the transverse crease of wrist. Regional anatomy: Between the humero-radial muscle and the long extensor muscle of thumb. There are the branches of the cephalic vein, radial artery and vein. The lateral cutaneous nerve of the anterior wall and the superficial branch of the radial nerve are distributed. Indications: Headache, cough, asthmatic breath, deviated mouth, swollen throat, swollen and painful teeth, stiff neck, pain in the elbow and arm, feverish sensation in the palms, Puncture: 1. 5—3 cm horizontally. Moxibustion of moxa cone or 5—10 minutes with warming moxibustion.

Lingdao (HT 4) 灵道 [líng dào] A point of Heart Meridian of Hand-*shaoyin*, the river-like (metal)point of the meridian. Location: At the palmar side of the forearm, at the radial edge of the ulnar flexor muscle of wrist, 4. 5 cm above the transverse crease of wrist. Regional anatomy: Running between the ulnar flexor muscle of wrist and the superficial flexor muscle of fingers, reaching at the deep flexor muscle of fingers. The ulnar artery passes through. The medial cutaneous nerve of the forearm is distributed. The ulnar nerve is in the deeper. Indications: Sudden aphonia, stiff tongue, palpitation with fear, headache, vertigo, profuse mense, metrorrhagia, pain in the lateromedial aspect of the shoulder, elbow and arm. Puncture: 1. 5—2. 5 cm

perpendicularly. Moxibustion: 1—3 moxa cones or 3—5 minutes with warming needling.

Liji 利机 [lì jī] An alternate term for Shimen (CV 5) and Huiyang (CY 1).

Liangshanmen 两扇门 [liǎng shàn mén] A point used in massage. A collective term for Yisanmen and Ersanmen. Located 1. 5 cm above the ends of the finger bilateral to the middle finger. Refer Yisanmen.

Liaoxue 髎穴[liáo xué]1. Generally referring to *shu* points, also called 'Liuxue'; 2. Specially referring to Baliao points.

lineiting 里内庭 [lǐ nèi tíng] An extra point. Located at the planter surface, at the suture between the 2nd and 3rd toes, opposite to Neiting (ST 44). Indications: Infantile convulsion, epilepsy, pain in the toes. Puncture: 1—1. 5 cm perpendicularly. Moxibustion: 3—5 moxa cones or 5—10 minutes with warming moxibustion.

liver 肝 [gān] One of the five storing viscera, Located at the hypochondriac region. Its function is to control the movement and to store blood, and is related to mind. If hepatic *qi* is weak, terror would occur; if overactive, anger would appear. This explains the relationship between blood and mind, and deficiency and excess symptoms resulted in. Liver Meridian of Foot-*jueyin* pertains to the liver, Gallbladder Meridian of Foot-*shaoyang* connects with the liver, and Kidney Meridian of Foot-*shaoyin* "upwardly penetrates through the diaphragm." Its back *shu* point is Ganshu (BL 18) and its anterior referred point, Qimen (LR 14).

Linghou 陵后[líng hòu]An extra point, located at the lateral aspect of the leg, in the depression below the posterior edge of the small head of fibula. Indications: Pains in the chest and hypochodrium, pain in the fibular nerve, inflammation of the knee joint, sciatica, numbness or paralysis of the lower limb. Puncture: 1. 5—3 cm perprndicularly. Moxibustion: 3—5 moxa cones or 5—10 minutes with warming moxibustion.

Lingxu (KI 24) 灵墟 [líng xū] A point of Kidney Meridian of Foot-*shaoyin*. Location: 6 cm lateral to Yutang (CV 18) at the midline of the chest, in the 3rd intercostal space. Regional anatomy: At the greater pectoral muscle. There is the artery and vein of the 3rd intercostal artery and vein. The anterior branch of the 3rd intercostal nerve is distributed. The 3rd intercostal nerve is in the deeper. Indications: Cough, asthmatic breath, profuse phlegm, distension and pain in the chest and hypochondrium, vomiting, breast carbuncle. Puncture: 1—1.5 cm obliquely. (It is not advisable to puncture it deep.) Moxibustion: 3—5 moxa cones or 5—10 minutes with warming needling.

lifting-thrusting method 抽添法 [chōu tiān fǎ] An acupuncture manipulation. First thrust the needle swiftly and lift it slowly at the times of the number of nine. after acquiring *qi*, slowly rotate the direction of the needle, by usually using lifting and thrusting (or to thrust while taking off air and lift it while taking air in) to make *qi* arrive at the affected area, then make the needle vertical and thrust it. It is used for treating paralysis, hemiplegia.

Li Shizhen 李时珍 (1518—1593) [lǐ shí zhēn] A medical expert in Ming Dynasty (1368-1644), born at Hubei province. He inherited his family learning, paid special attention to practice, referring 300 medical books and literatures concerned and experienced 27 years' efforts, wrote Outline of Nateria Medica, which is the treasury legacy of the treasure house in Chinese medicine and pharmacology. Li also had a deep study on basic theories of Chinese medicine. In 1577 he wrote Study on Eight Extra Meridians, and textually and systematically studied the literatures of eight extra meridians. The books he wrote are On the Picture of Five Storing Viscera, Answering Difficult Questions of Triple Energizer and Study and Textual Study on Mingmen, all of which had been lost.

Liufeng 六缝 [liù fèng] An extra point, located on the palmar side. Each has a one, plus one at the midpoint and the transverse crease of the metacarpophalangeal segment, 6 in each hand, 12 in both hands. Indication: Deep-rooted sore, infantile malnutrition. Puncture: 0.3—0.6 cm perpendicularly or prick to cause little bleeding with a triangular needle.

LI diseases 手阳明大肠经病 [shǒu yáng míng dà cháng jīng bìng] They are mainly dry mouth, stuffy nose, epistaxis, toothache, swelling neck, sore throat, pains in the anterior shoulder, arm and index finger, hotness and swelling or cold in the region where the meridian passes through, colic pain, borborygmus, diarrhea.

Liangguan 梁关 [liáng guān] I. e., Guanliang, an laternate term for Jinmen (GB 25).

LI points 手阳明大肠经穴 [shǒu yáng míng dà cháng jīng xué] According to Miraculous Pivot they are Shangyang (LI 1) (well-like), Erjian (LI 2) (spring-like), Sanjian (LI 3), Hegu (LI 4), Yangxi (LI 5) (river-like), Pianli (LI 6) (connecting), Wenliu (LI 7) (gap-like), Xialian (LI 8), Shanglian (LI 9), Shousanli (LI 10), Quchi (LI 11) (dea-like), Zhouliao (LI 12), Shouwuli (LI 13), Binao (LI 14), Jianyu (LI 15), Qugu (LI 16), Tianding (LI 17), Futu (LI 18), Kouheliao (LI 19), Yingxiang (LI 20), 20 in total, as well as Dachangshu (BL 25) pertaining to foot-*taiyang* meridean; the anterior-referred point of the large intestine meridian, Tianshu (ST 25), the lower joining point of the large intestine, Shaongjuxu (ST 37) pertaining to foot-*yangming* meridian.

Ligou (LR 5) 蠡沟 [lí gōu] A point of Liver Meridian of Foot-*jueyin*, the connectiong point of the meridian, also termed Jiaoyi. Location: 15 cm directly above the tip of the medial ankle, in the centre of the medial aspect of tibia. Regional anatomy: There is the medial cutaneous branch of the proper nerve of the posterior tibial artery and the muscular branch of the tibial nerve. Indications: Irregular menstruation, leukorrhea, prolapse of utenme, itch in the pubic region, hernia, dysuria, fullness in the lower abdomen, stiffness of the waist and back, pain in the tibia region. Puncture: 1. 5—2. 5 cm borizontally. Moxibustion: 1—3 moxa cones or 3—5 minutes with warming moxibustion.

Lingtai (GV 10) 灵台 [líng tái] A GV point, also, called Feidi. Location: At the midline of the back, between the spinal processes of the 6th and 7th thoracic vertebrae. Regional anatomy: Passing through the fasciae of the waist and the back, the supraspinal ligament and the interspinal ligament. Ther is the posterior branch of the 6th intercostal artery. The medial branch of the posterior branch of the 6th thoracic nerve is distributed. The spinal cord is in the deeper. Indications: Cough, asthmatic breath, pain in the back, stiff nape, general fever, deep-rooted sore. Puncture: 1. 5—3 cm obliquely. Moxibustion: 3—5 moxa cones or 5—10 minutes with warm needling.

lifting-thrusting manipulation 提插法 [tí chā fǎ] Referring to the action of lifting and thrusting the needle after inserting the needle.

Ling Yun 凌云 [líng yún] An acupuncture expert in Ming Dynasty (1368—1644). He was very skillful for needling, and was highly praised by Wang Ji in his Questions and Answers about Acupuncture. The book he wrote, Solving the Puzzling Problems about Ebb-Flow has not been found. The copies he wrote and handed down are Complete Book of Essentials of Acupuncture and Points on the Illustrations, Rhythmed Articles of Meridian Points. His needling techniques have been handed down by his desciple Nie Ying, and his grandsons, Ling Qianyi, Ling Xuan, Ling Zhenhou, etc.

Linquan 淋泉 [lín quán] An extra point, located 3 cm above the tip of the coccyx and 1. 5 cm bilateral to it. Indication: Abnormalities of micturition. Moxibustion: 3—5 moxa cones or 5—10 minutes with warming moxibustion.

lifting the needle 起针 [qǐ zhēn] I. e., withdrawing the needle.

liver meridian of foot-*jueyin* 肝足厥阴之脉 [gān zú jué yīn zhī mài] The original name of Liver Meridian of Foot-*jueyin*.

lifting manipulation 提法 [tí fǎ] Contrary to thrusting manipulation, referring to the action of withdrawing the needle.

limbs and joints 支节 [zhī jié] Referring to four extremities and joints, also generally referring to the acupuncture points.

liver and kidney have the same source 肝肾同源 [gān shèn tóng yuán] There exists a close relationship of mutual nourishment between the liver and the kidney.

lift-press and push-search 举、按、推、寻 [jǔ àn tuī xún] In pulse diagnosis, "lift-press" means a variation of the up-and-down pressure of the fingers, and "push-search" (means the side-way movements of the fingers).

Liuhua 六华 [liù huá] I. e., the upper six-points of Bahua points. (Fig 64)

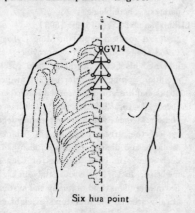

Six hua point

Fig 64

Linqi 临泣 [lín qì] A meridian point. There are two: One is located at the head, called Toulinqi (GB 15), the other at the foot, called Zulingi (GB 41)

Liu Wansu 刘完素 [liú wán sù] (Approx. 1120—1200) A famous medidcal expert in Jin Dynasty (266—420 B. C.) born at Heijian, Hebei Provicnce. He wrote the book in which the theories of Internal Classic were expounded and special attention was paid to acupuncture treatment. Another book was written by him in the name of Zhang Yuansu.

Locating the point 点穴 [diǎn xué] 1. Referring to locating the point on the human body; 2. To press the point.

lower abdomen 小腹 [xiǎo fù] I. e. , the lower abdomen.

lower joining points of six emptying viscera 六腑下合穴 [liù fǔ xià hé xué] Briefly termed lower corresponding points. The corresponding points of the six emptying viscera on the three yang meridians of foot. "The stomach corresponds with Sanli, the large intestine with Juxushanglian, the small intestine with Juxuxialian, the triple energizer with Weiyang (BL 39), the bladder with Weizhong (BL 40), and the gallbladder with Yanglingquan (BG 34)." Among them Zusanli (ST 36), the corresponding point of stomach, Weizhong (BL 40) that of the bladder, and Yanglingquan (GB 34) all are at the meridian, Shangjuxi (ST 37) the lower corresoponding point of the large intestine, and Xiajuxu (ST 39)that of small intestine all are below Zusanli (ST 36). Their main indications are disorders of the six emptying viscera. E. g. , for stomach trouble Zusanli(ST 36)is selected, for trouble of the large intestine Shangjuxu (ST 37) is selected. (Fig 65)

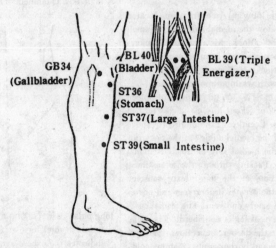

GB34 (Gallbladder)

BL 40 (Bladder)

BL 39 (Triple Energizer)

ST36 (Stomach)

ST37(Large Intestine)

ST 39(Small Intestine)

Fig 65

local selection of point 局部取穴 [jú bù qǔ xué] One of point-selected methods. That is to select the point concerned at the area where a desease or pain is located. This is the application of the point-selected principles, such as "where there a pain there is a point""along and reinforcing,"etc. In Internal Classic. E. g. , Zhouliao (LI 12) is selected for pain in the elbow, Xiyan (EX-LE 5) is selected for pain in the knee, Jingming (BL 1) is selected for pain in the eyes, Yingxiang (LI 20) is selected for stuffy nose, Zhongwan (CV 12) is selected for stomachahe, Zhongji (CV 3) and local tender spot, etc. are selected for enuresis. If there is an inflammatory focus, traumatic injury, scar or there are the important internal organs under them, it can be changed into proximal point-selection.

Locating the Point according to Time and Date of Midnight-noon Ebb-flow in Rythm 子午流注逐日按时定穴歌 [zǐ wǔ liú zhù zhú rì àn shí dìng xué gē] A rhythmed acupuncture article written by Xu Fengcuo in Ming Dynasty (1368—1644), recorded in compendium of Acupuncture. It contains the description of applying the points of 10 dates and time of midnight-noon ebb-flow.

Lower zone of cortex 皮质下区 [pí zhí xià qū] An ear point located at the medial aspect of the lower zone.

Lower Patate 下腭 [xià è] An ear point located at the medial 1/3 of the upper line of Zone$_2$.

Louyin 漏阴 [lòu yīn] An extra point, located 2.5 cm below the medial ankle on the small artery. Indications: Metrorrnagia, leukorrhea. Puncture: 1—1.5 cm perpendicularly. Moxibustion: 3—7 moxa cones or 5—10 minutes with warming moxibustion.

Lougu (SP 7) 漏谷 [lòu gǔ] A point of Spleen Meridian of Foot-*taiyin*, also termed Taiyinluo. Location: 1.8 dm directly above the tip of the medial ankle, at the posterior edge of the medial side of tibia. Regional anatomy: Passing through the soleus muscle, reaching at the long flexor muscle. There is the greater proper vein and posterior tibial artery and vein. The medial cutaneous nerve of leg is distribetd. The tibial nerve is in the deeper. Indications: Abdominal distension, borborygmus, clammy cold, numbness of the legs and knees, distension and pain in the ankles, dysuria. Puncture: 3—4.5 cm perpendicularly. Moxibustion: 3—5 moxa cones or 5—15 minutes with warming moxibustion.

longhan 龙颔 [lóng hàn] An extra point, longtou. Located on the midline of stern, 3—4 cm directly above the sternal xiphoid pro-

cess. Indications: Coldness and pain in the epigastrium, asthmatic breast, thoracalgia. Puncture: 1—2 cm horizonatally. Moxibustion: 3—5 warming moxa cones or 5—10 minutes with warming moxibustion.

Longtou 龙头 [lóng tóu] An alterate term for Nonghan.

Longquan 龙泉 [lóng quán] I. e., longyuan, an alternate term for Rangu (KI 2).

Longyuan 龙渊 [lóng yuān] Another name of Rangu (KI 2).

Longxuan 龙玄 [lóng xuán] An extra point, located at the vein 1.5 cm above Lieque (LU 6), 6 cm above the tranverse crease of the radial side of the forearm. Moxibustion: 3—5 moxa cones or 5—10 minutes with warming moxibustion.

Longmen 龙门 [lóng mén] 1. An extra point, located at the anterior commissure of labia; 2. I. e., Quanmen. (Fig 66)

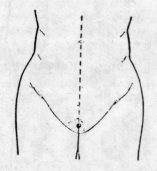

Fig 66

long pulse 长脉 [cháng mài] The pulse that is felt beyond its own location. It usually indicates the excess syndrome. It may also be seen in a healthy and robust person.

long needle 长针 [cháng zhēn] One of the needles in ancient times. Also termed *huantiao* needle in latter generations. Being long in its body, it is suitable for deep puncture, so as to treat the disorder in the deepr part of the body. In modern times it has been developed into the elongated needle.

loss of *qi* 失气 [shī qì] 1. Referring that anti-pathogenic *qi* is injured due to improper acupuncture; 2. Referring to disappearing of sensation of acquiring *qi* during acupuncture.

lower eyelid 目下纲 [mù xià gāng] Pertaining to myotendinous meridian of foot-*yangming*, also termed *mu xia wang*.

lower joining points 下合穴 [xià hé xué] A brief term for the lower joining points of six emptying viscera.

loose stools 泄泻 [xié xiè] The former (xié) refers to recurrent loose and watery stools and the latter (xiè), sudden evacuation of stools.

Lower abdomen 下腹 [xià fù] An ear point above the medial aspect of the external antrum auris.

lower selectioin for upper disease 上病下取 [shàng bìng xià qǔ] Select the point at the lower part of the body to treat the disease at the upper. "Select the point at the lower part of the body for treating the disease at the upper, select the point at the upper for treating the disease at the lower; select the point at the foot for treating the disease at the waist." (Miraculous Pivot).

Lower segment of rectum 直肠下段 [zhí cháng xià duàn] An ear point at the helix, at the level with Large Intestine.

Lower back 下背 [xià bèi] An ear point located near the lower edge of the protruding auricular concha on the back of ear.

lower bo 下膊 [xià bó] The forearm.

lungs concerned with purification and descendance 肺主肃降 [fèi zhǔ sù jiàng] Pulmonary *qi* should be fresh and descending. If it ascends or is obstructed, the symptoms with cough and dyspnea will result.

Lumbar vertebra 腰椎 [yāo zhuī] An ear point in the 2nd equivalent zong above Cervical Vertebra.

lung meridian of hand-*taiyin* 肺手太阴之脉 [fèi shǒu tài yīn zhī mài] The original name *of shou tai yin fei jing*.

Luxi (TE 19) 颅息 [lú xī] A point of Triple Energizer Meridian of Hand-*shaoyang*, also termed Luxin. Location: Posterior to the auricle, at the crossing point of the upper 1/3 and lower 1/3 of the line connecting Yifeng(TE 17)and Jiaosun(KI 8). Regional anatomy: There is the posterior artery and vein of ear. The anastomotic network of the greater aural nerve and the lesser aural nerve are distributed. Indications: Headache, tinnitus, ocular pain, infantile convulsion, vomiting up frothy saliva. Puncture: 1—1. 5 cm horizontally. Moxibustion: 1—3 moxa cones or 3—5 minutes with warming moxibustion. (Fig 67)

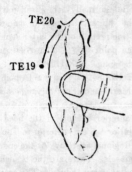

Fig 67

Luxin 颅颏 [lú xīn] I. e., Luxi (TE 19).

Lu Shouyan (1903—1969) 陆瘦燕 [lù shòu yàn] A contemporary acupuncture expert, born at Kunshan, Jiangshu Province. He once created Acupuncture Research Institute of New China before liberaton and its affiliated correspondence school. After liberation he was Dean of the Acupuncture Department of Shanghai College of Traditional Chinese Medicine, President of Shanghai Acupuncture Research Institute, Member of National Science &. Technology Committee. In 1959 he once went to the pre-Soviet Union to have a short-term investigation. He was ingaged in doing medial, teaching and scientific research work of acupuncture for a long period of time. His chief works are Illustration of Acupuncture Meridians and *Shu* Points, Illustrated Descriptions of Meridian Science, Introduction to *Shu* Points Science, General Description of Acupuncture-Moxibustion Techniques.

lu 膂 [lǚ] Referring to the muscle bilateral to the spinal column approximately at the sacrospinal muscle.

lujin 膂筋 [lǚ jīn] Referring to the muscles bilateral to the spine.

lungs concerned with air 肺主气 [fèi zhǔ qì] The lungs control the defensive *qi* of the body as well as the air of breathing.

lungs reflect their brilliance on the hair 肺其华在毛 [fèi qí huá zài máo] When the lungs function normally, they transmit nutrients to the skin and hair and to maintain luster and fine texture of the latter structures.

Luozhen point 落枕穴 [luò zhěn xué] I. e., Wailaogong. (EX-UE 8).

Luoque (BL 8) 络却 [luò què] A point of Bladder Meridian of Foot-*taiyang*, also termed Qiangyang, Naogai. Location: 16. 5 cm into the anterior hairline of the head, 4. 5 cm lateral or 4. 5 cm posterior to Tongtian (BL 7). Regional anatomy: At the end of occipital muscle. There are the branches of the occipital artery and vein. The branch of the greater occipital nerve is distributed. Indications: Vertigo, timnitus, stuffy nose, deviated mouth, mania, epilepsy, blurred vision, swollen neck, goiter. Puncture: 1—1. 5 cm horizontally. Moxibustion: 1—3 moxa cones or 3—5 minutes of warming moxibustion.

Luo Zao ju (1888—1945) 罗兆琚 [luó zào jù] An acupuncture expert in contemporary times, born at Liuzhou, Guangxi Province, once learned medicine from Luo Zhechu, etc, and was very special in acupuncture. During the Anti-Japanese War he once taught at Wuxi Acupuncture Institute. Later he returned to Liushou to practice medicine and received the desciple to hand down his acupuncture techniques. The book he wrote are Newly-written Chinese Acupuncture Surgical Treatment and Handbook of Practical Acupuncture.

Luo Zhechu (1878—1938) 罗哲初 [luó zhé chū] An acupuncture expert in contemporary times, born at Guilin, Guangxi Province. He was very interested in formulary, and read a lot of medical books, particularly had a deep study on Minraculous Pivot.

Lung 肺 [fèi] An ear point in the Lung Zone at 1/3 of the slightly medial side.

Lumbago point 腰痛点 [yāo tòng diǎn] An ear point 0. 2 mm inferomedial to the Sacrococcyx Vertebra.

Lumbago 腰痛 [yāo tòng] The pain is in the spine or at one side or bilateral side. It is one of the commonly seen symptom complexes, and frequently seen in injury of the softlessness at the waist, muscular rheumatism as well as pathologic change of the spinal column. It can be divided into lumbago caused by pathologic cold-dampness, lumbago caused by lumbar sprains and lumbago caused by weakness of the kidney.

lung 肺 [fèi] One the five storing viseera. located in the chest at the highest place of all viscera in charge of *qi* of the whole body. Various meridians meet at the lungs. It is due to the action of pulmoary *qi*. The refined principle is transported to various regions of the body, so as to make aquous liquid excreted. Heart Meridian of Hand-*shaoyin* ascends to the lungs. Pericardium Meridian of Hand-*jueyin* "internally connects with the heart and lungs"; Kidney Meridian of Foot-shaoyin enters into the lungs. Liver Meridian of Foot-*jueyin* irrigates the lungs. Lung Meridian of Hand-*taiyin* pertains to the lungs, Large Intestine Meridian of Hand-*yangming* connects with the lungs. Its back *shu* point is Feishu (BL 3) and its anterior referred point is Zhongfu (LU 1).

Lung Meridian of Hand-*taiyin* (LU) 手太阴肺经 [shǒu tài yīn fèi jīng] One of the twelve meridians. The course: Starting from the middle energizer (stomach), descending and connecting with the large intestine, turning back and running along the upper opening of the stomach to pass through the diaphragm, then merging into the lungs, emerging transversely from the pulmonary connection (esophagus) to the inferior axilla, descending along the medial (radial) side of the upper arm, running in front of hand-*shaoying* and hand-*jueyin* meridians, descending to the middle of the elbow, entering into the '*cunkou*' (the pulsation portion of the radial artery) along the inferial radius at the medial side of the forearm, ascending to greater *Yuji*, running along the edge, and emerging from the end of the thumb. A branch runs from the posterior wrist to the medial (tadial) side of the index finger, and emerging from its end (to connect with Large Intestine Meridian of Hand-*yangming*).

lushang 闾上 [lǘ shàng] An extra point, located one middle finger above the tip of the coccyx; the other two are 1/2 of the middle finger bilateral to the first point, three in total. Indications: Hemorrhoids, melena due to intestinal affection. Moxibustion: 3—7 moxa cones or 5—10 minutes with warming moxibustion.

lungs closely related to skin and hair 肺合皮毛 [fèi hé pí máo] The lungs are closely related to skin and hair (including sweat glands). They may influence each other physopathologically.

Lu points 手太阴肺经穴 [shǒu tài yīn fèi jīng xué] They are Zhongfu (LU 1) (meeting with foot-*taiyin* meridian), Yunmen (LU 2), Tianfu (LU 3), Jiabai (LU 4), Cize (LU 5) (joining), Kongzui (LU 6) (gap), Lieque (LU 7) (connecting), Jingqu (LU 8) (river-like), Taiyuan (LU 9) (stream-like) (source), Yuji (LU 10) (spring-like), Shaoshang (LU 11) (well-like), 11 in total. Feishu (BL 13) pertains to the foot-*taiyang* meridian; Zhongfu (LU 1) the anterior-referred point pertains to Lung Meri-

dian (Fig 68).

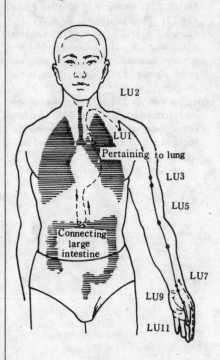

Fig 68

LU diseases 手太阴肺经病 [shǒu tài yīn fèi jīng bìng] They are mainly fullness and depression in the chest, distension of lung, asthmatic breath, cough, anxiety, short breath, pain in the shoulder and arm, pain and cold in the region the meridian passes through, and feverish sensation in the palm.

LR points 足厥阴肝经穴 [zú jué yīn gān jīng xué] They are Dadun (LR 1) (well), Xingjian (LR 2) (spring), Taichong (LR 3) (stream), Zhongfen (LR 4) (river), Ligou (LR 5), Zhongdu (LR 6) (gap-like), Xiguan (LR 7), Ququan (LR 8) (sea), Yinbao (LR 9), Wuli (LR 10), Yinlian (LR 11), Jimai (LR 12), Zhangmen (LR 13), Qimen (LR 14), 14 in total. The points where the meridian crosses other meridians are Snyin-jiao(BL 22), Chongmen (SP 12), Fushe (SP 13) (foot-*taiyin*), Qugu (CV, 2), Zhongji (CV 3), Guanyuan (ST 22). There is Ganshu (BL 18) pertaining to foot-*taiyang* meridian; The aterior referred point, Qimen (LR 14), pertaining to the meridian.

lying position 卧位 [wò wèi] One of the acupuncture body positions, subdivided into supine lying position (for puncturing the head, face, neck, chest, abdomen, and inte-rior side of the upper and lower limbs), side lying position (for puncturing one side of the face, temple, nape, back and hip, and posterolateral side of the lower limb) and prone lying postion. (for puncturing the points at the waist, back, hip and posterior side of the lower limb).

lying needle 卧针 [wò zhēn] To withdraw the needle to the subcutaneous region and to make it deviated just liking lying for further horizontal puncture or needle reten-tion.

M

maintenance of *qi* 守气 [shǒu qì] To administer proper acupuncture manipulation after acquiring *qi* by acupuncture, so as not let acquired *qi* disappear.

manipulation of the needle 运针 [yùn zhēn] During acupuncture, a variety of techniques of manipulations to maintain and strengthen needling sensation, such as twirling, thrusting and lifting needle, etc. Also termed *xin zhen*. It can be done intermittently or for a long period of time.

man stratum 人迎 [rén yíng] Alternately named Tianwuhui, Wuhui. Location: 4.5 cm lateral to the Adam's Apple, at the crossing point of the anterior sternocleidomastoidous muscle and the superior edge of the thyloid artilage. Indications: Closejaw, deviated mouth, swelling cheek, toothache, puffy face, scrofula, pain in the neck. Puncture: 1.5 cm perpendicularly. (avoiding the artery)

meridianal phenomena 经络现象 [jīng luò xiàn xiàng] Referring to some special phenomena of sensation conduction appearing along the course of the meridian, some of which produce after puncturing, pressing electric wave, and moxibustion stimulate the point, some others spontaneously appear under certain pathological states. After the *qigong* exerciser becomes quiet and his or her mind retained at *Dantian* there may appear the phenomena such as a special sensation conductiong along GV, which is generally called the propagated sensation along the meridian(PSM). There is also the change of the histometaphology appearing along the meridian, including distribution of skin rash, variation of pigment, etc., also called the visible meridian phenomena.

metrorrhagia 崩漏 [bēng lòu] A collective term for profuce metrorrhagia (copious vaginal bleeding between menstrual periods) and continuous uterine bleeding (continuous vaginal bleeding of small amounts between menstrual periods).

meridians and their collaterals 经络 [jīng luò] A collective term for the meridians and their collaterals. They contain the twelve meridians, eight extra vessels, twelve branch meridians, fifteen collateral meridians, twelve myotendinous meridians, twelve cutansous region.

midnight-noon thrustiong-inserting 子午捣白 [zǐ wǔ dǎo jiù] An acupuncture manipulation. Midnight-noon refers to rotating the needle left and right; *Daojiu* refers to thrsting and inserting the needle. This is the acupuncture manipulation by combining needle rotation with needle thrusting-inserting. (Fig 69)

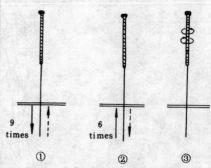

① Swift thrusting and slow lifting
② Swift lifting and swift thrusting
③ Left and right rotation

Fig 69

meridian points zone 经络穴区带 [jīng luò xuè qū dài] Referring to the sensitive zone of the body surface where the diseases are reflected. Its location accords with the meridian point is somewhat wide. In clinic the sensitive spot (point) can be found from

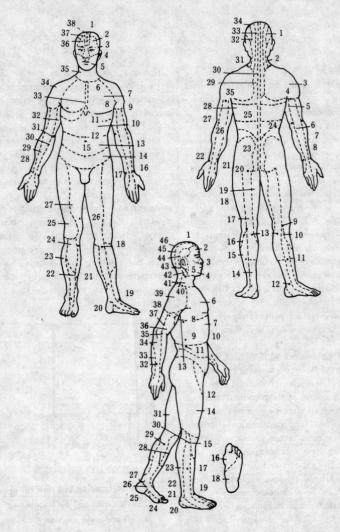

Fig 70

the concerning point zone for treatment of acupuncture and moxibustion. Hence it is called therapy of meridian-point zone. (Fig 70)

Manuscripts Dealing with Meridians 帛书经脉[bó shū jīng mài]One of the manuscripts

unearthed from Mawangdui Han Tombs at Changsha (168 A. D.). It is the therefore called Manuscripts Dealing with Meridians or Moxibustion Classic of Eleven Meridians because there was no name originally, which was divided into Moxibustion Classic of Eleven Meridians on Feet and Arms and Moxibustion Classic of Eleven Meridians of Yin and Yang.

magnetic needle 磁针 [cí zhēn] 1. Practising acupuncture with a magnetic iron needle or steel needle; 2. I. e. , the magnetic needle.

major-auxiliary and source-connecting points combination 主客原络配穴法 [zhǔ kè yuán luò pèi xué fǎ] One of point-composed methods. According to the diseases and syndromes the various meridians pertain to the source point of the meridians is selected as the 'host'. The connecting point of the meridian externally-internally related with the meridian it pertains to is called the 'guest'. A host and a guest are applied in cooperation.

Mangchang point 盲肠穴 [máng cháng xué] An extra point, located at the right side of abdomen, in the midpoint of the line connecting the anterosuperior ilium and the umbilical hole. Indications: Intestinal carbuncle, abdominal diarrhea. Puncture: 3—4. 5 cm perpendicularly. Moxibustion: 3—5 moxa cones or 5—10 minutes with warming moxibustion.

mai 脉 [mài] 1. The blood vessed; 2. The pulses.

medicinal vesculation 自灸 [zhì jiǔ] 1. Self moxibustion; 2. Drug-dressed blistering method.

Mammary gland poin 乳腺点 [rǔ xiàn diǎn] An ear point above Thoracic Vetebra to form an equivable triangle together with Thoracic Vertebra.

Meichong (BL 3) 眉冲 [méi chōng] A point of Bladder Meridian of Foot-*taiyang*, also termed Xiaozu. Location: At the medial end of the eyebrow, directly above Zanzhu (BL 2) 1. 5 cm into the hairline, at the midpoint of the line connecting Shengting (GV 24) and Qucha (BL 4). Regional anatomy: In the frontal muscle. There is the frontal artery and vein. The medial branch of the frontal nerve is distributed. The frontal muscle is below the point. Indications:

Epilepsy, headache, vertigo, blurred vision, stuffy nose. Puncture: 1—1. 5 cm horizontally. Moxibustion: 3—5 minutes with warming moxibustion.

meridian tunnels 经隧 [jīng shuì] Referring to the pathway of the meridians, internally communicated with the viscera and externally communicated with the limbs and trunk, or they are explained as the branch collaterals in the deep and superficial areas.

meridian-connected method 接经法 [jiē jīng fǎ] One of point-combined methods. It refers that several points on the same meridian are selected and connected mutually to strengthen their actions.

meridians 经脉 [jīng mài] The main pathways in which *qi* and blood circulates. Jing means the straight lines and the main stems, contrary to *luo* (their collaterals). The twelve meridians and eight extra vessels are the important consitutuents of the meridians.

meridian point examined apparatus 经穴测定仪 [jīng xué cè dìng yí] An apparatus used to examine skin resistance at the meridian point, so as to observe the changes of the functions of the meridians and the internal organs.

meridianal puncture 经刺 [jīng cì] 1. Referring to puncturing the biger meridian, contrary to collateral puncture. One of the nine needlings; 2. Referring to crossing puncture of the meridian; 3. Referring to selection of the point according to the meridian.

medial thigh 股阴 [gǔ yīn] Referring the medial side of the thigh.

meridian water 经水 [jīng shuì] Referring to a large and long water flow likened to the meridian.

medial ankle 内踝 [nèi huái] An outward protuberance of the lower end of tibia.

meridian qi 经气 [jīng qì] Referring to *qi* flowing in meridians, pertaining to antipathogenic *qi* in the human body.

Medical Secret of an Official 外台秘要 [wài tái mì yào] Also termed *waitai miyao* *fang*, written by Wang Tao in Tang Dynasty(618—907 A. D.), 40 volumes in total, chiefly recording the prescriptions and drugs for various diseases, consisting of 10,104 categories, recording over 6,000 presrciptions, 40 volumes, 39 cones recorded and discribed moxibustion techniques and meridian points.

Meitou 眉头 [méi tóu] Referring Zanzhu (BL 2).

meilenggu 眉棱骨 [méi léng gǔ] The bone forming the upper ridge of the orbit, corresponding to the supra-orbital ridge of the frontal bone.

medical needle 医工针 [yī gōng zhēn] Referring to the medical needling instrument, differring from other needling instruments.

medulla 髓 [suǐ] Including the brain, spinal cord and bone marrow. In traditional Chinese medicine. The kidney is supposed to produce medulla, probably implying a neuriohumoral mechanism.

Medial ear 内耳 [nèi ěr] An ear point located slightly above the centre of Zone.

Medial nose 内鼻 [nèi bí] An ear point located 1/2 below the medial aspect of the tragus.

merinian points 经穴 [jīng xué] 1. An abbreviation of the points of the fourteen meridians; 2. One of the five *shu* points, the river-like poins.

meridian-point diagnostic technique 经穴诊断法 [jīng xué zhěn duàn fǎ] To diagnose diseases and symptoms by examining the meridians and points. It contains palpation on body surface, electric examination of skin(examination of the meridian point)and examination of heat-sensation on the skin, of which the former one is the main. Variation of temperature at the meridian point and condition of *qi* and blood (deficiency or exceess) are judged by inspecting the body surface, finger press, touching, and press, etc. In clinic the plantar part of the thumb is used to slightly move along the meridian location or the thumb and index finger are used to slightly pinch it, so as to explore

the reactive spot at the surperficial stratum; The somewhat heavy press and kneading movement are used to explore the abnormal reaction in the deeper stratum. It is required to use the even power and note the comparison between the left and right sides. It is commonly used to examine the meridians at the chest, abdomen and four limbs, including the locations of *shu*, *mu* (anterior referred), *xi* (gap) and *he* (joining) points. The abnormal reaction seen in palpation is the node or the rope-like thing touched in the subcutaneous region, called the positive reactive thing; The sensitive reactions, such as local pain or sore and distension are called the tender points; There is also the local skin where the protrusion, hard node or depresion, loose and variations of color and temperature appear. Accoriding to different phenomena, the disease and symptom of the internal organ concerned can be predicted and analysed. The reaction often appears in Feishu (BL 13), Zhongfu (BL 1), and Kongzui (LU 6). In combination with other abnormal reaction of other points, that the patient suffers from certain disease can be predicted. These reactive spots that have the diagnostic action can also be selected for acupuncture and moxibustion treatment. In addition, the examinations of point electricity and heat sensation are the contemporary development of this method.

melancholia 郁证 [yù zhèng] The symptom-complex caused by mental depression and stagnation of *qi*. The clinical manifestations are mental depression, distress and pain of the chest and hypochondrium, feeling a lump in the throat, loss of appetite, trance, etc.

Mingtang Illustration 明堂图 [míng táng tú] A general term for ancient illustrations of acupuncture meridians and points in ancient China.

Miraculous Classic 神应经 [shén yìng jīng] A book written by Chen Hui in Ming Dyansty

(1368—1644) and edited by Liu Jun. In the book 548 symptoms and 211 points were recorded. The author added 64 empirical symptoms and 154 points of his own, and selected 119 points from them to compile them into rhythmed articles and illustrations and appended with the method of, reinforcing-reducing and illustrating explanation of point selection, point combination for varieties of diseases as well as acupuncture prohibitions, etc. It was completed in 1425.

Mingguang 明光 [míng guāng] An alternate term for Zanzhu (BL 2).

middle-finger *cun* 中指寸[zhōng zhǐ cùn]One of proportional *cun* for locating the point. The length of the middle segment of the middle finger is taken as the standard of measurement. 1. The length of the 3rd segment of the middle finger is taken as one *cun*. 2. The distance between the two transverse creases of the 2nd segment of the middle finger is taken as one *cun*.

Mianyan 面岩 [miàn yán] An extra point, located at the two parallel sides of the protuberances of ana lasi, superiorly opposite to the crossing point of the lateral 1/4 and medial 3/4 of the infraorbital edge. Indication: Facial deep-rooted sore. Puncture: 1—1. 5 cm perpendicularly.

Mianliao 面窌 [miàn liào] An alternate term for Chengqi (ST 1).

mingtang 明堂 [míng táng] 1. Referring to the nose; 2. Rerferring to the books of acupuncture, meridians and points. E. g., Mingtang Illustrations, Mingtang Classic, also referring to the model marked with meridians and points; 3. I. e., Shangxing (GV 3).

Mianwang 面王 [miàn wáng] An alternate term for Suliao (GV, DU 25).

Mianyu 面玉 [miàn yù] The wrong form of Mianwang.

Mianzheng 面正 [miàn zhèng] I. e., Mianwang. An alternate term for Suliao (GV, DU 25).

midline of head and face 头面正中线 [tóu miàn zhèng zhōng xiàn] The place that GV and CV pass through. Shenting (GV 24), Shangxingd (GV 23), Xinhui (GV 22), Qianding (GV 21), Baihui (GV 20), Houding (GV 19), Qiangjian (GV 18), Naohu (TE 13), Fengfu (GV 16), and Yamen (GV 15) are distributed over the midline of the head (in the hairline), Suliao (DU 25), Shuigou (DU 26), Duiduan (GV 27), Yinjiao (GV 28), and Chengjiang (CV 24) are distributed over the midline of the face.

midline of back 背正中线 [bèi zhèng zhōng xiàn]A line for locating the meridian point, also called the posterior midline, where GV passes through and Dazhui (GV 14), Todao (GV 13), Shenzhu (GV 12), Shendao (GV 11), Zhiyin (GV 10), Zhiyang (GV 9), Jinsuo (GV 8), Zhongshu (GV 7), Jizhong (GV 6), Xuanshu (GV 5), Mingmen (GV 4), Yangguan (GV 3), Yaoshu (GV 2), and Changqiang (GV 1) are distributed over.

migu 髊骨 [mí gǔ] Referring to the upper angle of the scapular bone, also called *fu gu*.

milk tumor 乳癖 [rǔ pǐ] Usually a collective term for the benign tumors of the breast. It may become maligment after a long period of time.

miraculous needling fire 神针火 [shén zhēn huǒ] A kind of moxibustion technique, also called *tao zhi jiu*. Ignite the peach branch rinsed with sesame oil, then blow out it and immediately put it on the affected area interposed by a cotton paper. Indications: Coldness and pain in the epigastric region, wind-cold-damp blockage.

miao 胮 [miǎo] Referring to the lateral loin, at the depression and the soft space between the hypochondrium and the crest of illium.

Middle ear 耳中[ěr zhōng]An ear point lateral to Diaphragm to form a right line with the interspace between Esophagus and Cardia.

midnight-noon ebb-flow 子午流注 [zǐ wǔ liú zhù] An ancient acupuncture theory of selecting acupuncture points. Essentially, the acupuncture points from the basis, and are related to the changes of the days and the hours in terms of the Heavenly Stems and Earthly Branches to predict the state of ebb and flow of *qi* and bood along the meridians, so as to select the appropriate points.

Middle back 中背 [zhōng bèi] An ear point at the protruding part of the auricular concha on the back of ear.

Miraculous Pivot 灵枢 [líng shū] A classic, also called *Lingshu Jing*, collectivelly called Internal Classic together with Plain Questions. Zhang Zhongjing called it Acupuncture Classic in his preface of Treatise on Cold Injury; Huangfu Mi called it Acupuncture Classic in his preface of Systematic Classic of Acupuncture; Wang Bin called it Miraculous Pivot in his preface of Plain Questions; It was also called *Jiu Ling*, *Jiu Xu*. It was divided into 24 volumes and 81 chapters in total after checking and approving the old edition stored in his family by Shi Song in Song Dynasty (420—479 A. D.). It mainly describes the nine needling techniques, meridians, storing-emptying viscera, points, puncturing techniques as well as diagnosis and treatment of diseases, etc. It is a classic of acupuncture science and also one of the earliest important acupuncture literatures.

midnight-noon reinforcing-reducing manipulation 子午补泻 [zǐ wǔ bǔ xiè] The reinforcing-reducing manipulation by left-right twirling of needle. The left rotation of the needle is the clockwise rotation, that is turning from the *zhi* position to the *wu* one; The right rotation is the counterclockwise one, that is turning from the *wu* position to the counter-clockwise one, that is turning from the *wu* position to the *zhi* one...

midnight-noon manipulation 子午法 [zǐ wǔ fǎ] Referring to rotation or reinforcing-reducing manipulation. Twirl the needle left and right to search for *zhi* and *wu* positions, while twirling the needle, pushing the thumb foreward is from *zhi* to *wu* position while withdrawing the thumb is from *wu* to *zhi* position...

Mingguan 命关 [mìng guān] 1. An extra point, located directly below the nipple, at the level with the spot 12 cm above the umbilicus. Moxibustion can be administered at it for treating abdominal distension, edema, anuria, asthmatc breath, vomiting and regurgitation, rest dyesntery, incontinence of defecation, malaria, persistent pain in the hypochondrium; 2. The point used for infantile massage and diagnosis, referring to the transverse crease of the palmar side of the last segment of the index finger.

Mingmen (GV 4) 命门 [mìng mén] A GV point also termed Shulei, Jinggong. Location: At the lumbar midline between the 2nd and 3rd lumbar spinal processes. Regional anatomy: There is the lumbar back fascia, the supraspinal ligament, the interspinal ligament, the posterior branch of the lumbar artery. The medial branch of the posterior branch of the lumbar nerve is distributed. Indications: Lumbago due to asthenia, stiff spine, unuresis, frequent ugination, diarrhea, spermatorrhea, impotence, premature ejaculation, leukorrhea, habitual abortion, injuries caused by five types of stains, dreaminess, tinnitus, epilepsy, cold clammy hands and feet. Puncture: 1.5—3 cm obliquely. Moxibustion: 3—7 moxa cones or 5—15 minutes with warm needling.

moxibustion fainting 晕灸 [yùn jiǔ] The fainting phenomenon suddenly occurring in the course of moxibustion treament. It is usually caused by weak constitution, mental stress and excessive moxibustion with mugwort. The manifestations and the dealing method are similar to those of acupuncture.

moxibustion with the handle of needle 针柄灸

[zhēn bǐng jiǔ] I. e. , warm needling moxibustion.

moxibustion doctor 灸师 [jiǔ shī] Referring to the doctor who specially administers moxibustion.

moxibustion with grub 蛴螬灸 [qí cáo jiǔ] A kind of indirect moxibustion. That is to moxibustion by using the grub as the interposing layer. The actions are removing malignant bloold, subsiding something stagnant, such as sore and furuncle, etc.

moxibustion sore 灸疮 [jiǔ chuāng] A sore formed by suppuration and erosion of the local area where moxibustion is done due to scorching injury, also called *jiǔ chuàng*. In ancient China after administering moxibustion various methods were used to promote moxibustion. In general, moxibustion sore heals by scarring 3—5 weeks later. During this period the surface of sore must be kept clean; The applied glu shoule be changed frequently lest infection should occur.

moxibustion and needling techniques 灸刺 [jiǔ cì] Referring to moxibustion and needling techniques, usually used in ancient books.

moxibustion-replaced plaster 替灸膏 [tì jiǔ gāo] One of the formularized drug for application.

moxibustion interposed by chilli paste 椒饼灸 [jiāo bǐng jiǔ] A kind of moxibustion inteprosed by paste. To prepare a thin paste with white powder mixed with flour and water. Put a small amount of cloves, bark of Chinese cassia tree and musk into the centre of the paste. Then, do moxibustion with moxa cone on it. Usually used for treating rheumatc blockage and pain, stomachache due to pathogenic cold.

Mobility Vessel of Yin 阴跷脉 [yīn qiāo mài] One of the eight extra vessels. The course: Splitting from foot-*shaoyin* meridian, originating from posterior Rangu (Zhaohai, KI 16), ascending to the Jiaoxin (KI 8), superfior to the medial ankle, directly ascending along the medial aspect of the thigh to enter into the pubic region, ascending along the inner chest in front of Renying (ST 9), entering into the lateral nose, pertaining to the inner canthus, joining Motility Vessel of Ying.

moderate moxibustion 温和灸 [wēn hé jiǔ] Also termed *wen-jiu*. A moxibustion method to make the local area warm but not scorch the skin. In general, moxibustion with moxa stick or direct moxibustion is usually used to do moxibustion till red spots appear. While using indirect moxibustion the interposing thing and moxa cone should be properly moved according to the condition of the patient's reaction. If direct moxibustion is used, burning moxa cone must be blown out before the fire burns the skin, Change it and then continue to do moxibustion till mild heat reaches.

movement of the fingers 移指 [yí zhǐ] In pulse diagnosis, according to the status of the patient's pulse, the physician moves the fingers for palpating the pulse.

moxibustion with sesame leaves 麻叶灸 [má yè jiǔ] One of moxibustion techniques, used for treating scrofula.

moxibustion with tube 筒灸 [tóng jiǔ] A kind of moxibustion technique. To moxibustion at one end of a small bamboo or reed tube of which the other end is put into the ear.

moxibustion with mice's stool 鼠粪灸 [shǔ fèn jiǔ] To do moxibustion with dried mice's stool.

moxibustion with sulphur 硫黄灸 [liú huáng jiǔ] A kind of moxibustion technique. "A piece of sulphur shaped as the opening of the sore. Use a small amount of sulphur and burn it, then use the burning sulphur to touch the one on the opening 3—5 times till the pus is dried. Used to treat the fistula formed by the sore that has not been healed for a long period of time.

moxibustion with wax 黄蜡灸 [huáng là jiǔ] A kind of moxibustion technique. First make a circle around swollen carbuncle or furuncle with rinsed flour that is 3 cm high, and touched the skin, like the opening of a well. Then put five pieces of wax within the circle, 0.9—1.2 cm in thickness, and scorch the wax with the mulburry wood and put into a branze laddle to make the wax smelt and boiling, and then add some pieces of wax till the 'well' is full. After moxibustion, pour some cold water on the wax, and finally take away the wax after it becomes cold. It is used for treating carbuncle or ceillulitis, malignant or stubborn sore.

movable cupping 推罐法 [tuī guàn fǎ] A kind of cupping method, also called cup-pushed method, cup-moved method. After the cup is absorbed on the skin, move the cup so as to widen the size of which it acts on. While applying it, first paint some vasilin or wax oil as lubricants on the opening of the cup and the therapeutic area, then after a few minutes, when the cup is absorbed on the skin, hold the body of the cup with the hand and slowly move, push and pull it to and for 6—8 times till the red spots appear locally. It is usually used at the waist and back, and suits rheumatic pain and gastroenteritic trouble. (Fig 71)

moxibustion with loes paste 黄土饼灸 [huáng tǔ bǐng jiǔ] A kind of moxibustion interposed with paste, made of loes for treating ear trouble.

moxibustion with fermented soyal beans paste 豉饼灸 [cǐ bǐng jiǔ] A kind of paste-interposed moxibustion. For lumbodorsal ceilulitis (or carbuncle), moxibustion with moxa cone can be done by putting a round paste made of powder of fermented soyal beans mixed with yellow wine, 0.6 cm in thickness to promote healing of the wound.

moxibustion for the sunken 陷下则灸之 [xiàn xià zé jiǔ zhī] One of therapeutic principles of acupuncture moxibustion. It is advisable to apply moxibustion treatment to warm the meridians and dissipate pathogenic cold in the case of deficiency-cold diseases and syndromes in which the vessels are sunken.

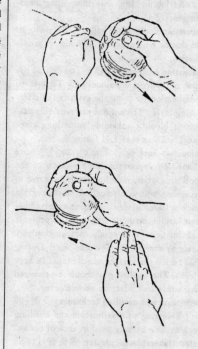

Fig 71

moxibustion shade 灸罩 [jiǔ zhào] A tool for moxibustion, cone-shaped with a hole on its top. It is used to cover moxa cone used to administer moxibustion.

moxibustion sensation 灸感 [jiǔ gǎn] A term of moxibustion. Referring to the patient's sensations, such as warm heat or numbness, insect-running, etc., due to administering moxibustion on the patient. Sometimes it can spread over or transfer to a certain direction.

moxibustion scar 灸瘢 [jiǔ bān] The scar formed due to moxibustion treatment.

moxibustion interposed by pokeberry-root paste 商陆饼灸 [shāng lù bǐng jiǔ] A kind of moxibustion interposed by paste, used to treat scrofula, etc.

moxibustion with mulberry wood 桑木灸

[sāng mù jiǔ] A kind of moxibustion to fumigate the point with an ignited mulberry branch.

moxibustion with mulberry branch 桑枝灸 [sāng zhī jiǔ] A kind of moxibustion. "For carbuncle and furuncle that have not yet swollen, and erossive, scrofula, and stuborn sore, egnite the mulberry branch and use it to do moxibustion on them immediately after browing out it twice daily." (Outline of Materia Medica, VOL. 7)

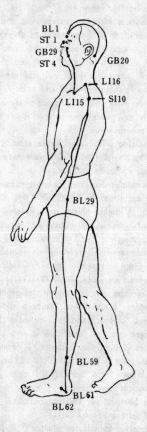

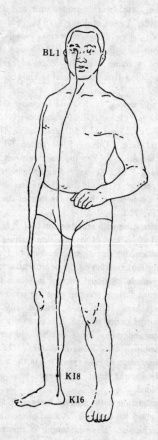

Fig 72

moxibustion with bottle gourd 苦瓠灸 [kǔ hú jiǔ] One of interposed moxibustion. According to Prescriptions for Universal Relief, for treating carbunele, the bottle gourd (fresh, bitter in taste) can be cut into small pieces and then put one piece on the sore, and do moxibustion on it for 2—7 moxa cones.

moxibustion with butlercup 毛茛灸 [máo qín jiǔ] A kind of drug-adressed blistering moxibustion. Pound the fresh herb into small pieces, then apply it on the point so that small blisters will occur next night, resembling fire moxibustion.

Moxibustion Techniques for Emergency 备急灸法 [bèi jí jiǔ fǎ] A medical book compiled by in Southern Song Dynasty (1127—1279). Carbuncles, furauncles, deep-rooted sores, abdominal pain diarrhea and vomiting, etc. were recorded in it.

Mobility Vessel of Yang 阳跷脉 [yáng qiāo mài] One of eight extra vessels. The course: Splitting from foot-*taiyang* meridian, starting from the centre of heel, ascending from the lateral ankle (Shenmai, BL 62), passing through (Pucan, BL 61, and Fuyang, BL 59) and Jingming (BL 1), the hip (Juliao, GB 29), shoulder (Naoshu, SI 10), Jugu (LI 16) and Jianyu (LI 15) and face (Dicang SJ4, Juliao ST3 and Chengqi, ST 1) to the inner canthus (Jingming, BL1), ascending together into Fengchi (GB 20), and entering into the brain between the two tendons of the nape. (Fig 72)

moxibustion with moxibustion tool 灸器灸 [jiǔ qì jiǔ] A kind of moxibustion technique. To administer ironing moxibustion or fumigating moxibustion on the point with a specially-made moxibustion tool in which ignited moxa floss is put can give the point warming heat stimulation continuously for a longer period of time. It is generally used at the abdomen, waist and back to treat abdominal pain, lubago, diarrea, abdominal distension of cold type. It has the action of dissipating cold and regulating *qi* and blood.

moxibustion with *yangsui* **lozenge** 阳燧锭炎 [yáng suí dìng jiǔ] A kind of moxibustion technique. *Yangsui* lozeng is prepared by mixing sulphur with other drugs. To administer moxibustion by igniting and putting it on the point. It is used for treating pain due to damp blockage, articular spasm, spasm of hand and foot.

moxa roll 艾卷 [ài juǎn] I. e., moxa stick.

moxibustion with moxa-roll 艾卷灸 [ài juǎn jiǔ] I. e., moxibustion with moxa stick.

moxa floss 艾茸 [ài róng] I. e., moxa floss.

moxa pill 艾圆 [ài yuán] I. e., moxa pill used for moxibustion.

moxa cone 艾炷 [ài zhù] A cone-shaped moxa is made with its tip sharp and base flat for application of moxibustion, also called moxa pill. Its shape is according to the needle of moxibustion treatment.

moxibustion with pittosporm root and fresh jinger 山栀生姜灸 [shān zī shēng jiāng jiǔ] A kind of indirect moxibustion. Break and decoct pittosporm root and take its thick juice, mix them with flour and lime, and stir them into past and paint it on the point. And then put a piece of fresh jinger on it, and put a moxa cone on it to administer moxibustion.

moxibustion with small moxa cone 小炷灸 [xiǎo zhù jiǔ] Moxibustioin treatment by using a smaller moxa cone.

moxibustion-substituted plaster-dressed on the umbilicus 代灸涂脐膏 [dài jiǔ tú qí gāo] A kind of plaster to be dressed on the point, which can substitute moxibustion with mugwort. "The moxibustion-substituted plaster dressed on the umbilicuss: Prepared aconite root, sweetiris seed, cnidium fruit, bark of Chinese cassia free, evodia rutaecarpa in equal amount and ground into powder, a sponful of flour, a sponful of drug, (or half a sponcer) mixed with fresh ginger into glu, distribute it on a piece of paper (9 cm in diameter), dress it at Guanyuan (CV 4), Qihai (CV 6) below the umbilicus from morning till night. It can substitut moxibustion 10 moxa cones. It can be used for treating umbilical pain." (Weisheng Baojian Buyi)

moxibustion-substituted plaster 代灸膏 [dài jiǔ gāo] A kind of formularized drug for dressing. It can be used for treating senile people's weakness, deficiency of primordial *qi* and cold, weak viscera, coldness, pain in the hand and foot that can not be tolerated, The prescription: Aconite root, evodia rutae carpa, bark of Chinese cassia trea, auklandia root, cnidium fruit, 2 geach, sweet iris flower. The above-mentioned drugs should be fine powder, half a sponful powder, half a sponful flour are given, half a sponful fresh ginger that are decocted as glu. Then distribute them over a piece of paper. When dressed on the umbilicus in clinic, cover it with a piece of oil paper, then wrap them with a cotton cloth, from night till morning, every night, as if the moxibustion with 100 moxa cones is down on the waist and abdomen. For expelling accumulating pathogenic cold and lumbago, dress it on Taodao (EX-B 7).

moxibustion with small moxa cone 小壮灸 [xiǎo zhuàng jiǔ] I. e., moxibustion with small moxa cone.

moxibustion with croton seed paste 巴豆饼灸 [bā dòu bǐng jiǔ] A kind of paste-interposed moxibustion.

moxibustion with Sichuan chilli-paste 川椒饼灸 [chūan jiāo bǐng jiǔ] Sichuan chilli is used to prepare as the drug paste and applied in moxibustion treatment.

moxibustion with fermented soya beans 豆豉灸 [dòu chǐ jiǔ] See *chi bing jiu.*

moxa floss 艾绒 [ài róng] The material used in moxibustion, also called *airong* (艾茸), which is prepared by processing moxa leaves.

mouth *cun* 口寸 [kǒu cùn] One of the proportional measurements for selecting the extra point. The distance between the two courses of the patient's mouth is taken as 3 cm.

moxibustion flower 灸花 [jiǔ huā] A term of moxibustion techique. Referring to the suppurative stage of moxibustion sore.

moxibustion plate 灸板 [jiǔ bǎn] An instrument for moxibustion.

Moxibustion Techniques of Gaohuangshu 膏肓俞穴灸法 [gāo huāng shū xué jiǔ fǎ] A book also named *gaohuang jiu fa* written by Zhuang Zuo in Southern Song Dynasty (1127—1279), one volume, in which the indications, location and different schools's selection of Gaohuangshu were introduced and the illustrations were appended. It was

completed in 1128, and is one of Four Acupuncture Books complied by Dou Guifang in Yuan Dynasty (1271—1368).

moxibustion technique 灸法 [jiǔ fǎ] A therapeutic technique by making use of mugwort floss, etc., to scorch or fumigate and iron the point. The application of moxibustion techniques in contemporary times are classified into moxibustion with moxa cone (direct moxibustion and indirect moxibustion), moxibustion with moxa stick, moxibustion with warming moxibustion tool, electrothermal moxibustion, and moxibustion with applied drug. (blistering by applying drug)

moxibustion interposed by prepared aconite root 附子灸 [fù zǐ jiǔ] A kind of indirect moxibustion. A drug paste can be prepared by using unripened aconite root (19), cloues (Q 59) that are ground into fine powders and mixed with concentrated honey, which is shaped like a corn, 0. 6 cm in thickness and a few holes are made in the middle of it, then a moxa cone is put on it.

mouth, the window of the spleen 脾开窍于口 [pí kāi qiào yú kǒu] Some of pahysiopathologic conditions of the spleen can be discerned and observed from the status of the mouth and lips.

Mouth 口 [kǒu] An ear point below the crus of helix laterosupperior to anti-antrum auris.

moxibustion Classic of Eleven Meridians 十一脉灸经 [shí yī mài jiǔ jīng] The medical manuscripts unearthed from Mawangdui Han Tombs at Changsha, China.

moxibustion with moxa cone 艾炷灸 [ài zhù jiǔ] A kind of moxibustion technique. To administer moxibustion by putting a moxa cone on the point. It can be divided into direct moxibustion and indirect moxibustion.

model of the human body marked with meridians and points 人体经穴模型 [rén tǐ jīng xué mó xíng] The instrument for acupuncture teaching, usually made of paper pulp and gypsum or plastic. The shape is reduced according to the proportion of the healthy person varied in norms. The sign for selecting the point is manifest at its surface and the locations and names of the points of the four meridians are marked. On the smaller one the names of the common points are marked for application of teaching meridian points.

moderate needling 平针法 [píng zhēn fǎ] The acupuncture manipulation that chiefly for acquiring *qi* without differentiating reinforcing and reducing manipulations after inserting the needle.

moderate manipulation 平补平泻 [píng bǔ píng xiè]1. Contrary to reducing manipulation, the reifnforcing-reducing manipulation with gentle manipulation and smaller volume of stimulation for some cases due to imbalanced yin and yang. It is no need to use greater reinforcing or reducing manipulsation, but only use that of lifting and thrusting the needle to regualte *qi*; 2. Referring to the prior reinforcing and later reducing manipulation. Through it pathogenic *qi* can be expelled and body resistance strengthened, yin and yang becomes harmonious; 3. Referring to the needling without differentiating reinforcing and reducing manipulations. Also termed regulating manipulation, similar to the *qi*-guided method in ancient times.

moxibustion with large moxa cone 大炷灸 [dà zhù jiǔ] Usually used in indirect moxibustion in modern times. If it is used in direct moxibustion and results in scar, it pertains to supperative moxibustion. The minimal diameter of a moxa cone is 1 cm, which was usually used for suppurative moxibustion in ancient China.

moxibustion with moxa stick 艾条灸 [ài tiáo jiǔ] A kind of moxibustion technique, to fumigate or do moxibustion or scorch the point with a specially-made moxa stick, including hanging moxibustion and touching moxibustion. Each moxibustion lasts 10—20 minutes till the skin becomes hot and a

red area appears. It is called moxibustion with medicinal moxa stick that drugs of pungent, warm and fragrant nature are added to moxa.

moxibustion 艾灸 [ài jiǔ] The major moxibustion technique. To administer moxibustion on the points directly or indirectly by putting the fuel moxa on the point. A small amount of fragrant and dry drug powder can be added into moxa to strengthen the action. It can be divided into moxibustion with moxa cone, moxibustion with moxa roll, moxibustion with an instrument, etc.

moxibustion with scar 瘢痕灸 [bān héng jiǔ] I. e. , suppurative moxibustion.

muscular puncture 分刺 [fēn cì] It refers to puncturing the muscle appending to the bone for treating muscular disorder.

moxibustion with lozenge 药锭灸 [yào dìng jiǔ] One of moxibustion techniques. To grind various kinds of drugs into powders and melt them with supsus to make the lozenge and put it on the point for moxibustion.

moxibustion interposed by drug paste 药饼灸 [yào bǐng jiǔ] A kind of indirect moxibustion. To put the drug paste made of drugs of pungent, warm and fragrant nature on the point, and then to put a moxa cone on it to administer moxibustion. It has the action of warming the middle energizer, dissipating pathogenic cold, and promoting circulation of *qi* and blood. In clinic it varies in moxibustion inperposed by aconite roat, moxibustion inperposed by chilli paste and moxibustion interposed by fermented beans cured paste , etc.

moxibustion with twisted drug powder 药捻灸 [yào niǎn jiǔ] One of moxibustion techniques. To weap drug powder closely with a piece of cotton paper and to twist it into a small threaad and then cut it into small segments, finally adhere it on the point for moxibustion, E. g. , *Ponglai* fire is a kind of twisted drug powder moxibustion.

moxa pill 艾丸 [ài wán] The pill formed by

rolling moxa, used for moxibustion. Refer moxibustion with moxa cone.

moxa holder 艾斗 [ài dǒu] A moxibustion instrument. It consists of the two parts. The upper part is formed by a springing holder winded with the metal thread and the lower is made of artifical leather and asbestos lining. By the side of the lining there is a silk ribon used to fix the moxa. It can be used for warming moxibustion after filling igniting moxa.

moxa stick 艾条 [ài tiáo] A moxa stick made of mugwort, also called moxa roll. In general, the latter is made by adding certain drug into the moxa while preparing it, make 20 g of pure moxa (If the medicinal moxa stick is prepared, add 6—8 g of drug powder into the moxa and stir them even) on cotton paper 9 dm in length and 15 cm in width, then fold the two ends of the cotton paper, and then roll it closely and seal its openings with egg white, then make it dry by putting it in sun and store it for use. Refer moxibustion with moxa stick. (Fig 73)

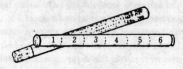

Fig 73

Muchuang (GB 16) 目窗 [mù chuāng] A point of Gallbladder Meridian of Foot-*shaoyang*, the confluence of foot-*shaoyang* meridian and Connecting Vessel of Yang. An alternate term for Zhiyin (BL 67). Location: With the eyes look forward directly above the pupil, 3—4 cm in the hairline, i. e. , 1 cm posterior to Toulinqi (GB 15). Regional anatomy: At the galea aproneuotica. There are the frontal branches of the superficial temporal artery and vein. The combined branch of the internal and external branches of the temporal nerve is distributed. Indication: Headache, vertigo, redness and pain in the eyes, myopia, puffiness of face,

swelling of the upper arms, infantile convulsion. Puncture: 1—2 cm hodrizontally. Moxibustion: 1—3 moxa cones or 3—5 minutes with warming moxibustion.

mud coin 泥钱 [ní qián] A moxibustion tool, made of mud, coin-shaped but thicker with a round hole in its centre. Moxibustion is done by putting a moxa cone on it.

mud moxibustion 泥土灸 [ní tǔ jiǔ] I. e. , moxibustion with a paste of yellow earth.

muqiao 目窌 [mù liào] An alternate term for Sizukong (TE 23).

Mulinqi 目临泣 [mù lín qī] I. e. , Toulingqi (GB 15).

muscle-touched moxibustion 着肉灸 [zháo ròu jiǔ] A kind of needling technique, i. e. , direction moxibustion.

mulberry needling 桑枝针 [sāng zhī zhēn] I. e. , moxibustion with mulberry branch.

muscular blockage 肉痹 [ròu bì] A blockage syndrome characterized by mainly with the symptoms of the muscles. The chief manifestations are numbness or pain and weakness of the muscles, generalized lassitude, easy sweating, etc.

musculadr node 肉节 [ròu jié] Referring to the node of the sinew.

meridian in the muscle 肉里之脉 [ròu lǐ zhī mài] The branch of foot-*taiyang* meridian at the leg.

mumps 痄腮 [zà sāi] An acute infectious disease characterized by swelling, distension and pain in the cheek below the ear, also termed epidemic parotitis.

musculocutaneous junction 腠理 [còu lǐ] Usually the junction between the muscle and skin.

myopia 近视 [jìn shì] An ocular trouble due to ametropia often seen in youngsters.

myotendinous meridian of foot-*yangming* 足阳明经筋 [zú yáng míng jīng jīn] One of the twelve myotendinous meridians. It starts from the middle three toes (2nd, 3rd and 4th), knots at the dorsal foot. One of the branches that runs obliquely to the lateral side, covers the fibula, ascends to knot at the lateral side of knee, directly ascends and knots at the hip joint (Pishu, BL 20), ascends along the hypochondrium, pertains to the vertebrae. The vertical one ascends along the tibia and knots at the knee, the branch knots at the fibular region, joins myotendinous meridian of foot-*shaoyang*. The other vertical one ascends along the quadraceps muscle of thigh, ascends and knots in front of thigh, joins at the pubic region, ascends and distributes itself over the abdomen and knots at the supraclavicular fossa, ascends to the neck, runs at the nose. Its upper part joins myotendinous meridian of foot-*taiyang*. Myotendinous meridian of foot-*taiyang* forms at the 'upper canthus and that of the foot-*yangming*,' the 'lower canthus.' Its branch knots in front of ear from the cheek.

myotendinous meridian of foot-*taiyang* 足太阳经筋 [zú tài yáng jīng jīn] One of the twelve myotendinous meridians. Starting from the small toe, ascending and knotting at the lateral ankle, ascending obliquely and knotting at the knee. The lower part runs along the lateral side and knots at the heel, the upper part ascends along the Achilles tendon and knots at the cubital fossa. The branch knots at the lateral calf, ascends to the medial side of the cubital fossa, runs in parallel to one branch in the cubital fossa, knots at the hip, ascends by the lateral spine to the neck. The branch enters and knots at the tongue proper. The vertical one knots at the occiput, ascends to the head, descends to the forehead, knots at the nose. The branch forms the upper eyebrow, descends to knot at the lateral nose, another branch runs from the posterior axilla to knot at the scapular region. The branch enters into the inferior axilla, ascends to emerge from the supraclavicular fossa, and knots at the mastoid process; Another branch emerges from the supraclavicular fossa, ascends obliquely and emerges from the lateral nose.

myotendinous meridian of foot-*taiyin* 足太阴经筋 [zú tài yīn jīng jīn] One of the twelve myotendinous meridians. Starting from the end of the medial aspect of the great toe, ascending and knotting at the medial ankle. The vertical one knots at the superior condyle of the tibia at the the medial knee along the medial thigh, knots at the thick, gathers at the pubic region, ascends to the abdomen, knots at the umbilicus, then it runs along the inner abdomen, knots at the hypochondrium, distributes itself over the inner chest and finally appends to the spinal vertebra.

myofascial meridian of hand-*taiyin* 手太阴经筋 [shǒu tài yīn jīng jīn] One of the twelve myofascial meridians, starting from the thumb, ascending along the thumb, knotting at the posterior *Yuji* (dorso-palmar boundary), turning over the lateral side of the artery at *cunkou* setion, running along the forearm and knotting at the elbow, running over the medial side of the upper arm, entering into the inferior axilla, ascending and emerging from the supraclavicular fossa, knotting at the anterior Jianyu (LI 15). Its upper part knots at the supraclavicular fossa, and the lower knots in the chest, passes through the diaphragm separately and joins at the inferior axilla and reaches at the hypochondrium.

myotendinous meridian of hand-*yangming* 手阳明经筋 [shǒu yáng míng jīng jīn] One of the twelve myofascial meridians. It starts from the tip of the index finger, knots at the wrist, runs along the arm, knots at the lateral side of the elbow, passes through the upper arm and knots at Jianyu (LI 15). The branch winds the scapula, runs along the lateral spine. The vertical one ascends to the neck from Jianyu (LI 15), the branch ascends to the cheek and knots at the lateral nose. The vertical one ascends and emerges in front of hand-*taiyang* meridian, ascends to the corner of head, connects with the head, descends to the mandible at the opposite side.

myotendinous meridian of hand-*shaoyang* 手少阳经筋 [shǒu shào yáng jīng jīn] One of the twelve myofascial meridians. It starts from the tip of the ring finger, knots at the wrist, ascends along the arm and knots at the elbow, runs over the lateral aspect of the upper arm, ascends to the shoulder, runs over the neck, meets the hand-*taiyang* myofascial meridian. The branch enters at the corner of the mandible and connects with the tongue proper; Then branches to ascend and descend the corner of the mandible, the outer canthus, ascends to the forehead and knots at the corner of the head.

myofascial meridian of hand-*shaoyin* 手少阴经筋 [shǒu shào yīn jīng jīn] One of the twelve myofascial meridians. Starting from the medial side of the small finger, knotting at the piseform bone, ascending and knotting at the medial side of the elbow, ascending and entering into the axilla, crossing that of hand-*taiyin*, merging into *Ruli* and knotting at the chest, descending along the diaphragm and connecting with the umbilicus.

myofascial meridian of hand-*taiyang* 手太阳经筋 [shǒu tài yáng jīng jīn] One of the twelve myofascial meridians. Starting from the upper part of the small finger, knotting at the wrist, running from the upper part of the small finger, knotting at the wrist, running upward along the medial side of the arm, knotting at the posterior part of the mediosuperior condyle of the humerus, entering into and knotting below the axilla. The branch runs toward the posterior side of the axilla, upward winds the scapula, and runs in front of the myofascial meridian of foot-*taiyang* along the lateral neck, knots at the posterior ear (the mastoid process). Another branch enters into the ear. The vertical one emerges from the superior ear, runs doward and knots at the mandible, ascends along the manidible and pertains to the corner of mandibe, runs along the anterior ear, pertains to the outernal canthus, ascends to the cheek, and knots at the corner of the head.

myotendinous meridians 经筋 [jīng jīn] The tendons and muscles of the whole body are similar to the twelve meridians, divided into the twelve myotendinous meridians.

myotendinous meridian of hand-*jueyin* 手厥阴经筋 [shǒu jué yīn jīng jīn] One of the twelve myofascial meridians. Starting from the middle finger, running together with hand-*taiyin* meridian, knotting at the medial side of the elbow, passing through the medial side of the upper arm, knotting below the axilla, descending and distributing over anteriyposteriorly, winding the hypochonndrium. The branch enters into the interior axilla, distributes over the chest, and knots at the diaphragm (cardia).

myotendinous meridian of foot-*shaoyin* 足少阴经筋 [zú shào yīn jīng jīn] One of the twelve myotendinous meridians. It starts at the inferior aspect of the small toe, runs in parallel to that of foot-*taiyin* and then runs obobliquely below the ankle, knots at the heel, joins that of foot-*taiyang*, ascends and knots below the medial condyle of tibia, runs in parallel to that of foot-*taiyin*, then as ends along the medial side of thigh and knots at the pubic region. Then it runs by the muscle along the verterbae, ascends and reaches the nape, knots at the occiput and joins with that of foot-*taiyang*.

myotendinous meridian of foot-*jueyin* 足厥阴经筋 [zú jué yīn jīng jīn] One of the twelve myotendinous meridians. It starts from the dorsum of the toe, ascends to knot in front of the medial ankle, ascends along the medial side of tibia, knots at the medial condyle of tibia, ascends to the medial side of the thigh, knots at the pubic region, and connects with various myotendinous meridians.

N

Naoshu (SI 10) 臑俞 [nào shū] A meridian point pertaining to Small Intestline Meridian of Hand-*taiyang*, the confluence of Hand-*taiyang* meridian, Connecting Vessel of Yang and Motility Vessels. Location: Directly above the posterior plica of axilla, in the hollow at the inferior edge of the spine of scapula. Regional anatomy: Posterior to the deltoid muscle, reaching at the infrospinal muscle. There is the posterior humeral circumflex artery and vein. The superoscapular artery and vein are distributed. The posterior cutaeneous nerve of arm and the axillary nerve are distributed. The superoscapular nerve is in the deeper. Indications: Soreness, pain and weakness of the shoulder and arm, swollen shoulder, cervical scrofula. Puncture: 3—4. 5 cm perpendicularly. Moxibustion: 3—7 moxa cones or 5—15 minutes with warm moxibustion.

Nanyinfeng 男阴缝 [nán yīn fèng] An extra point. Located in the centre of the place where the root of penis meets the scrotum. Indications: Jaundice, testes. Moxibustion: 3—5 maxa cones or 5—15 minutes with warming moxibustion.

naogai 脑盖 [nǎo gài] An alternate term for Luoque (BL 8).

Naokong (GB 19) 脑空 [nǎo kōng] A point of Gallbladder Meridian of foot-*shaoyang*, the confluence of foot-*shaoyang* meridian and Connecting Vessel of Yang, also termed Nienao. Location: Directly above Fengchi (GB 20). At the level with the superior edge of the external occipital protuberance. Regional anatomy: At the occipital muscle. There is the branches of the occipital artery and vein. The greater occipital nerve is distributed. Indications: Headache, vertigo, stiffness and pain in the neck, congestion, swelling and pain of the eyes, pain in the nose, deafness, epilepsy, palpitation with fright, febrile disease. Puncture: 1—1. 5 cm horizontally. Moxibustion: 3—5 moxa cones or 5—10 minutes with warming moxibustion.

Naohu (GV 17) 脑户 [nǎo hù] A GV point, the confluence of GV and foot-*taiyang* meridian, also termed Zafeng, Huie, Helu. Location: At the midline of the posterior head, 4. 5 cm directly above Fengfu (GV DU 16) on the external occipital muscle. There is the left and right occipital artery and vein. The branch of the greate occipital nerve is distributed. Indications: Heaviness of the head, congestive eyes, yellow complexion, vertigo, facial pain, aphonia, stiffness in the neck, mania, epilepsy, goiter, bleeding of the tongue propper. Puncture: 1—1. 5 cm obiquely. Moxibustion: 3—5 minutes with warming moxibustion.

nature and man correspond to each other 天人相应 [tiān rén xiāng yīng] The tissues and structures, physiologic phenomena and pathologic changes of the human body correspond with the changes of the nature. In diagnosis and treatment, due attention must be paid to the influence of the evironmental factors, such as the climate of the four seasons on pathologic changes. The patient must be managed properly according to the seasons, environments and individual himself.

nazi method 纳子法 [nà zǐ fǎ] I.e., nazhi method.

nazhi method 纳支法 [nà zhī fǎ] One of the contents of needling techniques of midnight-noon ebb-flow, referring to combination of the twelve meridians with the twelve earthly branches, also called *na zi fa* because in the earthly branches 'zi' is the first one.

name of the acupuncture point 穴名 [xué míng] The name of the *shu* point. The nomenclature of the *shu* point is of certain significance. " ··· the points of which the meanings are near wood relate to the livers, those of which the meanings are near wind relate to the heart, those of which the meanings are near wind relate to the heart, those of which the mainings are near metal relate to the lungs, those of which the meaning of which are near water relate to the kindeys ··· " (Plain Questions)

najia method 纳甲法 [nà jiá fǎ] I. e., *na gan fa.*

Naoliao 臑窌 [nào liào] I. e., Naohui (TE 13).

Naoliao 臑交 [nào jiāo] An alternate term for Naohui (TE 13).

Naohui (TE 13) 臑会 [nào huì] A point of Triple Energizer Meridian of Hand-*shaoyang*. Location: At the inferior edge of the deltoid uscle, 9 cm directly below Jianliao (TE 14). Regional anatomy: Between the long head and the lateral head of the brachial triceps muscle. There is the middle accessory artery and vein. The dorsal cuntaeous nerve of the arm and the muscular branch of the radial nerve are distributed. The radial nerve is in the deeper. Indications: Pains in the shoulder and arm, goiter, scrofula, ocular trouble, swelling and pain in the scapular negion. Puncture: 2.5—3.5 cm perpendicularly. Moxibustion: 3—7 moxa cones or 5—15 minutes with warming moxibustion.

Nangdi 囊底 [náng dǐ] An extra point, located in the crossing crease posterior to the male's scrotum. Indications: Hernia of the small intestine, thoracalgia, closejaw, dampness and itch of the scrotum, testitis. Moxibustion: 3—5 moxa cones or 5—10 minutes with warming moxibustion.

nasal needling 鼻针 [bí zhēn] Referring to the therapeutic method to treat diseases by puncturing the specific points at the nasal region. It was seen in 1960. The points used are based on Miraculous Pivot, differring from the location of the facial needling, not

widely in clinic. Refer the appended Figure and Chart. (Fig 74)

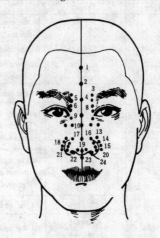

Fig 74

Neiyangchi 内阳池 [nèi yáng chí] An extra point, located 3 cm above the transverse crease of the posterior palm. Indications: Stomatitis, sore throat, tinea unguium, infantile convulaion. Puncture: 1—2 cm perpendicularly. Moxibustion: 5—7 moxa cone or 10—15 minutes with warming moxibustion.

Neiguan (PC 6) 内关 [nèi guān] A point of Pericadium Meridian of Hand-*jueyin*, the connecting point of the meridian it pertains to, one of eight confluential points, communicated with Connecting Vessel of Yin. Location: At the palmar side of the forearm, 6 cm above the transverse crease of the elbow between the long palmar muscle and the flexor radial muscle of wrist. Select it by making the hand supine. Regional anatomy: Passing through the superficial-deep flexor muscle of finger, reaching at the quadrate pronator muscle. There is the central artery and vein of forearm. The palmar interosseous artery and vein of forearm are in the deeper. The medial cutaneous nerve of forearm, the lateral cutaneous nerve of

Division	Name of	Location
Line	Point	
The 1st Line	Head-face	In the centre of forehead, i. e. , at the midpoint of the line connecting the midpoint between the two eyebrows and the front hair line.
	Throat	At the midpoint of the line connecting Toumian and Lung.
	Lung	At the midpoint of the line connecting the medial ends of the two eyebrows.
	Heart	At the midpoint of the line connecting the two inner canthi.
	Liver	Below the highest point of the nose bridge, at the crossing point of the line connecting the two zygomatic bones and the midline of the nose, the line connecting Heart and Spleen.
	Spleen	At the midline of the upper edge of Zhuntou at the end of the nose, at the end of the nose, at the midpoint of the line connecting heart and External Genitalia.
	Kidney	At the midpoint of the line connecting Spleen and External Genitalia.
	External Genitalia	At the tip of the end of nose.
	Testicle ovary	At the bilateral tip of nose, at the medial edge of ala nasi.
The 2nd Line	Gallbladder	Below the inner canthus, at the lateral spect of Liver.
	Stomach	Below Gallbladder, at the lateral aspect of Spleen.
	Small Intestine	At the upper 1/3 of ala nasi, below Stomach.
	Large Intestline	At the centre of ala nasi, below Small Intestline.
	Bladder	At the end of the wall of ala nasi, below Large Intestine.
The 3rd Line	Ear	At the end of the medial aspect of the eyebrow.
	Chest	Below Meilingu, above the supraorbiful fossa.
	Breast	Above the medial aspect of the inner canthus, below Chest.
	Neck -Back	Below the medial aspect of the inner canthus, below Breast.
	Lumbar Vertabra	At the medial aspect of zygoma, at the level with liver.
	Upper Line	At the level with the upper edge of *zhuntou* of the end of nose and Spleen, below Lumbar Vestebra.
	Hipbone-Femur	At the upper edge of ala nasi, below upper limb.
	Knee-tibia	At the lateral aspect of the midpoint of ala nasi, above the nasolabial groove, below Hipbone-Femur.
	Toe	Below Knee-Tibia, at the level with Bladder.

forearm, and the palmar cutaneous nerve of the central nerve are distributed. Indications: Palpitation, cardialgia, pains in the chest and hypochondrium, vomiting, hiccup, stomachache, malaria, nental confusion, mania, epilepsy, insomnia, pains in the elbow and arm, numb hands. Puncture: 1. 5—2 cm perpendicularly. Moxibustion: 3—5 moxa cones or 5—10 minutes with warming moxibustion.

Neizhiyin 内至阴 [nèi zhì yīn] An extra point. Located at the medial aspect of the small toe, approx. 0. 3 cm to the corner of the fingernail, opposite to Zhiyin (BL 67). Indications: Infantile convulsion, syncope. etc. Puncture: 0. 3—0. 6 cm perpendicularly, or pricking to cause a little bleeding with a triangular needle.

neifu 内辅 [nèi fǔ] The condye of the medial aspect of tibia.

Neijin 内筋 [nèi jīn] Referring to Jiaoxin (KI 8)

Neijingming 内睛明 [nèi jīng míng] An extra point. Located on the lacrimal carbuncle of the inner canthus. Indications: Congestive, swelling and painful eyes, blurred vision, atrophy of the visual nerve, retinal hemorrhage, conjunctivitis. Puncture: 1—2 cm along the wall of the medial side of the orbit with no twirling and thrusting and inserting the needle.

Neiting (ST 44) 内庭 [nèi tíng] A point of Stomach Meridian of Foot-*yangming*, the spring-like (water) point of the meridian it pertains to. Location: At the end of the transverse crease between the 2nd and 3rd toes at the midpoint between the metatarsophlangeal joint and the edge of foot. The medial cutsaneous nerve of the dorsal foot is distributed. Indications: Foothchache, deviated mouth, sore throat, epistaxis, abdominal pain, abdominal distension, diarrhea, dysentery, swelling and pain in the dorsal foot, febrile diseases. Puncture: 1—2 cm perpendicularly or obliquely. Moxibustion: 3—5 moxa cones or 5—10 minutes

with warming moxibustion.

needle handle pinched technique 夹持押手 [jiá chí yā shǒu] One of the ways to holding the needle during acupuncture. See *nie qu jin zhen*. (Fig 75)

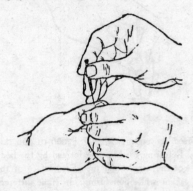

Fig 75

needle-lifted manipulation 提针法 [tí zhēn fǎ] I. e., *qi*-lifted manipulation.

needle and mugwort 针艾 [zhēn ài] The needle applied in acupuncture while mugwort is applied in moxibustion. So 'needle and hand' deals with the tool while 'puncture and moxibustion' deals with their application.

needle-insertion by finger press 指压进针 [zhǐ yā jìn zhēn] One of needle insertions. The procedure: Hold the needle with the right hand, pinch the root of needle with the thumb and index finger, touch the point directly with the middle and ring fingers, make the body of needle closely adhere to the lateral finger, and then insert the needle swiftly into the point by applying pressure of the thumb and index finger. It suits insertion of the short needle. It can be operated by a single hand with no need of pressing and holding with the left hand. (Fig 76)

needling at the affected area 散针法 [sǎn zhēn fǎ] Referring to selecting the point at the diseased area for acupuncture.

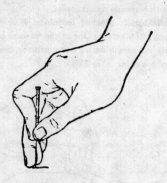

Fig 76

needling angle 针刺角度 [zhēn cì jiǎo dù] Referring to the angle formed by the body of the needle and the skin surface of the point while puncturing. In clinic different angles are selected for inserting the needle according to the anatomical characteristics of the punctured area and requirement of needling technique. For most of the perpendicular puncture (approx. 90°) is adopted. If the perpendicular puncture can not be adopted at certain locations, oblique puncture (30°—60°) or horizontal puncture (10°—20°) is adopted, as was said in "*Zhenjiu Neibian*," "Horizontal puncture can be done deep while perpendicular puncture should be suferficial." (Fig 77)

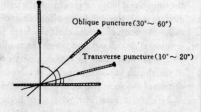

Perpendicular puncture(80°~ 100°)

Oblique puncture(30°~ 60°)

Transverse puncture(10°~ 20°)

Fig 77

needle box 针盒 [zhēn hé] An instrument for storing the needles, usually made of metal. Its inner part is divided into several square boxes for putting the needles of different norms, convenient for sterilization and application.

needle-insertion with a casing pipe 套管进针 [tào guǎn jìn zhēn] One of needle-insertions. To put a small vaccum tube pipe on the point vertically which is somewhat shorter than the filiform needle, then to put a filiform needle of which its handle is flat into the pipe, and swiftly tap the exposed handle of the needle to make the tip of the needle swiftly puncture into the subcutaneous region, and then to take off the pipe. This method can relieve pain caused by needle insertion.

needle-stored apparatus 藏针器 [cáng zhēn qì] In order to carry the needling instruments conveniently, it was usually wrapped with cloth or silk, called the 'needling bag' in ancient China. There was also the 'needling sylinder' made of metal. In contemporary times, there is the 'needle-stored wallet' made of the 'needle-stored tube' just like a pen, etc.

needle insertion by pinching up the skin 捏起进针 [niē qǔ jìn zhēn] One of the needle inserted methods. Also called *jia chi ya shou*. That is to pinch up the skin where the point is located with the thumb and index finger of the left hand and to puncture the point horizontally with the neddle held by the right hand. It is suitable for the location where the skin and muscle are superficial and thin and can not be punctured deep. E. g., Dicang (ST 4) at the corner of the mouth and Yintang (EX-HN 3) /between the two eyebrows. (Fig 78)

needle insertion by stretching the skin 撑开进针 [chēn kāi jìn zhēn] One of needle insertions, also called *shu zhang jia shou*. To make the skin proximal to the point tense with the left thumb and index finger, and to insert the needle into the point with the right needle held by the right. It suits the region where the skin is loose and needs to be punctured perpendicularly. E. g., various points at the abdomen. (Fig 79)

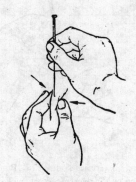

Fig 78

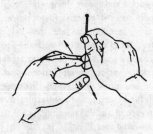

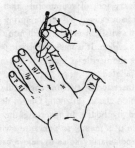

Fig 79

needle 针 [zhēn] It originally implied the tool used for sewing. Later it was called the medical needle. It can be known that from the construction of the characters and unearthed relics that there had been the bamboo needle first and then the metal needle. The needling tools recored in Internal Clas-

sic were divided into nine kinds, collectively called the nine needles. In 1968 four medical gold needles and five silver needles were excavated from Liu Shen's Tomb unearthed at Mancheng in Hebei Province, which are silmilar to the sharp prismatical needle, round needle and sharp round needle in ancient nine needles. Most of the modern needling tools are made of stainless steel, which are firm and smooth, not being easily erosive, fine in process, a few of them were made of gold and silver. Refer nine neeldes, gold needle, silver needle.

needle retention 置针 [zhì zhēn] I. e. , needle retention.

Newly-compiled Acupuncture Science 新编针灸学 [xīn biān zhēn jiǔ xué] A book compiled by Lu Zhijun. In this book the effects and technical operation of acupuncture were technical operation, and few common treatment of diseases were introduced. Publishe in 1950, played an active role in propopularizing acupuncture.

Neihuaiqianxia 内踝前下 [nèi huái qián xià] An extra point, located one transverse finger width, anterior to the midpoint of the inferior edge of the medial ankle.

Neihuaishangyicun 内踝上一寸 [nèi huái shàng yī cùn] Located on the posterior edge of the medial side of tibia, 3 cm above and at the level with the extra point, Neihuaijian. .

New Acupuncture Science 新针灸学 [xīn zhēn jiǔ xué] A book written by Zhu Lian, repsectively pulished by People's Publisher and People's Health Publisher in 1951 and 1954. It was republised by Guangxi People's Publisher after being revised. In this book acupuncture knowledge was prescribed in viewing with modern medicine. Including acupuncture techniques, acupuncture points and diseases and treatment. It brought out that the principle of treatment of diseases by acupuncture is mainly to regulate and irrigate the nervous system, particularly the function of cerebral cortex, and correspondingly classified acupuncture manipulations into the excitment and inhibition classifications of points and medical records.

needling stone 箴石 [zhēn shí] 1. Referring to *bian* (sharp) stone; 2. Respectively referring to the needle and stone.

Neck 颈 [jǐn] An ear point slightly at the medial side between Cervical Vertebra and Thoracic Vertebra.

Neihuaishang 内踝上 [nèi huái shàng] An extra point, Same with Neihuaijian in locatiion. "Administer moxibustion on Neihuaishang with 40 moxa cones for the tenson of the medial ankle in the case of wind affection." (Psesriptions Worth a Thousand Gold)

New eye point 新眼点 [xīn yǎn diǎn] An ear point, located among Esophagus, Cardia and Lung.

needling techniques 刺法 [cì fǎ] 1. Generally referring to the methods of acupuncture treatment; 2. A name of the ancient literature; 3. A book written by an unknown person, one volume, lost.

needle insertion by gripping the needle 夹持进针 [jiá chí jìn zhēn] One of the needle-inserted methods. After sterilizing the fingers, grip the lower segment of the needle with the thumb and index finger of the left hand, with the tip of the needle exposed to appoint the point, hold the handle of the needle with the right hand. Then, exert the power of the two hands in cooperation to swiftly insert the needle into the point. It is suitable for perpendicular puncture with a long needle. (Fig 80)

needling exercises 练针法 [liàn zhēn fǎ] Referring to some methods to practice acupuncture manipulations. Since a filiform needle is comparatively soft, it can not be applied skillfuly if one does not do some exercises. While learning the finger power needs to be exercised and the manipulation skillful. It can not be used in clinical treatment before one masters the skill. Common

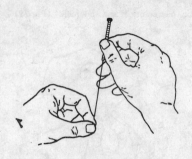

Fig 80

needling exercises are: 1. Practicing needling on the overlapped paper: To fold a piece of rough paper into a small square, then rotate and insert the needle into it repeatedly so as to exercise finger power. 2. Practicing needling on a cotton ball or a plaster: Wrap a small ball with the cotton, etc. or use a small piece of plaster repeatedly practice various manipulations, such as needle-insertion, lifting and thrusting the needle, and twirling the needle, etc. to reach the degree of skillful needling. (Fig 81)

needle-inserted tool 进针器 [jìn zhēn qì] An accessary tool of acupuncture that can relieve pain caused by needle spring apparatus to swiftly insert the needl into the cutaneous region. It is made of plastic or metal. After the needle is inserted, the needle is manipulated.

needle insertion by twirling the needle 捻转进针 [niǎn zhuǎn jìn zhēn] One of needle-inserted methods. In inserting the filiform needle it is mainly to puncture swiftly and perpendicularly, so as to relieve pain when it penetrates through the skin. If the body of the needle is soft (e. g., the filiform needle made of gold and silvrer) or the local skin is so hard that the needle can be inserted swiftly, the twirling method is used. The amplitude of rotation should be narrow and the body of the needle should be kept vertically straight and the action of the two hands should be cooperated, so as to benefit

needle insertion. (Fig 82)

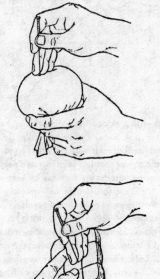

Fig 81

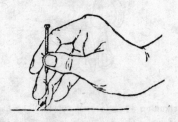

Fig 82

needle-inserted method 进针法 [jìn zhēn fǎ]
A method to insert the needle into the subcutaneous region. According to the depth,

the punctured location and the length of the
needle, the method to insert the needle can
be grasped flexibly. In general, it is required to penetrate through the skin quickly, so as to reduce painful sensation. After
penetrating the skin, needling sensation is
required to be explored carefully according
to needling techniques. The needle-inserted
techniques commonly used are the filiform
needle inserted technique, the needle-inserted technique by fingernail, pinching, the
technique by rotating the needle, the swift
needle-inserted technique by rotating the
needle, the swift needle-inserted technique,
the needle-inserted by holding the needle
with two fingers, the needle-inserted by
pinching the needle, the needle-inserted by
stretching the skin, etc. In addition, there
is the technique by adopting the needle-in-
sereted tube or the needle-springing instrument.

needle-inserted tube 进针管 [jìn zhēn guǎn]
An accessary tool of acupuncture. A small
round tube made of metal or plastic,
through which the filiform needle can pass.
Its length should be somewhat shorter than
that of the filiform needle. While using it,
press the tube in the point with the left
hand, spring the right hand, so as to make
the needle swiftly insert into the cutaneous
region. It can avoid painful sensation caused
by needle insertion. (Fig 83)

Neilongyan 内龙眼 [nèi lóng yán] An extra
point, i. e., Neixiyang (EX-LE 4). Located
on the edge of the medial side of the pattela
of the knee joint, in the depression at the
level with the inferior edge of patella, one
transverse finger width to the edge of the
medial side of the patella ligament. Indication: Inflammation of the knee. Puncture:
1. 5—2 cm perpendicularly. Moxibustion:
3—5 moxa cones or 5—10 minutes with
warming moxibustion.

needle insertion with a pressing hand 爪切押
手 [zǎo qiè yá shǒu] One of the ways of
pressing hand during acupuncture. That is

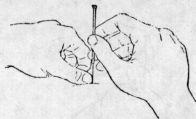

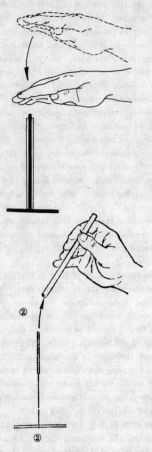

Fig 83

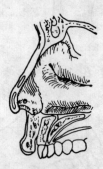

Fig 84

hole with a dry cotton ball with one hand, to turn the body of the needle slightly and gently withdraw it with the other hand. As to the needle that has been inserted deeper, it can be withdrawn segment by segment. Do not do it too swiftly and violently lest hemorrhage and pain should result.

Neiyingxiang 内迎香 [nèi yíng xiāng] An extra point, located at the mucoid membrance of the lateral side of the mediosuperior nostril. Indications: Congestive, swelling and painful eyes, itch and stuffiness of nose, swelling and sore throat, sunstroke, headache, pricking to cause little bleeding. (Fig 85)

Fig 85

to use the finger of one hand, press the point and the other hand (puncturing hand) to hold the needle and by making the tip of the needle adhere the edge of the finger to insert it into the point. (Fig 84)

needle-withdrawn technique 出针法 [chū zhēn fǎ] A technique to withdraw the inserted needle from the point, also termed *qizhen*, *bazhen*, *paizhen*, and *fazhen*. In general, to press the skin by the needling

Neikunlun 内昆仑 [nèi kūn lún] 1. I. e., Taiyuan (KI 3); 2. Xiakunlun, the extra point. "Xiakunlun is also called Neikunlun, located 3 cm below the lateral ankle. "(Prescriptions of Peaceful Holy Benevolence)

needle retention 留针 [liú zhēn] After inserting the needle into the point, the duration of retaining the needle is decided according to the characteristics of the disease condition and way of needling. While the filiform needle is retained, the needle can be administered intermittently or warming needling or electroacupuncture can be used. According to Miracutous Pivot it can be used in treating febrile or cold diseases.

Nephritis point 肾炎点 [shèn yān diǎn] An ear point located inferolateral to Clavicle.

Neihuaijian 内踝尖 [nèi huái jiān] An extra point, also termed Huaijian. Located at the highest point of the medial ankle. Indications: Spasm, foot *qi*, toothache, etc.

nianshou 年寿 [nián shòu] The middle segment of the nose bridge between the root of tongue and the end of nose, also called *nianshang, shoushang.*

nianying **moxa-stick** 捻盈药条 [niǎn yíng yào tiáo] A kind of moxa stick. Made of moxa

floss mixed with cinnamon twig, Sichuan aconite root, realgar, orange peel, sandawood, red sage root, nutgrass flatsedge rhizome, dahurian anqelica root, cablin, pacholi, dalbergia wood, galangal zhizome.

nine indications 九宜 [jiǔ yí] The application of the nine needles has their appropriate scale according to their special shapes.

Nine *Ling* 九灵 [jiǔ líng] I. e., Miraculous Pivot.

nine needles 九针 [jiǔ zhēn] The needles of nine different varieties used by ancient acupuncturists. Their names are as follows: the arrowhead needle, round needle, blunt needle, sharp needle, three-edged needle, sword-like needle, sharp needle, round needle, filiform needle, long needle and large needle. The round needle and the blund needle can be used for massage on the body surface and the sword-like one for cutting to evacuate pus. (Fig 86)

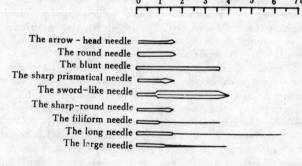

Fig 86

nine yang revigorating points 回阳九针穴 [huí yáng jiǔ zhēn xué] The nine first-aid points that have the action of reviving yang, I. e., Yamen (GV 15), Laogong (PC 8), Sanyinjiao (BL 22), Yongquan (KI 1), Taixi (KI 3), Zhongwan (CV 12), Huantiao (GB 30), Sanli (ST 36) and Hegu (LI 4). Clinically used for treating syncope, fainting, cold limbs, hidden pulse, weakness of yang that collapse would oc-

cur, closejaw and aphasia.

Niaoxue 尿血 [niào xuè] An extra point. Located 15 cm lateral to the spinal process of the 7th thoracic vertebra. Indication: Hematuria. Puncture: 1.5—3 cm obliquely. Moxibustion: 3—5 moxa cones or 5—10 minutes with warming nedelling.

Niaobao 尿胞 [niào bāo] An alternate term for Quguduan.

nine-six reinforcing-reducing 九六补泻 [jiǔ

liù bǔ xiè] The reinforcing-reducing manipulation in association with the numbers of nine and six.

nineth vertebra 第九椎 [dì jiǔ zhuī] Referring to the nineth thoracic vertebra.

Nizhu 逆注 [nì zhù] An alternate term for Wenliu (LI 7).

nienao 颞颥 [niè nào] 1. Mainly referring to the upper part of the temporal hair; 2. An alternate term for Naokong (GB 19); 3. Nienao, an extra point, located at the midpoint of the line connecting the lateral end of the eyebrow and the outer canthus. Indications: Seasonal pathogenic *qi*, cold injury, headache, vertigo, eye trouble, facial paralysis. Puncture: 1—1.5 cm horizontally.

nine needlings 九刺 [jiǔ cì] The nine ancient acupuncture techniques, viz., *shu*-point puncture, distant puncture, meridian puncture, collateral-meridian puncture, crack puncture, evacuation pouncture, shallow puncture, contralateral puncture and fire puncture. *Shu*-point puncture (selecting the five-*shu* and back-*shu* points), distant puncture (selecting the points in the lower part of the body to treat the disease in the upper), meridian puncture (puncture small blood vessels), crack puncture (puncture the muscle), evacuation puncture (evacuating pus), shallow puncture (puncture the skin), contralateral puncture (selecting the points in a cross way), fire puncture (puncture after burning the needle).

Niwangong 泥丸宫 [ní wán gōng] 1. Referring to the cerebral region; 2. Referring to Baihui (GV 20).

non-suppurative moxibustion 非化脓灸 [fēi huà nóng jiǔ] Generally referring to warm-heat moxibustion, also including moxibustion with moxa cone of which a small amount of little moxa cone is used to do moxibustion till a red area appears locally but without scorching injury.

non-heat moxibustion 无热灸 [wú rè jiǔ] I. e., the drug-applied blistering technique.

non-scar moxibustion 无瘢痕灸 [wú bān héng jiǔ] I. e., non-suppuration moxibustion. The moxibustion technique that there is no suppuration and ulceration and no scar is left after moxibustion. Generally referring to warm-heat moxibustion.

nose, the opening for the lungs 肺开窍于鼻 [fèi kāi qiào yí bí] The lungs are concerned with breathing, and the nose is the portal for respiration. Hence, the nose is the opening of the lungs.

norm of filiform needle 毫针规格 [háo zhēn guī gé] The modern filiform needle is usually made of stainless steel, also of gold, silver or other high-alloy steel. It consists of the five portions: The part held by the hand is called the handle, which is winded with copper wire (silver-plated) or aluminium (oxidized). The shape varies with the dragon-winded handle, the budder shandle, (circling handle), the flat handle and tube-like handle; The upper end of the handle is called the tail of needle; The sharp part of the anterior end of the needle is called the tip of needle, shaped as a pine leave; The part between the tip and the handle is called the body; The connective part between the body and handle is called the root. The length of the needle varies in 15 mm, the old norm, 25 mm, 40 mm, 50 mm, 65 mm, 75 mm, 100 mm, 125 mm, and 150 mm, etc. The diameter varies in 0.45 mm (No 26), 0.42 mm (No 27), 0.38 mm (No 28), 0.34 mm (No 29), 0.32 mm (No 30), 0.30 mm (No 31), 0.28 mm (No 32), 0.23 mm (No 34), 0.20 mm (No 36). (Fig 87)

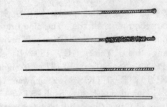

Fig 87

Notes to Meridians 经络笺注 [jīng luò qiān

zhù] A book compiled by Wei Qinpu in Ming Dynasty (1368—1644). It contains two volumes, and the body shape was taken as its guide line. The whole body is divided into 66 guidelines from head to foot.

Nuxi 女膝 [nǚ xī] An extra point, also termed 女须. Location: At the midpoint of the heel bone at the calcaneus. Indications: Vomitting, diarrhea and charley horse, osteomyelitis of the maxillary bone, gigivitis, fright with palpitation. Puncture: 1 cm perpendicularly. Moxibustion: 3—7 moxa cones or 5—15 minutes with warming moxibustion. (Fig 88)

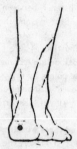

Fig 88

nutritional *qi* 营气 [yíng qì] Refined *qi* derived from cereals circulates in the meridians, and has the nourishing action on the whole body.

nutrition, defence, *qi* and blood 营卫气血 [yíng wèi qì xuè] A collective term for nutrients, defense, *qi* and blood.

needle-twirled manipulation 捻法 [niǎn fǎ] A needling manipulation by twirling the needle forward and backword. (Fig 89)

***nu* manipulation** 努法 [nǔ fǎ] Originally it refers that before administering acupuncture the doctor flicks the point to promote fullness and flourishing of *qi* and blood. Now it is called '*nu*' that the body of the needle is laterally pressed by the doctor's middle finger during administering acupuncture. (Fig 90)

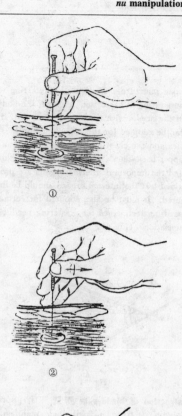

Fig 89

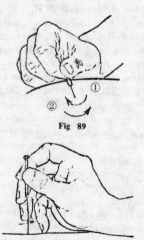

Fig 90

O

oblique puncture 斜刺 [xié cì] Referring to puncturing at a 30°—60° angle of the body of the needle with the skin of the point. It can be adopted for the area with thin muscles and the chest and hypochondrium and upper back etc., where the muscle is thin and the important internal organs are proximal lest the internal organs should be injured. It must be also adopted for certain needling techniques for mastering needling sensation. (Fig 91)

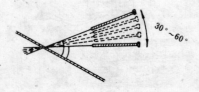

Fig 91

obstruction of bladder *qi* 膀胱气闭 [páng guāng qì bì] The pathologic manifestations of distension and fullness of hypogastrium, dysuria or uroschesis as a result of impairment functions of the bladder.

obstruction of the lungs by phlegm and dampness 痰湿阻肺 [tán shì zhǔ fèi] The pathologic manifestations due to accumulation and retention of pathogenic dampness and phlegm in the lungs. The main symptoms are fever, cough with copious whitish sputum, fullness and distress of chest and hypochondrium, rough or whitish and slippery coating of tongue, stringy and smooth pulse, etc.

Occiput 枕 [zhěn] An ear point at the edge of the cartillege of the antitragus where the upper zone is opposite to Brain Spot.

occipital bone 枕骨 [zhěn gǔ] Same as occi-

pitl bone in anatomy.

ocular connection 眼系 [yǎn xì] Also called *mu xi*, referring to the tissue connecting with the posterior eye and brain.

obstruction of the lungs by phlegm 痰阻肺络 [tán zhǔ fèi luò] The pathologic manifestations due to retention of phlegm and fluids in the lungs. The major symptoms are cough, dyspnea, copious sputum, etc.

ocular *cun* 目寸 [mù cùn] One of the propertional measuements of selecting the extra point. The distance between the patient's inner corner of the eye and the outer is taken as 3 cm.

oil-rinsed moxibustion 油捻灸 [yóu niǎn jiǔ] A kind of moxibustion technique. To moxibustion at the points by using a twisted paper that is rinsed with plant oil and ignited.

one yin 一阴 [yī yīn] Referring to *jueyin* meridian.

one insertion and three withdrawals 一进三退 [yī jìn sān tuì] To insert the needle directly to the deep stratum, then withdraw it gradually from the deep to the middle and then to the superficial. It can be administered repeatedly. (Fig 92)

one yang 一阳 [yī yáng] Referring to *shaoyang* meridian.

onion-interposing moxibustion 隔葱灸 [gé chōng jiǔ] A kind of indirect moxibustion. 1. To smash the onion white into small pieces and put them on the point at the abdomen, then to do moxibustion by putting a moxa cone on it. Used for treating collapse, abdominal distension, abdominal pain due to cold affection, abnormal micturition; 2. To bound a bunch of onion white with a thread, which is 6 cm in length, then put it vertically on the point, and then put a moxa cone on the top of it to do moxibustion, used for treating carbuncle and rheumatic pain.

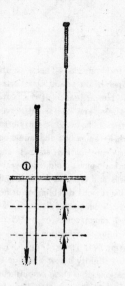

Fig 92

open moxibustion 明灸 [míng jiǔ] I. e. , direct moxibustion.

opening, closing and pivoting 开阖枢 [kāi hé shū] See *guan he shu*.

opening-closing reinforcing-reducing 开阖补泻 [kāi hé bǔ xiè] One of reinforcing-reducing manipulations in acupuncture. Reinforcing and reducing manipulations are differentiated by opening or closing (by kneading) the needling holes while withdrawing the inserted needle.

Origin of Acupuncture 针灸逢原 [zhēn jiǔ féng yuán] A book written by Li Xuechuan in Qing Dynasty (1644—1911), 6 volumes. The 1st and 2nd volumes select the doctrines of Internal Classic concerning acupuncture; The 3rd collects acupuncture treatments and rhythmed articles of various schools in succeeding dynasties, the 4th deals with a textual study on the meridian points, records 361 meridian points and 96 extra points, the 5th and 6th contain the individual treatment of diseases. It is simple and direct in viewpoints, and was completed in 1815.

osseous blockage 骨痹 [gǔ bì] A blockage syndrome characterized with the symptoms of pain in the bones, heavy feeling and lameness of the body and limbs.

out of the fingernail 去爪 [qù zhǎo] The name of needling technique. Refferring to applying the *shu* points at the lumbar spine and points of four limbs.

Ovary 卵巢 [luǎn cáo] An ear point located anterinferior to the interior cortex.

Outer abdomen 腹外 [fù wài] An ear point at the lateral side of the antihelix at the level with Kidney.

outer canthus 目外眦 [mù wài zì] Referring to the outer corner of the eye.

outer canthus 目锐眦 [mù ruì zì] Referring to the outer corner of the eye.

P

palpation and feeling pulse 切诊 [qiè zhěn]
The technique to feel the pulse of the radial
artery proximal to the carpal joints, or to
examine other parts of the body by palpation with the tips of the fingers.

palpation 触诊 [chù zhěn] To examine the
body excluding pulse by touching or com-
pression with the finger tips.

painful point taken as a _shu_ point 以痛为俞
[yǐ tòng wéi shū] A term used in selecting
the point. '_Tong_' here refers to disease or
tenderness, that is to take the affected area
or pathological reactive point as the _shu_
point to treat disease.

pain in the face 面痛 [miàn tòng] Referring
to contraction and pain of the cheek, usually occurring unilaterally frequently seen in
people at the age of over 60.

palpitation 心悸 [xīn jì] Self consciousness
of the unpleasant heartbeat, usually proxismal in occurrence, and induced by emotional disturbance or overexertion.

Pancreas-gallbladder 胰胆 [yí dǎn] An ear
point between Liver and Kidney.

pairing the opposites 对待 [duì dài] The
classifying method to simplify the multitute
pulse by pairing the opposites. For instance, floating and sinking, slow and
rapid, smooth (slippery) and rough, and de-
fcienct and substantive. These eight paired
pulses are regarded as guides to recognize
the nature of a disease, being exterior or interior, cold or hot, deficient or substantive,
and following or reverse (favourable or un-
favorable).

Pangguangshu (BL 28) 膀胱俞 [páng guāng
shū] A point of Bladder Meridian of foot-
taiyang, the back _shu_ point of the bladder.
Location: At the posterior foramen of the
2nd sacrum, 4.5 cm lateral to the midline
of the sacral region. Regional anatomy: Between the iliospinal muscle and the greatest

gluteal muscle. There is the posterior
branch of the lateral sacral artery and vein.
The lateral branch of the posterior branch
of th 1st and 2nd sacral nerves are distributed. Indications: Scanty urine, spermatorrhea, enuresis, abdominal pain and diarrhea, constipation, stiffness and pain in the
lumbar spine, cold and weakness of the
knees and feet, destension and pain in the
pubic region, dribbling of urine. Puncture:
3—4.5 cm perpendicularly. Moxibustion:
3—7 moxa cones or 5—15 minutes with
warming moxibustion.

Pangting 旁廷 [páng tíng] An extra point located slightly below Yuanyue (GB 22). Indications: Full chest, vomiting and asthmatic breath, dry throat and painful hypochondrium. Puncture: 1—1.5 cm obliquely
Moxibustion: 3—5 moxa cones or 5—10
minutes with warming moxibustion.

Pangting 旁庭 [páng tíng] I.e., 旁廷.

Pancreasitis point 胰腺炎点 [yí xiàn yán
diǎn] An ear point at the lower 2/3 of
Dueodnum and Pancreas-Gallbladder.

paper-interposing moxibustion 隔纸灸 [gé
zhǐ jiǔ] A kind of indirect moxibustion.

paste of prepared aconite root 附子饼 [fù zǐ
bǐng] A kind of drug paste of moxibustion. Refer moxibustion with prepared a-
conite root.

**pai zhen** 排针 [pái zhēn] 1. Withdrawing the
needle; 2. The needling technique with multiple needles that tense and arranged in a
row.

Parotid gland 腮腺 [sāi xiàn] An ear point at
the highest point of the middle zone.

Palate 上腭 [shàng é] An ear point located at
the lower 1/4 of the lateral line of Zone₂.

PC points 手厥阴心包经穴 [shǒu jué yīn xīn
bāo jīng xué] According to Systematic
Classic, they are Tianchi (PC 1), Tianquan
(PC 2), Quze (PC 3) (sea-like), Ximen

(PC 4) (gap-like), Jianshi (PC 5) (river-like), Neiguan (PC 6) (connecting), Daling (PC 7) (stream-like), Laogong (PC 8) (spring-like), Zhongchong (PC 9) (well-like), 9 in total. There is also Jueyinshu (BL 14), pertaining to foot-*taiyang* meridian and anterior-referred point, Danzhong (CV, DU 17) pertaining to CV.

PC diseases 手厥阴心包经病 [shǒu jué yīn xīn bāo jīng bìng] They are mainly palpitation, anxiety, cardialgia, distension and fullness in the chest and hypochondrium, flushed face, abnormall laugh, discomfort at the area where the meridian passes through.

Pelvis 盆腔 [pén qiāng] An ear point at the crossing point of the upper anti-helix and the lower anti-helix.

Pericardium Meridian of Hand-*jueyin* (PC) 手厥阴心包经 [shǒu jué yīn xīn bāo jīng] One of the twelve meridians. The coures: Starting from the chest, emerging and joining the pericardium, passing through the diaphragm and going over the upper, middle and lower energizers and connecting with triple energizer. The branch emerges at the hypochondriac region along the inner chest, ascending from the lateral nipple to reach at the inferior axilla, running along the medial side of the upper arm, running between hand-*taiyin* and hand-*shaoyin* meridians, entering into the elbow, descenging to the forearm, going between the radial flexor muscle of wrist and long palmar muscle, entering into the palm, running along the medial edge of the radial side of the middle finger, and emerging from the tip of the middle finger. One branch splits from the palm, runs along the ring finger and emerges from it. (connects with Triple Energizer Meridian of Hand-*shaoyang*.)

penetrating puncture 透刺 [tòu cì] To puncture the point according to certain direction to penetrate through certain point or region. The opposite points at the lateral aspect of the four imbs or the anterior and posterior aspects of the four llimbs can be penertrated through. The points at the upper and lower parts of various portions or the proximal (anterior, posterior) can be penetrated obliquely or horizontally. E. g. , puncture from Neiguan (PC 6) through Waiguan (TE 5), puncture from Yanglingquan (GB 34) through Yinlingquan (SP 9), etc. , which are straight deep penetrating methods.

pericardium meridian of hand-*jueyin* 心主手厥阴之脉 [xīn zhǔ shǒu jué yīn zhī mài] The original name of Pericadrdium Meridian of Hand-*jueyin*.

pericardium 心包 [xīn bāo] The external membrane of the heart. The hand-*jueyin* meridian pertains to the "pericardium" while the hand-*shaoyang* meridian "distributes itself over the pericardium."

perpendicular puncture 直刺 [zhí cì] To puncture the point with the body of the needle formed a 90° angle with the skin surface of the point. It suits the points at the waist, hip, abdomen and four limbs where the muscles are thicker. As the point where the muscle is thinner and approaches the important region, perpendicular puncture must not be done deep but oblique or horizontal puncture can be adopted. (Fig 93)

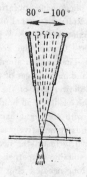

80° − 100°

Fig 93

peripheral arthritis 漏肩风 [lòu jiān fēng]

Also termed *jian nizhen*. The patients suffering from it are usually about 50 years old. It is mainly manifested as soreness, heaviness and pain of the unilateral or bilateral shoulder joints and limited movement.

Peaceful Holy Benevolent Prescriptions 太平圣惠方 [tài píng shèn huì fāng] A medical book compiled by Wang Huaiyin in Song Dynasty (960—1279), 100 volumes, accomplished in 992 A. D. , *Mingtang* Moxibustion Classic and Infantile *Mingtang* Moxibustion Classic were recorded in the 100th volumes.

Phyllostachys nigra (Lodd.) 竹茹 [zhú rú] One of materials used in moxibustion. The shin of bamboo.

'phoenix extends its wings' 凤凰展翅 [fèng huáng zhǎn cì] An acupuncture manipulation, same as flying manipulation. Contrary to the hungry horse shakes the bell. While twirling the needle, take off the finger immediately after twirling the needle just like the phonix's extending its wings. It pertains to reducing manipulation because the needle turns to left while it is twirled, and turns right while it is rotated.

phenomenon of propagated sensation along the meridian (PSM) 循经感传现象 [xún jīng gǎn chuán xiàn xiàng] Some special propagated phenomena appearing along the meridians. Refer meridianal phenomema.

pinching insertion of needle 夹持进针 [jiá chí jìn zhēn] One of the needle-inserted techniques. That is after sterilization, use the thumb and index finger of the left hand to pinch the lower part of the needle with the tip of the needle, and hold the shift of the needle with the right hand and make the two hands cooperatively simultaneously, then swiftly insert the needle into the point. It is suitable for perpendicular puncture of the long needle. (Fig 94)

Pingyi 平翳 [píng yì] I. e. , Pingyi (屏翳).

Pingyi 屏翳 [píng yì] An alternate term for Huiyin (CV 11).

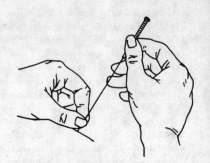

Fig 94

Pianjian 偏肩 [piān jiān] An alternate term for Jianyu (LI 15).

Piangu 偏骨 [piān gǔ] An alternate term for Jianyu (LI 15).

pinching manipulation 掐法 [qiā fǎ] To press the skin with the fingernail while needling.

Piba 琵琶 [pí bā] An extra point approx. at the anterior edge of the lateral side of the clavicular bone, in the depression at the superior edge of the coracoid process. Indications: Piain in the shoulder, inability of the upper limb to raise. Puncture: 1—1. 5 cm perpendicularly. Moxibustion: 5 moxa cones or 5—10 minutes with warming moxibustion.

pharynx 咽 [yān] Same as in Western medicine.

phlegm 痰 [tán] 1. The secretion of the respiratory tract; 2. The pathologic mucoid or solid substance collected in some diseased organs or tissues; 3. A concept of pathogenesis of certain symptoms, such as mania, epilepy, coma, dizziness, distress of the chest, vomiting, etc. , as related to phlegm.

phlegm and excess exudate 痰饮 [tán yǐn] 1. In a broad sense, it is a general term for diseases caused by disturbance of water metabolism and accumulation of fluids in the body cavity and extremities, etc. , and 2, in a narrow sense, it is one of *shuiyin* diseases, a disease of water retention in the

stomach and intestines. It is mainly mani-
feted as splashing sound in the upper abdomen with watery vomitus or diarrhea,
epigastric distension which is temporarily
slightly relieved after moving the howels
but recurs immediately and marked borborygmus, etc.

phlegm-damp 痰湿 [tán shí] 1. Dampness
and turbid pathognens, after prolonged stay
in the body may become phlegm. Since they
are sometimes hard to be distinguished
from each other, they are collectively called
phlegm-dampness. 2. The phlegm-dampness syndrome. The clinical manifestations
are large amounts of thin whitish suputm,
distress of the chest, nausea, asthmatic
cough, whitish glossy or slippery glossy
coating of tongue, etc.

Pianli (LI 6) 偏历 [piān lì] A point of Large
Intestine Meridian of Hand-*yangming*, the
connecting point of the meridian. Location:
At the radial side of the dorsal forearm, on
the line connecting Yangxi (LI 5) and
Quchi (LI 11), 9 cm above Yangxi (LI 5)
or at the end of the middle finger with *hukou* of the two hand crossed. Regional anatomy: Between the radial extensor muscle of
wrist and the long adductor muscle of
thumb. There is the cephalic vein at the radial side. There is the lateral cutaneous
nerve of the forearm and the superficial
branch of the radial nerve at the ulnar side.
There is the dorsal cutaneous nerve of the
forearm and the dorsal nerve of interosseous nerve of the forearm. Indications: Epistaxis, congestive eyes, tinnitus,
deafness, deviated mouth and eyes, sore
throat, pains in the shoulder, elbow and
wrist, edema, epilepsy. Puncture: 1.5—
2.5 cm perpendicularly. Moxibustion: 3—
5 moxa cones or 5—10 minutes with warming moxibustion.

**planning treatment in accordance with syn-
drome differentiation** 辨证论治 [biàn
zhèng lùn zhì] In traditional Chinese
medicine, *bianzheng* means that the pa-

tients, symptoms and signs are analyzed
and summaried in order to identity the etiology, the location of the lesion, the pathologic changes and the body condition, etc.
Lunzhi menas that a proper therapeutic
program is determined according to the result of the diagnosis. *Bianzheng* is the way
of traditional Chinese medicine to analyze
and recognize diseases while *lunzhi*, to
forulate a definitive therapeutic program,
for instance, at the initial stage of a disease, the patient may experience fever and
chills, no sweating, headache, general
ache, no thirst, thin whitish coating of
tongue, supericial and tense pulse, etc.
These symptoms and signs may be recognized as the exterior symptome of wind and
cold according to traditional Chinese
medicine. Hence, the therapeutic principle
of relieving such symptoms is to apply di-
aphoretics of pungent and hot nature. This
is the general principle of planning treatment in accordance with syndrome differentiation.

plum needle 梅花针 [méi huā zhēn] A kind
of cutaneous needle. Its head is formed by
the five thready needles, used to superifi-
cally puncture the skin. Refer cutaneous
needle.

Pigen 痞根 [pǐ gēn] An extra point, located
9—15 lateral to Xuanshu (GV 5). There is
the branch of the lumbar artery, the posteriror branch of the waist and the thoraco-
back nerve. Indications: Abdominal masses, lumbago, stomachache, enlargement of
the liver and spleen, hepatitis, gastritis, enteritis, renoptosis. Puncture: 1.5—3 cm
perpendicularly. Moxibustion: 5—7 moxa
cones or 10—15 minutes with warming
moxibustion.

Pingchuan 平喘 [píng chuǎn] An ear point
appox. 0.2 mm anteroinferior to the parotid
gland.

Pishe 脾舍 [pí shè] An alternate term for
Diji (SP 8).

Pishu (BL 20) 脾俞 [pí shū] A point of Bladder Meridian of Foot-*taiyin*, the back *shu* point of the spleen. Location: 4. 5 cm lateral to the Jizhong (GV 6) between the spinal processes of the 11th and 12th thoracic vertebrae. Regional anatomy: Between the broadest muscle of back and the longgest muscle and the interiliocostal muscle. There is the medial branch of the posterior lateral branch of the 11th intercostal artery and vein. The medial cutaneeous branch of the posterior branch of the 11th thoracic nerve is distributed. The lateral branch of the posterior branch of the 11th thoracic nerve is in the deeper. Indications: Hypochondriac pain, distension, jaundice, vomiting, diarrhea, dysentery, hematuria, indigestion, edema, pain in the back. Puncture: 1. 5—2. 5 cm obliquely (It is not advisable to puncture deep). Moxibustion: 5—7 moxa cones or 10—20 minutes with warming moxibustion.

Plain Questions 素问 [sù wèn] A medical book collectively called Internal Classic together with Miraculous Pivot, the earliest work of traditional Chinese medicine science. The original contains 9 volumes, the 7th volume had been lost. Plain Questions wroted by Wang Bin contains 81 chapters, 24 volumes in total, in which yin-yang, visceral manifestations, meridians and their collateral meridians, etiology, pathogenesis, diagnostics, general rules for treament, etc. , were expounded. Corresponding with Miraculaus Pivot, many of the chapters deal with acupuncture treatment of diseases, prohibitions in application of the points, etc. It is an important reference book for study on acupuncture moxibustion.

point-combined method 配穴法 [pèi xué fǎ] A method to combine the points for acupunture treatment. In clinic it can be divided into superficial-deep point-combination, yin-yang point-combination, upper-lower point-combination, anterior-posterior point-combination, left-right point combination, distal-proximal point combination,

etc. In ancient litereatures there is also the host-guest and source-connecting point combination, eight-meridians and eight-points combination, maternal offspring reinforcing-reducing, reducing-south and reinforcing-north. In addition, midnight-noon ebb-flow, eight miraculous turtle techniques are special point-combinations according to time.

point selection from the proximal segment 近节段取穴 [jìn jié duàn qǔ xué] A classification of the point-selected methods. It refers that the point selected in clinical treatment and acupuncture anesthsia and the trouble or the location of the operation are controlled by the same or proximal segement of the spinal cord. Local selection of the point called usually and proximal selection of the point are classified into this classification. Another example, selection of the point at the upper limb for the trouble of the thoracic cavity or the operation and selection of the points at the lower limb for the trouble of the abdominal cavity or the operation are also classified into this classification. In acupuncture anesthesia, Quanliao (SI 18) is selected for the craniocerebral operation, Futu (LI 18) is selected for the thyroidectomy, Hegu (LI 4) and Neiguan(PC 6) are selected for the cervical and thoracic operations. (Fig 95)

points of the fourteen meridians 十四经穴 [shí sì jīng xué] The *shu* points of the fourteen meridians, briefly called the meridian points. The single points on the meridian (CV and GV) are 49, and double ones on the bilateral sides (the twelve meridians) are 300, 349 in total. They were gradually added in the latter works of acupuncture and moxibustion. According to Origin of Acupuncture, the unilateral points on the midline were 52, the bilateral 309, 361 in total. They are respectively 28 of GV, 24 of CV, 11 of the Lung Meridian, 9 of Pericardium Meridian, 9 of Heart Meridian, 20 of Large Intestine Meridian, 23 of

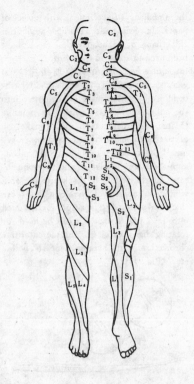

Fig 95

Triple Energizer Meridian, 19 of Small Intestine Meridian, 45 of Stomach Meridian, 44 of Gallbladder Meiridian, 67 of Bladder Meridian, 21 of Spleen Meridian, 14 of Liver Meridian, and 27 of Kidney Meridian.

porcelain needle 陶针 [táo zhēn] To puncture with a piece of porcelain in ancient China. At precent there is still the application of porcelain needle in the Zhuang people in China. In general, the pieces of porcelain are washed and broken into small pieces and respectively used according to different sharpness. The rough one can be used for blood letting by heavy puncture; The thinner one for children. In general, the moderate one is usually taken.

porcelain needle 陶瓷针 [táo cí zhēn] In ancient China, the pieces of porcelain were used for puncture.

points of taiyang meridian selected for acute diseases 暴病者取之太阳 [bào bìng zhě qǔ zhī tài yáng] One of the therapeutic principles in Internal Classic. That is to treat acute diseases by selecting the points at the *taiyang* meridians.

postpartum anemic fainting 产后眩晕 [cǎn hòu xuán yūn] Sudden conset of dizziness and vertigo, unable to sit up or epigastric distress, nausea and vomitting or dyspnea with copious sputum, or even, mutual confusion, lockjaw, unconsciousness, and other critical postpartum symptoms.

polio 小儿麻痹证 [xiǎo ér má bì zhèng] An infectious disease caused by seasonal pathogens, clinically similar to common cold, e. g., fever, vomiting, diarrhea, pain in limbs, then paralysis of limbs. At the late stage muscular atrophy and malformation of the joints can be seen.

postpartum abdominal pain 产后腹痛 [cǎn hòu fù tòng] After delivery the parturient suffers from pain in the lower abdomen.

points of three portions 三部穴 [sān bù xué] Referring to Dabao (SP 21), Tianshu (ST 25) and Diji (SP 8).

point selection according to the muscle group 按肌群取穴 [àn jī qún qǔ xué] One of point-selected methods to select the point at the muscle or muscle group where the pathological change occurs. Often used for muscular paralysis of the hip muscle. Futu (ST 32) is selected for paralysis of the quadriceps muscle of thigh.

point-selected method 选穴法 [xuǎn xué fǎ] A method to select the point in clinical treatment, also called *qǔ xué fǎ*.

point magnetic therapy 穴位磁疗法 [xué wèi cí liáo fǎ] A therapy by making use of the action of the magnetic object or the point to treat diseases. Nowadays, the quiet magnectic therapy, motion magnetic therapy, and electric therapy are mainly used. In quiet magnectic therapy, the permanency of the magentic field is mainly to dress the magnetics on the point. The moving of the magnetic field vary along with the change of time, so it must be spiralled. The electric magnetic therpay is mainly to apply the low-frequent alternately-changing magnetic field, generated by magnetic materials. In general, the strength of the magnetic field is 100—4,000G. As to the way of dressing is to fix the magnetic object on the point, usually used for treating hypertention, sprains, thecal cyst, etc. The rotating therapy is to carry on treatment by putting the magnetic object on the surface of the point to rub and rotate, usually used for treating headache, herpes zoster, etc. The electric magnetic therapy is to select the appropriate magnetic head and put it on the point, usually used for bronchitis, peumonia, lumbar muscle strain, arthritis, etc. It must not be used for the one who is hypersensitive to magnetic therapy or has the severe side-effects, such as fatigue, amnesia, insomnia, etc. It is prohibited to use it at the pregnant woman's lower abdomen, or at the anterior cardiac region of the infant and of the patient with severe heart disease.

point-absorbed tool 穴位吸引器 [xué wèi xī yǐn qì] A kind of the cupping tool that can absorb air. It is made of the rubberized ball and the specially-made glass cup of which there is an opening at its bottom. The two parts are connected with a rubberized tube. To form the negatice pressure (approx. 240 mm) by pinching the rubberized ball with the hand to absorb the air within the cup, so as to use it in air-absorbed cupping technique.

point-cold stimulation therapy 穴位冷激法 [xué wèi lěng jí fǎ] A therapeutic method by giving the point cold stimulation. "For obstruction of defecation and micturition, fill in the umbilicus with alum powder, then drip water on to it. The patient may feel cold penetrating into the abdomen. The illness will be spontaneously cured. In case the umbilicus is flat, circle it with a piece of paper. In recent years, a proper amount of chloethane or carbondioxide, etc., have been used to spray to the point.

point suture embedment 穴位埋线法 [xué wèi mái xiàn fǎ] To treat disease by embedding the suture made of chromium into the subcutaneous area where the point is located or deeper muscle and to make use of its continuous stimulating action. In general, the needle specially made for embedding the suture is adapted and the point located at the abdomen, back and the area where the muscle of the four limbs are thick and selected. The suture is embedded into 1—2 points once. It can be used for treating digestive ulcer, chronic enteritis, chronic branchitis, asthma, neurosis, polio, etc. (Fig 96)

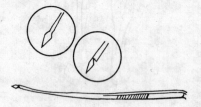

Fig 96

point ultrasonic stimulation therapy 穴位超声刺激法 [xué wèi cāo shēng cì jí fǎ] A therapeutic method to make highly-frequent sound energy with certain strength penetrate through the point by the head that can launch sound energy. Its volume can be controlled according to the distance between the head and the point as well as the regulated strength and time of action.

point radiation therapy 穴位照射法 [xué wèi zào shè fǎ] A therapeutic method by making use of the action of light radiating energy on the point. In Yellow Emperor's Toad Classic administering moxibustion by igniting moxa was recorded. In Hunmai's Chronic of Yi Jian in Southern Song Dynasty (1127—1279), the moxibustion technique that the abdomen was covered with moxa and was exposed in sunshine was recorded. In modern times, the diseases are treated by radiating the point with the infrared ray, ultrared ray, laser, etc.

point selection according to syndrome differentiation 辨证取穴 [biàn zhèng qǔ xué] One of the point selections. According to the principle of syndrome differentiation, the relevent points are selected by analysing the relationship between the diseases (and syndrome) and the viscera and meridians. E. g. , for insomnia pertaining to weaknesses of heart and spleen, Shenmen (HT 7) and Sanyinjiao (BL 22) can be selected; For that due to flaring fire of liver-gallbladder fire, Yanglingquan (GB 34) and Taichong (LR 3) can be selected; For that due to dissociation between heart and kideys, Shenmen (HT 7) and Taixi (KI 3) can be selected again; For blurred vision Ganshu (BL 18) can be selected to nourish the eyes and the liver, and brighten the eyes to promote vision; For toothache due to yin deficiency and excess fire, Taixi (KI 3) can be selected to nourish yin and reduce fire.

point-pressed diagnosis 压诊 [yā zhěn] Also called *an zhen*. The diagnostic technique of searching for the abnormal change of the meridian point by press, palpation, etc. , so as to associate the diagnosis. In clinic the ventral thumb is used to palpate or the thumb and index finger are used to pinch, so as to explore the abnormal reaction of the subcutaneous superficial stratum. The thumb used to press and knead, the finger power should be used evenly, and compare that of the left with that of the right. While examining the waist, the thumbs of the two hands may be used to closely adhear the bilateral side of the styloid process of the vertebra and compress them from the lower to the upper, segment by segment, and attention should be paid to the bilateral iliac crest and the edge of the medial aspect of the scapula. The main points to be pressed by point-pressed diagnosis are Jiaji (EX-B2), back-*shu* point, anterior-referred points, gap-like point, joining point, etc. The subcutaneous node, loop-like thing, tender point, numb region as well as protruding, hard node, hollow, looseness, varied color, abnormal temperature. The result got by examination must be analyised synthetically in combination with the four diagnostic techniques and the general condition of the body, so as to select the point according to syndrome differentiation.

point-exuded by the drug ion of direct current 直流电药物离子穴位透入法 [zhí liú diàn yào wù lí zǐ xué wèi tòu rù fǎ] An abbreviation of *yao wu li zi xue wei tou ru fa*. The method to make the drug ion exude the point by making use of the electrolystic action for treating disease. Put the rough electrode of the direct current therapeutic apparatus and the padding rinsed with fresh drug liquid on the point, once within six points. The nature of the electrode of the drug must accord with the electrode, i. e. , the drug of the positive electrode is guided by the yang positive electrode while that of the negative ion by the negative electrode. For the one of which the nature of the electrode is not clear, it can be guided from the two electrodes, the strength of the current is proper for the patients' tolerance, the time for connecting electricity is approx. 10—20 minutes. It can be used for treating neuralgia, neuritis in the surrounding nerve, dysfunction of the vegetative nerve, neuroschies, hypertension, hemorrhage from the base of the eye.

point-selected method 定穴法 [dìng xué fǎ] A method to locate and select the location of the *shu* point.

point selection according to the nerve 按神经取穴 [àn shén jīng qǔ xué] One of point-selected methods. To select the point concerned according to the distribution of the meridian, usually to select paravertebral points that correspond with the spinal nerve and certain points that are distributed over the pathways of the nerve plexus or nerve stem. E. g. , for numbness of finger, select Neiguan(PC 6) on the central nerve, Quchi (LI 11) on the radial nerve or some points on the brachial plexus; For pain in the leg,select Yanglingquan(GB 34) on the peroneal nerve, Weizhong (BL 40) on the tibial nerve as well as sciatica or some points on the sacral plexus.

point-selection according to disease location 看部取穴〔kàn bù qǔ xué〕One of the point selected methods. For disorders at the head and trunk,the relevant points can be selected according to the meridian. In general,for disorders of the upper part of the body, the points of hand-*yangming* meridian are selected, for those of the middle, those of foot-*taiyin* meridian, for those of the lower, those of foot-*jueyin* meridian. For disorder of the anterior body, the points of foot-*yangming* meridian are selected, for those of the posterior body, those of foot-*taiyang* meridians are selected.

point-selected method 取穴法〔qǔ xué fǎ〕1. Referring to the method of locating and selecting the point. For details,see bone-measurement method,finter-*cun* method; 2. Referring to selection of the point before acupuncture treatment.

pole bone 柱骨〔zhù gǔ〕1. Explained as the clavicular bone; 2. Explained as the cervical vertebrae, also called *tianzhu gu*.

popliteal fossa 腘〔guó〕Referring to the popliteal fossa.

protruding muscle 腘肉〔jiǒng ròu〕Referring to the protruding muscle.

posterior yin 后阴〔hòu yīn〕Referring to anus. It is so called because it is contrary to anterior yin (external genitalia).

posterior eye 目本〔mù běn〕Referring to the posterior part of the eye.

pokeberry root 商陆〔shāng lù〕A drug for external applying and moxibustion. The root of phytolacca acinosa Roxb.

Pomen 魄门〔pò mén〕Referring to anus.

Pohu（BL 42）魄户〔pò hù〕A point of Bladder Meridian of Foot-*taiyang*. Location：Below the spinal process to the 3rd thoracic vertebra, 9 cm lateral to Shenzhu (GV, DU 12). Regional anaotomy：Passing through the trapezius muscle, and rhomboid muscle, reaching at the iliocostal muscle. There is the posterior branch of the 3rd intercoatal nerve and the descending branch of the transverse artery of neck. The medial cutaneous branches of the posterior branches of the 2nd and 3rd thoracic nerves and the dorsal scapular nerve are in the deeper. Indications：Pulmonary tuberculoses, cough, asthmatic breath, stiffness of neck,pains in the shoulder and back. Puncture：1. 5—2. 5 cm obliquely(It is not advisable to puncture deep). Moxibustion：3—5 moxa cones or 5—15 minutes with warming moxibustion.

Prescriptions for Emergency 肘后备急方〔zhǒu hòu bèi jí fāng〕A book originally named *Zhou Hou Cui Xiao Fang*, briefly called *Zhou Hou Fang*, written by Guo Hong in Jin Dynasty （265—420 A. D.）. The original was divided into three volumes, later supplemented as the eight volumes by Tao Hongjing in Liang Dynasty （502—557 A. D.）and Yang Yongdao in Jin Dynasty (1265—420 A. D.). It records the prescriptions and drugs used for diseases of various specialites, such as internal medicine, surgery, gynecology, pediactircs and ophthalmology, which are mostly comon and simple prescriptions in folk and empirical prescriptions in folk, simple and easily-got. In the book over 100 acupuncture prescriptions were introduced, of which most of them are moxibustion techniques. More pages were used for recording application of techniques of moxibustion for critical diesaeses and symptoms.

pressing the point 按跷〔àn qiào〕A therapeutic method by pressing and pinching the point.

Prescriptions Worth a Thousand Gold 千金要方 [qiān jīn yào fāng] A medical book, originally called Important Presscriptions Worth a Thousand Gold for Emergencies, briefly called Prescription Worth a Thousand Gold, written by Sun Simiao in Tang Dynasty (618—907 A. D.), 30 volumes, the first famous formulary book of Tang Dynasty preserved. It widely collected a large amount of medical findings before Tang Dynasty (618—907 A. D.) and enumerated the symptoms, treatments and formulas and drugs of gynecology, pediactrics, dietetic nutrition, health preservation, acupuncture, etc. Besides moxibustion various diseases acupuncture and moxibustion were recorded, pariticularly many moxibustion techniques. In the 29th and 30th volumes acupuncture and moxibustion were mainly described. Three hundred and forty-nine points were enumerated and acupuncture-moxibustion prohibitions of the viscera, examples for practising acupuncture, as well as selection of the points for various diseases recorded.

press manipulation 切法 [qiē fǎ] An auxiliary manipulation in acupuncture. That is to press the point with the fingernail before insertion of the needle, so as to disperse *qi* and blood.

pressing hand 押手 [yá shǒu] While inserting the needle, press and pinch the point with the left hand to assist needle insertion. It is respectively called fingernail-pinching insertion of needle, *zhi qie jia shou*, needle insertion by widening the skin (*shu zhang jia shou*), needle insertion by pinching up the skin, (*jia chi jia shou*), needle insertion of holding the needle (*ping zhi jia shou*), etc.

pressing-closing manipulation 扪法 [mén fǎ] The auxiliary manipulation in acupuncture. It refers to torch and press the point with the finger after the inserted needle is withdrawn. "While administering reinforcing manipulation, use the finger to close the point while withdrawing the inserted needle so that it does not flow outside. " (Miraculous Pivot)

pregnant reactions 妊娠恶阻 [rèn shēn è zǔ] Pregnant reaction of different severities, such as nausea, vomiting, chest distress, perversion for sour food, anorexia, etc. , during the first trimester of pregnancy.

Prescriptions *Taiyi* Moxa stick 太乙神针方 [tài yí shén zhēn fāng] A medical book. Checked up by Feng Zuohuai in Qing Dynasty (1016—1911) accomoplished in 1862—1874. Compiled by Chen Buichou in Qing Dynasty (1616—1911).

prolapse of uterus 阴挺 [yīn tǐng] Prolapse of certain genital structures in or out of the vagina, usually of the uterus, but possibly of the bladder or rectum.

proxismal selection 近取 [jìn qǔ] An abrreviation of *jindao quxue*.

proxismal selection of the point 近部取穴 [jìn bù qǔ xué] I. e. , *jindao quxue*.

proxismal selection of the point 近道取穴 [jìn dào qǔ xué] One of point-selected methods, also called *jinbu quxue*, *jiujin quxue*, briefly called *jinqu*, opposite to distal selection of the point.

prohibited point 忌穴 [jì xué] Referring to the point that can not be puncture at certain time or day. There was the theory of choosing the date for acupuncture in ancient China and though that a certain date is proper for acupunctue or not proper for acupuncture of certain part can not be punctured.

proxismal selection of point 邻近取穴 [lín jìn qǔ xué] One of the point-selected methods. Referring to selecting the point concerned in the surrounding affected area to carry on treatment. Its scale is larger than that of local selection of point. E. g. , select Taiyang (EX-HN5) for eye trouble, select Waiguan (TE, SJ 5) for pain in the wrist, select Yinshi (ST 33) and Yanglinquan (GB 34) for pain in the knee, etc.

Prostate 前列腺 [qián liè xiàn] An ear point at the medical aspect of Bladder, inferior to Sympathetic.

prolonged palpation 久持 [jiǔ chí] The time of feeling the pulse is relatively long for about several minutes.

proportional *cun* 同身寸 [tóng shēn cùn] The proportioinal measurement used for selecting the point. 1. Referring to the bone-length measurement; 2. referring to proportional *cun* of the middle finger.

proximal selection of point 就近取穴 [jiù jìn qǔ xué] I. e., *jin dao qu xue.*

pressing manipulation 按法 [àn fǎ] An acupuncture manipulation. There are two meanings: One is to press the point with the hand before acupuncture, the other is to thrust the needle while puncturing. Also called *cha fa.*

pricking treatment 挑治法 [tiāo zhì fǎ] Also called *tiao zhen* or *zhen tiao.* To prick out the white fibrous thing from the point or the special rash spot of squeeze some fluid so as to treat disease. In clinical pricking treatment, the rash spots are usually found from the back, e. g., for sty the rash spot is searched at the scapular region; For esophagea varicosis the rash spot is searched at the bilateral chest and back; For hemorrhoids, the rash spot is searched at the lumbosacral region. The rash is slightly protruded on the skin surface and its color may be grey, bronze or pinkish, and is not faded. (It must be differentiated from that of folliculitis, pigmented spot.) Prick 1—2 spots once. The point concerned can also be selected for pricking according to the disease condition. Sterilization must be strict and the pricked local rea after pricking must be covered and protected by sterilized gauze.

pricking 挑刺 [tiāo cì] A needling technique. To prick the skin of the point by a triangular needle, then to break its superficial tissue by pricking it.

pricking treatment for hemorrhoids 挑痔法 [tiāo zhì fǎ] A therapeutic method to prick the special rash spot (hemmoroisal spot) or point at the lumbosacral region with a tri-

angular needle for treating hemorrhoids.

principle of *shu* **points** 俞理 [shū lǐ] It implies that acupuncture treatment must adhere to the speculated law and must not be against the principle of the *shu* point.

primordial *qi* 元气 [yuán qì] The primary motive force of activities of life.

promoting circulation of meridian *qi* 飞经走气 [fēi jīng zǒu qì] A term of acupuncture technique. Some acupuncture manipulations used to promote circulation of meridian *qi.*

prolapse of rectum 脱肛 [tuō gāng] Prolapse of the rectal mucosa or all the layers of the rectal wall out of the anus.

prone postion 俯卧位 [fǔ wò wèi] A body position for acupuncture.

protube rance of small head of ulna 两手研子骨 [liǎng shǒu yán zǐ gǔ] Referring to the protruding part of the small head where Yanglao (SI 6) is located.

proximal selection from the surrounding 四周取穴 [sì zhōu qǔ xué] I. e., selecting the point proximal to disease.

pruritic vulva 阴痒 [yīn yǎng] Itching, sometimes unbearable itching and pain in the vulva or vagina.

Pucang (BL 61) 仆参 [pú cān] A point of Bladder Meridian of Foot-*taiyang*. The confluencee of foot-*taiyang* meridian and Motility Vessel of Yang. Also termed Anxue. Location: Directly below Kunlun (BL 60) between the lateral ankle and Achilles tendon at the dorsoventral boundary in the depression of calcaneous. Regional anatomy: There are the lateral branch of the femoral artery and vein. The lateral branch of calcaneous of the femoral vein nerve is distributed. Indications: Atrophy and weakness of the lower limb, pain in the heel, cramp in cholera morbus, epilepsy, foot *qi* and swelling of the knees. Puncture: 1—2 cm perpendicularly. Moxibustion: 3—5 moxa cones or 5—10 minutes with warming moxibustion.

puncturing collateral meridians 刺络 [cì luò] A needling technique, to dot or discentrally puncture the superficial collateral with a triangular needle or plum needle, so as to let a proper amount of blood bleed. It is used for acute tonsilitis, acute conjunctivitis, acute sprains, sunstroke, coma due to apoplex, erysipelas, acute gastroenteritis, headache, hypertension, pulmonary edema, etc. Care must be taken of injurying the artery. It is not advisable to use it for the person weak in constitution, hypotension, hyloglyemia, and blood-disease patients as well as the pregnant woman.

puncture and moxibustion 刺灸 [cì jiǔ]Referring to acupuncture and moxibustion, also called *jue ci*.

pulse as reflector of disease 脉象主病 [mài xiàng zhǔ bìng] A certain combination of pulse with symptoms and signs. In the clinical manifestation, the pulse taken should be reviewed together with symptoms and signs with reference to each other, analyzed in detail, and summed up, comprehensive so as to estimate the status of the illness.

puffiness treated by selecting meridian points 浮肿者治其经 [fú zhǒng zě zhì qí jīng] One of the principles of selecting the point in Internal Classic. It refers that the five *shu* points of the meridian concerned can be selected for treating facial puffiness.

pulse with tense yin and yang 脉阴阳俱紧 [mài yīn yáng jù jǐn] The tense and forceful pulse at *cun* and *chi* sections, i. e., the superficial and tense pulse. It indicates yin cold syndrome or excessive exterior syndrome.

puncturing hand 刺手 [cì shǒu] While inserting the filiform needle, the two hands operate the needle simultaneously. The hand holding the needle (right) is generally called the puncturing hand while the hand (lift) that cooperates with the other to press and pinche the point is called the pinching hand.

pulse indications 脉象 [mài xiàng] The changes of the pulse as felt by the fingers, including its frequentcy, rhythm, fullness,

smoothness and amplitude.

pulmonary connection 肺系 [fèi xì] The connecting tissue of the lungs, referring to the throat, including Adam's Apple and esophgus.

pushing and pressing 推而纳之 [tuī ér nà zhī] Pushing and thrusting the needle administering manipulation, reinforcing manipulation, contrary to 'moving and extending'.

pulse with superficial yin and yang 脉阴阳俱浮 [mài yīn yáng jù fú] The pulses at *cun* and *chi* sections are both superficial. It indicates the exterior syndrome.

puncture of Baxie to cause little bleeding 八关大刺 [bā guān dà cì] The technique to puncture Baxie (EX-UE 9) to cause a little bleeding.

pulse without gastric *qi* 脉无胃气 [mài wú wèi qì] The pulse loses its slow, moderate and rhythmic character. It is often regarded as a critical sign.

purified *qi* 清气 [qīng qì] 1. The thin and clear part of the refined materials of water and grain; 2. Air inhaled into the lungs.

pulmonary tuberculosis 肺痨 [fèi láo] A chronic infectious consupmptive disease with clinical manifestations of progressive emaciation, cough, hemoptysis, low-grade fever, night sweating, etc. 1. Excess syndrome: Cold excess fluid hiding in the lungs: Lieque (LU 7), Chize (LU 5), Fengmen (BL 12), Feishu (BL 13); 2) Obstruction of the lungs by phlegm heat, Hegu (LI 4), Dazhui (GV 14), Fenglong (ST 40), Danzhong (CV 17), Zhongfu (LU 1), Feishu (BL 13), Quchi (LI 11), Dazhui (GV 14). 2. Cough due to internal injury: Feishu (BL 13), Pishu (BL 20), Taiyuan (LU 9), Taibai (SP 3), Fenglong (ST 40), Hegu (LI 4); 3. Scorching of the lungs by hepatic fire: Feishu (BL 13), Ganshu (BL 18), Jingqu (LU 8), Taichong (LR 3).

pylorus 幽门 [yōu mén] The lower opening of the stomach, one of the seven important portals.

Q

Qizhiyinxi 气之阴郄 [qì zhī yīn xī] An alternate term for Changqiang (GV, DU 1).

Qizhong 气中 [qì zhōng] An extra point, also termed Qichong (ST 30).

Qiuxu 丘虚 [qiū xū] I. e., Qiuxu (GB 40).

Qiuxu (GB 40) 丘墟 [qiū xū] A point of Gallbladder Meridian of Foot-*shaoyang*, the source of the meridian. Location: In the depression to the lateral side of the long extensor muscle of toe, anteroinferior to the lateral ankle. Regional anatomy: There is the branch of the anterior artery of the lateral ankle. The branch of dorsal intermediate nerve of foot and the superficial peroneal nerve are distributed. Indications: Pain in the neck, pain in the chest and hypochondrium, atrophy of the lower limbs, swelling and pain in the lateral ankle, malaria, hernia, congestive and painful eyes, nebula, paraplegia due to apoplxy. Puncture: 1. 3—3 cm perpendicularly. Moxibustion: 1—3 moxa cones or 5—10 minutes with warming moxibustion.

qi-promoted method 行气法 [xíng qì fǎ] Referring to various methods that can promote propagation and conduction of needling sensation. In Miraculous Pivot, the conduction of needling sensation is promoted by adopting needle rotation, etc. In compendium of Acupuncture, the importance of promoting flow for treatment was pointed out. In Golden Needle in Rhythm, for making *qi* ascend, twirl the needle right, for making *qi* descend, twirl the needle left. In Dragon-tiger ascending techniques there is the press method of pressing it anteriorly to make *qi* flow posteriorly; Press it posteriorly to make *qi* flow anteriorly for the purpose of controlling needle sensation. If one wants to make the induction upward, the finger may be used to press the inferior of the point closely to make *qi* ascend; if the induction is required to descend, the finger may be used to press the superior of the point to make *qi* descend. It is also called *qi*-regulated method.

qi-promoted manipulation 进气法 [jìn qì fǎ] Also called *yun qi fa* in Compendium of Acupuncture. While puncturing first puncture perpendicularly and swiftly thrust and slowly insert the needle at the times of digit number of 'six'. After acquiring *qi*, make the needle obliquely appoint the affected area. After promoting *qi* flow, let the patient inhale 5—7 breaths so as to aid in *qi* flow. It is used for various pain symptoms. (Fig 97)

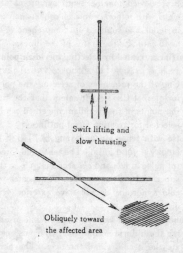

Swift lifting and
slow thrusting

Obliquely toward
the affected area

Fig 97

qi-gong (Chinese deep breathing exercises) 气功 [qì gōng] The system of exercises for physical fitness and the treatment of diseases by making use of deep-breathing and conscious control of mind in order to tranquilize mental activities or in combination with the harmonious and slow movements of limbs and trunk.

Qiguan 气关[qì guān]A point used for infantile massage diagnosis, referring to the transverse crease of the palmar side of the middle segment of the index finger.

Qizhen 气针[qì zhēn]1. Referring to the filiform needle, contrary to fire needle; 2. A method to inject sterilized air or oxygen into the point.

qi **received from the triple energizer** 气纳三焦 [qì nà sān jiāo] A term used in acupuncture techniques of midnight-noon ebbflow, contrary to blood received from the pericardium.

Qishe (ST 11) 气舍 [qì shè] 1. A point of Stomach Meridian of Foot-*yangming*. Location: In the depression between the head of sternal bone of sternocleidomastoidous muscle and that of the scapular bone on the superior edge of the scapula, directly below Renying (ST 90)on the anterolateral side of the neck. Regional anatomy: Passing through the cervical broader muscle, reaching between the two ends of sternocleidomastoidous muscle. There is the anterior cervical vein. The common cervical artery is in the deep. The cervical cutaneous muscle is distributed. The sympathetic stem of the vagus nerve is in the deeper. Indications: Sore throat, asthmatic breath, hernia, goiter, scrofula, stiffness and pain in the neck, swelling shoulder. Puncture: 1—2 cm perpendicuarly. Moxibustion: 3—5 moxa cones or 5—10 minutes with warming moxibustion; 2. Another name of Shenque (CV 18).

Qifu 气府 [qì fǔ] An alternate term for Jingmen (GB 25).

Qishu 气俞 [qì shū] An alternate term for Jingmen (GB 25).

Qiyuan 气原 [qì yuán] An alternate term for Zhongji (CV 3).

Qimen 气门 [qì mén] An extra point. located 1 dm lateral to Guanyuan (CV 4). Indications: Sterility, metrorrhagia, prolapse of uterine, *lin* syndrome, enuresis, hernia of the small intestine, testitis. Puncture: 3—4 cm perpendicularly. (prohibited in the case of pregnant woman.)Moxibustion: 3—5 moxa cones or 5—15 minutes with warming moxibustion. (Fig 98)

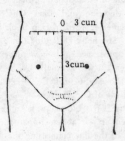

Fig 98

Qianding (GV 21) 前顶 [qián dǐng] A GV point, Location: At the midline of the frontal head, 9—10 cm to the anterior hailine, i. e., 4. 5 cm antrior to Baihui (GV 20). Regional anatomy: In galea aponeurotica. There is the anastomotic network of the left and right temporal superficial artery and vein. The branch of the greater occipital nerve is distributed. Indications: Epilepsy, dizziness, vertigo, vertical pain, rhinitis, congestive, swollen and painful eyes, infanfile convulsion. Puncture: 1—1. 5 cm horizontally. Moxibustion: 3—5 moxa cones or 5—10 minutes with warming moxibustion.

Qianshencong 前神聪 [qián shén cōng] One of Shencong located 3 cm anterior to Baihui (GV, DU 20)

Qianfaji Point 前发际穴 [qián fà jì xué] An extra point, located 9 cm directly above Taiyang (EX-HN 5). Indications: Deeprooted sore at the face. Puncture: horizontally. Moxibuston: 1—3 moxa cones or 5—10 minutes with warming moxibustion.

Qianguan 前关 [qián guān]An laternate term for Tongziliao (GB 1).

Qin Yueren 秦越人 [qín yuè rén] A medical expert during the Warring Periods. He learned medicine from Chong Shangjun. In lengendary he was the creator of Pulse-feeling, good at acupuncture, moxibustion, drug decoction, massage, heat ironing, etc. He travelled many places to treat people's diseases, and was highly skillful in acupuncture-moxibustion. Bian Que's Internal Medicine and Bian Que's external Medicine recorded in Han Book have been lost. The book Difficult Classic that have been preserved till now described Qin Yueren. It was acutually by the persorn in Han Dynasty (206 B.C. —220 A.D.) in the name of Qin Yueren.

Qiankong 钱孔 [qián kǒng] An extra point, located at the abdomen, at the crossing point of the line connecting the nipple and the umbilicus and the inferior edge of the costal arc. Indication: Jaundice. Moxibustion: 3—5 moxa cones or 5—10 minutes with warming moxibustion.

Qi Bo 岐伯 [qí bó] An anceint medical expert, the teacher of Yellow Empiror. His name is seen in Internal Classic that have been preserved now. Internal Classic written by adopting the form of questions and answers between Huangdi (Yellow Empiror) and Qi Bo. Qi and Huang are called in latter generations, representing medicine.

Qibojiu 岐伯灸 [qí bó jiǔ] The extra point, "When bladder qi upward rushes to the hypochondria and below the umbilicus and then into the abdomen, administer moxibustion at the point 18 cm below and 4.8 cm bilateral to the umbilicus (Qibojun) with 3—7 moxa cones."

Qingling (HT 2) 青灵 [qīng líng] A point of Heart Meridian of Hand-*shaoyin*. Location: At the anteromedial side of the upper arm, 9 cm above the transverse crease of elbow, at the medial sulsus of the biceps muscle of arm. Regional anatomy: There is the basilic vein and the superior ulnar accessary artery. The ulnar nerve, the medial cutaneous nerve of arm and the medial cutaneous nerve of forearm are distributed. In-

dications: Yellow eyes, headache, chills, hypochondriac pain, pain in the shoulder and back. Puncture: 1.5—3 cm perpendicularly. Moxibustion: 3—7 moxa cones or 5—10 minutes with warm needling.

Qinglingquan 青灵泉 [qīng líng quán] I.e., Qingling (HT 2).

qi-held manipulatioin 纳气法 [nà qì fǎ] First swiftly thrust and slowly lift the needle nine times or swiftly lift and slowly thrust the needle six times. After *deiqi* make the tip of the needle appoint the affected region obliquely and make *qi* ascend, then make the needle stand erect, and then press it downward so that *qi* can not flow back. It is to promote circulation of *qi* and eliminate something stagnant.

Qiangu (SI 2) 前谷 [qián gǔ] A point of Small Intestine Meridian of Hand-*taiyang*, the spring-like (water) point of the meridian. Location: At the ulnar side of the small finger. In the depression anterior to the 5th metacarpophalangeal point. When a fist is formed, it is at the dorso-parlmar boundary at the end of the transverse crease before the joint. Reginal anatomy: There is the dorsal digital artery and vein coming from the ulnar artery and vein. The dorsal digital nerve of the ulnar nerve and the proper palmar digital nerve are distributed. Indications: Febrile disease with no sweat, malaria, mania epilepsy, tinnitus, ocular pain, nebula, aches in the head and neck, swollen cheek, stuffy nose, sore throat, postpartum shortage of lacation, pain in elbow, numbness of the fingers. Puncture: 1—1.5 cm perpendicularly. Moxibustion: 3—5 moxa cones or 5—10 minutes with warming moxibustion.

Qinglengquan 清冷泉 [qīng léng quán] I.e., Qinglengquan (TE 11).

Qinglengyuan (TE 11) 清冷渊 [qīng léng yuān] A point of Triple Energizer Meridian of Hand-*shaoyang*, an alternate term for Qingling. Location: With the elbow flexed, at the dorsal side of the upper arm, 6 cm directly above the tip of the elbow (olecranon). Regional anatomy: At the triceps muscle, there is the terminal branch of the accessary artery and the brachial vein. The dorsal cutaneous nerve of arm and the muscular branch of the radial nerve are distributesd. Indications: Headache, yellow eyes, pains in the shoulder and arm. Puncture: 2.5—3.5 cm perpendicularly. Moxibustion: 3—7 moxa cones or 5—15 minutes with warming moxibustion.

***qi*-lifted manipulation** 提气法 [tí qì fǎ] It means to swiftly lift the needle and slowly thrust the needle with the number of 'six'. After acquiring *qi*, slightly twirl and lift the needle so as to strengthen needling sensation. Used for local numbness and coolness. (Fig 99)

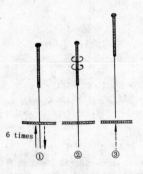

6 times

①Swift lifting and slow thrusting
②Slight twirling
③Slight lifting

Fig 99

Qizuma 骑竹马[qí zhú mǎ]An extra point located at the back. To measure straightly from the tip of the coccyx with the length from the patient's tip of the middle finger to the midpoint of the transverse crease of the elbow. It is located one proportional *cun* bilateral to the end of the coccyx. Indications: Nameless swelling and poison, cellulitis, toothache, scrofula, carbuncle and deep-rooted sore in the lower part of the

lower limbs. Moxibustion: 3—7 moxa cones or 5—15 minutes with warming moxibustion.

Qiangyang 强阳 [qiáng yáng] An alternate term for Luoque (BL 8).

Qiangjian (GV 18) 强间 [qiáng jiān] A GV point, also termed Dayi. Location: 24 cm to the anterior hairline of the midline of the vertex. I. e., 9 cm posterior to Baihui (GV, 20). Regional anatomy:At galea aponenrotica. There is the left and right occipital artery and vein. The branch of the greater occipital nerve is distributed. Indications: Headache, vertigo, stiffness and pain in the neck, insomnia, , anxiety, epilepsy, deviated mouth. Puncture: 1—1.5 cm horizontally. Moxibustion: 1—3 moxa cones or 3—5 minutes with warming moxibustion.

***qi*-retained method** 流气法 [liú qì fǎ] See 留气法.

Qimen(LR 14)期门 [qī mén]A point of Liver Meridian of Foot-*jueyin*, the anterior referred point of the liver, the confluence of foot-*taiyin*, foot-*jueyin* meridians and Connecting Vessel of Yin. Location: Directly below the nipple, in the 6th intecostal space. Regional anaotomy: There is the 6th intercostal artery and vein. The 6th intercostal nerve is distributed. Indications:Distension, fullness and pain in the chest and hypochondrium,vomiting,hiccup,diarrhea, acid regurgitation, cough and asthmatic breath, malaria, pathogenic heat invading the blood chamber, injury of cold. Puncture: 1.5—2.5 cm obliquely or horizontally (It is not advisable to puncture deeply). Moxibustion: 3—7 moxa cones or 5—15 minutes with warming moxibustion.

***qi*-retained method** 留气法 [liú qì fǎ]First insert the needle 2 cm deep then swiftly thrust and slowly lift the needle at the number of times of 'nine'; After acquiring *qi* insert the needle 3 cm deep, then slightly lift the needle and then withdraw it to the original area. Do like this repeatedly for the purpose of breaking up *qi* and dissipating

stagnation. (Fig 100)

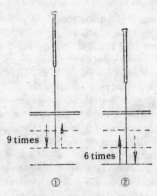

9 times

6 times

① ②

①Swift thrusting and slow lifting
②Swift lifting and slow thrusting

Fig 100

qi regulation 调气 [tiáo qì] It refers that acupuncture has the action of regulating meridianal *qi*. In regulating *qi* it can be said that the induction is properly regulated on the basis of obtaining to the induction, so as to regulate the body function and reinforcing body resistance.

qi-regulated method 调气法[tiáo qì fǎ]Referring various methods of regulating needling sensation, including rotation, lifting and thrusting, respiratory cooperation, searching and pressing by fingers, as well as 'ascent of the tiger and dragon', reception of *qi*, the 'dark-green dragon sways its tail', the 'white tiger shakes its head', the 'dark-green turtle explores the point', the 'red phoenix', etc.

qi can not be properly disposed of 气化不利 [qì huà bú lì] Dysfunction of kidney and bladder leads to patholoigic manifestations of edema, impairment of urination and the like.

Qiuhou 球后 [qiú hòu] An extra point located at the crossing point of lateral 1/4 and medial 1/4 of the inferior edge of the infrorbital edge, lateroinferior to the inferior tarsal plate in the orbicular muscle of eye. The branch of the facial nerve and the branch of the temporzygomatic and facial nerve are in the superfical. There is the infrorbital artery and vein and the inferorbital nerve in the deeper. Indications: Atrophy of the visual nerve, optic neuritis, glaucoma, myopia, vitreous opacity, pigmentary degeneration of retina, internal strabismus. During acupuncture, advise the patient look upward, fix the eyeballs gentlly with the finger, puncture with the tip of the needle toward the mediosuperior direction toward the visual nervous foramen 3—4.5 cm perpendicularly, with no rotating, lifting and thrusting the needle. After withdrawing the needle slightly press the local area 2—3 minutes lest little bleeding should occur. (Fig 101)

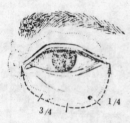

1/4

3/4

Fig 101

qi as the commander of blood 气为血帅 [qì wéi xuè shuài]*Qi* can lead the blood to circulate through the whole body as a commander leads the army. That is, blood circulation depends upon *qi* as its motive force.

Qishangxia 脐上下 [qí shàng xià] An extra point 1.5 cm superior and inferior to the umbilicus. Indications: Sunken fotannel, disclosure of fantanel, abdominal distention and borborygmus, edema, hernial pain, dysentery, enteritis. Puncture: 1.5 cm perpendicularly. Moxibustion: 3—5 moxa cones or 5—15 minutes with warming moxibuston.

qi-promoted method 运气法 [yùn qì fǎ] See

jin qi fa.

Qishu 奇俞 [qí shū] 1. Referring to the extra point; 2. Referring to 59 *shu* point for febrile diseases.

Qixialiuyi 脐下六一 [qí xià liù yī] See Qi Bo's moxibustion.

qiugu 䪼骨 [qiú gǔ] Referring to the zygomatic part by the nose.

qigu 歧骨 [qí gǔ] The bone where the two bones branch off.

qiaoxue 窍穴 [qiào xué] Referring to the aperture, same with *shu* point in meaning.

Qihaishu (BL 24) 气海俞 [qí hǎi shū] A point of Bladder Meridian of Foot-*taiyang*. Location: 4. 5 cm lateral to the spinal process of the 3rd lumar vertebra and the 4th. Regional anatomy: Passing through the lumbar and back fascia, reaching between the longest muscle and the iliocostal muscle. There are the posterior branches of the 3rd lumbar artery and vein. The lateral cutaneous branch of the posterior branch of the 2nd lumbar nerve are distributed. Indications: Lumbago, immovable legs and knees, dysmenorrhea, hemorrhoids. Puncture: 1. 5—3 cm perpendicularly. Moxibustion: 3—7 moxa cones or 5—15 minutes with warming moxibustion.

Qitang 气堂 [qì táng] An alternate term for Qichong (ST 30).

qi **pathway** 气街 [qì jiē] 1. A pathway of meridian *qi*. Its range exceeds the main trunks of the meridians. It is divided into four pathways of *qi* in the four regions: the head, chest, leg, abdomen and leg; 2. Referring to qichong (ST 30).

qi 气 [qì] 1. Referring to the refined material which is highly nutritious and circulates in the body. It is analogous to the essence of virtue *qi*; 2. Referring to functional activities of the viscra and tissues; 3. Respiratory gases, etc.

Qishangxiawufen 脐上下五分 [qí shàng xià wǔ fēn] I. e., Qishangxia.

Qizhong 脐中 [qí zhōng] I. e, Shenque (CV 8).

Qizhongsibian 脐中四边 [qí zhōng sì biān] An extra point located at the centre, and 3 cm above, below, left and right of the umbilicus, five in total. Indications: Acute-chronic gastroenteritis, gastric spasm, edema, indigestion. Puncture: 3—4. 5 cm perpendicularly. Moxibustion: 5—7 moxa cones or 5—15 minutes with warming moxibustion. For Qizhong point salt-interposing moxibustion or warming moxibustion can be used. (Fig 102)

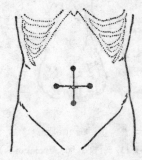

Fig 102

Qihai (CV 6) 气海 [qì hǎi] A point of CV, also termed Boyang, Xiahuang. Location: 3—15 cm below the umbilicua, on the abdominal midline. Regional anatomy: In the white abdominal line, there are the branches of the superifical abdominal artery and vein and those of the hypogastric artery and vein. The anterior branch of the 11th intercostlal nerve is distributed. Indications: Pain in the surrounding umbilicus, edema and tympanite, epigastric distension, indigestion, constipation, diarrhea, uroschesis, enuresis, spermatorrhea, impotence, prolapse of uterine, retention of placenta, emaciation and weakness of the four limbs. Puncture: 3—4 cm perpendicularly. (Be cautious in the case of the pregnant woman.) Moxibustion: 1. 3 —7 moxa cones or 15—30 minutes with warming moxibustion; 2. One of the 'four seas', referring to Danzhong (CT 17).

Qiduan 气端[qì duān]An extra point, located at the ends of the ten toes. Indications:Foot *qi*, paralysis of the toes, congestion and swelling of the dorsal foot, first aid. Puncture:0. 3—0. 6 cm perpendicularly or pricking to cause little bleeding with a triangular needle. Moxibustion:1—3 moxa cones or 3—5 minutes with warming moxibustion. (Fig 103)

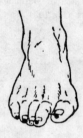

Fig 103

Qihu (ST 13) 气户[qì hù]A point of Stomach Meridian of Foot-*yangming*. Location:12 cm lateral to Xuanji(CV 21)on the thoracic midline between the scapular bone and the 1st rib. Regional anatomy:At the starting point of the broadest muscle of chest. The infraclavicular muscle is below. There are the branches of the thoraco-acromial artfery and vein. The clavicular vein is above. The branch of anterothoracic nerve is distributed. Indications:Asthmatic breath, cough, distension and chest and hypochondrium, hiccup, pains in the chest, back and hypochondrium. Puncture:1—2 cm obliquely. Moxibustion:3—5 moxa cones or 5—10 minutes with warming moxibustion.

Qixue 气穴[qì xué]A point of Kidney Meridian of Foot-*shaoyin*, the confluence of Vital Vessel and foot-*shaoyin* meridian, also termed Baomen, Zhihu. Location:1. 5 cm lateral to Guanyuan(CV 1),1 dm below the umbilicus. Regional anatomy:In the artery of the hypogastric artery and vein. The infracostal nerve is distributed. Indications:

Irregular menstruation, leukorrhea, sterility, flatulence, diarrrhea, pain in the lumber spine, enteritis, infection of the biliary duct. Puncture:3—4 cm perpendicularly. Moxibustion:3—5 moxa cones or 5—10 minutes with warming moxibustion.

Qisibian 脐四边[qì shì biān]I. e., Qizhongshibian.

Qipang point 脐旁穴 [qì páng xué] I. e., Shanqi Point.

quya 曲牙[qū yá]1. The superior area of the corner of the mandible; 2. Jache (ST 6).

Quchi 曲尺[qu chǐ]An extra point. Location: In the depression between the anterial tibial muscle and the long extensor muscle of thumb, anteroinferior to the medial ankle, on the medial side of the dorsal foot. Indications: Pain in the lower bilateral abdomen, nocturnal emission and hernia. Puncture:1—2 cm perpendicularly. Moxibustion: 3—5 moxa cones or 5—15 minutes with warming moxibustion.

Qujie 曲节 [qū jié] An alternate term for Shaohai (HT 3).

Qufa 曲发 [qū fā] I. e., Qubin (GB 7), an alternate term for Lieque (Lu 7).

Quchi (LI 11) 曲池 [qū chí] A point of Large Intestine Meridian of Hand-*yangming*, the sea-like (earth) point of the meridian. Location: At the midpoint of the end of the radial side of the transverse crease of superolateral condyle of humerus. Select it with the elbow flexed. Regional anatomy:At the starting part of the long extensor lateral muscle. There is the branch of the recurrent artery and vein. The dorsal cutaneous nerve of forearm is distributed. The radial nerve is in the deeper stratum at the medial side. Indications:Fever,headache,red eyes, toothache, sore throat, pain in the elbow and arm, paralysis of the upper limb, insanity, scrofula, goiter, deep-rooted sore, abdominal pain,diarrhea and vomiting, dysentery, hypertension, etc. Puncture:3—4. 5 cm perpendicularly. Moxibustion:3—5 moxa cones or 5—10 minutes with warming moxibustion.

Quze(PC 3)曲泽[qū zé] A point of Pericardium Meridium of Hand-*jueyin*, the sea-like (earth) point of the meridian. Location: On the transverse crease of the elbow, at the edge of the ulnar side of biceps muscle of arm. Select it when the elbow is slightly flexed. Regional anatomy: Passing through the ulnar side of the biceps muscle of arm, reaching at the humeral muscle. There is the humeral artery and vein. The primary stem of the medial nerve is distributed. Indications: Cardialia, palpitation, stomachache, anxiety, febrile diseases, vomiting, spasm and pain of the ellbow and arm, tremor of the upper limb, cough. Puncture: 1.5—2.5 cm perpendicularly, or prick to cause little bleeding. Moxibustion: 3—5 minutes with warming moxibustion.

Quyuan (SI 13) 曲垣 [qū yuán] A point of Small intestine Meridian of Hand-*taiying*. Location: In the depression at the end of the medial side of the superior fossa of the spine of scapula. Refional anatomy: Passing through the trapezius muscle, reaching at the supraspinous muscle. There is the descending branch of the transverse cervical artery and vein. the muscular branches of supraspinal artery and vein are in the deeper. The posterior and lateral branches of the accessary nerve of the 2nd thoracic nerve are distributed. The muscular branch of the supraspinous nerve is in the deeper. Indications: Pain in the shoulder, contracture and pain in the arm, inflammation of supraspinous muscle, suprohumeral periarthrites, Puncture: 1.5—3 cm perpendiculully. Moxibustion: 3—5 moxa cones or 5—10 minutes with warming moxibustion.

Qugu 屈骨 [qū gǔ] I.e., 曲骨, Qugu (CV 2).

Quguduan 屈骨端 [qū gǔ duān] An extra point, also termed Henggu, Niaobao. Located at the midpoint of symphysis pubis. Indications: Weakness and failure of the five storing viscera, nocturnal emission, fre-

quent urination, difficulty abnormal urination, distension and fullness in the abdomen, diarrhea. Puncture: 1—1.5 cm obliquely. Moxibustion: 3—7 moxa cones or 5—15 minutes with warming moxbustion.

Qihui 气会 [qì huì] One of eight confluential points.

Qihe 气合 [qì hé] I.e., Qishe (ST 11), an alternate term for Shenque (CV 8).

Qichong (ST 30) 气冲 [qì chōng] 1. A point of Stomach Meridian of Foot-*yangming*. Location: 6 cm lateral to Qugu (RN 2), 1.5 dm below the umbillicus. Regional anatomy: Passing through the peritendineum of the external trapezius muscle of abdomen and the internal trapezius muscle of abdomen, reaching at the lower part of transverse abdominal muscle. There are the branches of the superficial abdomenal artery and vein, and its external side is the hypogastric artery and vein. The ilioinguinal nerve is distributed. Indications: Distension and pain in the extenal genitalia, abdominal pain, hernia, irregular menstruation, infertility, impotence, pain in the penis. Puncture: 1.5—3 cm perpendicularly. Moxibustion: 3—5 moxa cones or 5—10 minutes with warming moxibustion; 2. An extra point, an alternate term for Qitang, located on the midline of the neck, at the midpoint of the line connecting the notch of the thyloid cartilege and that of the supracervical thoracic presternum. Indications: Cough, asthma. Puncture: 1 cm perpendicularly. Moxibustion: 3—7 moxa cones or 10 minutes with warming moxibustion; 3. Qizhong, an alternate term for Qizhong.

quintuple puncture 杨刺 [yáng cì] One of the twelve puncture techniques. It is to puncture the centre of the affected area with one needle and four superficially arround it. The puncture is comparatively supercifical and wide for treating cold blockage in a large scale, etc. Together with triple puncture, it pertains to the needling technique of simultaneously using the multiple needles.

Quanliao 权髎 [quán liáo] I.e., Quanliao (SI 18).

Qujiao 曲角 [qū jiǎo] The part forwardly protruding at the upper part of the hair on the temples, where Hanyang (GB 4), Xuanlu (GB 5) and Xuanli (GB 6) are located.

Quzhou 曲周 [qū zhōu] I.e., *qujiao.*

Quanjian 拳尖 [quán jiān] An extra point, located at the higher spot of the small head of the 3rd metacarpal bone of the dorsal hand. Select it when a fist is formed. Indications: Congestive eyes, ocular pain, vitiligo, wart. Moxibustion: 3—5 moxa cones.

Quezhong 阙中 [què zhōng] Referring to the interspace between the two eyebrows.

Questions and Answers of Acupuncture 针灸问对 [zhēn jiǔ wèn duì] A book compiled by Wang Ji in Ming Dynasty (1368—1644). The whole book was written by adopting the form of questions and answers, divided into 3 volumes. The 1st volume introduces the basic theories of acupuncture and meridians, the 2nd, needling techniques; the 3rd, moxibustion techniques and appended rhythmed articles dealing with meridian points. Its contents are mainly from Plain Questions, Miraculous Pivot, and the acupuncture books that were common at that time. The author kept the different viewpoints to acupuncture manipulations that were popular in Yuan and Ming dynasties (1368) and mid-night-noon ebb-flow. Quite a few that can not be seen in Compendium of Acupuncture are preserved in the book. It was completed in 1530.

Qu Liang 瞿良 [qú liáng] A medical expert in the folk in Ming and Qing dynasties (1368—1911), born at Yidu (in Shandong Province). He wrote varieties of medical books. Of them Compilation of Meridians further put forth the concepts, such as *xiluo*, *chanluo*, and *sunluo*, etc.

Quanliao (SI 18) 颧髎 [quán liáo] A point of Small Intestine Meridian of Hand-*taiyang*, the confluence of hand-*shaoyin* meridian and hand-*shaoyang* meridian, also

termed Duigu, Duiduan. Location: Direcltly below the outer canthus, in the depression posteroinferior to zygoma. Regianal anatomy: The zygoamtic musle and the masseter are below. There are the branches of the facial transverse artery and vein. The facial nerve and the infroaorbital nerve are distributed. Indications: Deviated mouth and eyes, tremor of eyelids, swollen cheek, toothache, yellow eyes, flushed face, swollen lips. Puncture: 1—1.5 cm perpendicularly, or 1.5—3 cm obliquely or horizontally.

Quepeng (ST 12) 缺盆 [quē péng] A point of Stomach Meridian of Foot-*yangming*, also termed Tiangai. Location: In the centre of the supraclavicular fossa, 12 cm lateral to midline of the chest, directly above the nipple. Regional anatomy: At the platysma and the lateral aspect of sternocleidomastoidous muscle. There is the transverse cervical artery in the upper. The middle branch of the supraclaviclarl nerve is distributed. The brachial plexus is just in the deeper. Indications: Cough, asthmatic breath, suffocating chest, pain in the supraclavicular fossa, scrofula, goiter, sore throat, numbeness of the upper limb. Puncture: 1—1.5 cm perpendicularly. Moxibustion: 3—5 moxa cones or 5—10 minutes with warming moxibustion, also referring to the supraclauicular fossa.

Quanmen 泉门 [quán mén] An extra point. Located at the superior rim of the anterior commissure of labia. Indications: Infertility, leukorrhea, irregular menstruation, amenorrhea. Puncture: 0.9—1.5 cm perpendicularly. Moxibuston: 1—3 moxa cones or 5—10 minutes with warming moxibustion.

Quanshengzu 泉生足 [quán shēng zú] An extra point, located in the centre of the Achilles tednon, at the midpoint of the superior transverse crease of the superior edge of calcaneus. Indications: Dystocia, lumbago, sapsm of esophagus. Puncture: 0.6—0.9 cm perpendicularly. Moxibustion: 3 moxa cones or 5—10 minutes with warming moxibustion.

Quanyin 泉阴 [quán yīn] An extra point, located at the abdomen, 9 cm lateral to the centre of symphysis of pubis. Indications: Hernia, testitis. Puncture: 1.5—3 cm perpendicularly. Moxibustion: 3—5 moxa cones or 5—10 minutes with warming moxibustion.

Quanye 泉液 [quán yè] I. e., Yuanye (GB 22).

Qucha (BL 4) 曲差 [qū chā] A point of Bladder Meridian of Foot-*taiyang*, also termed Bichong. Location: At the 1st lateral line of the head, 4 cm lateral to Shenting (GV 24), in the centre of the hairline, 1.5 cm inside the hairline. Regional anatomy: There is the frontal artery and vein in the frontal muscle. The lateral branch of the frontal nerve is distributed. Indications: Headache, vergio, stuffy nose, epistaxis, nasal sore, reduced vision, rhinitis. Puncture: 1—1.5 cm horizontally. Moxibustion: 1—3 moxa cones or 3—5 minutes with warming moxibustion.

Qumei 曲眉 [qū méi] I. e., Yintang (EX-HN 3).

Qujia 曲颊 [qū jiá] Referring to the corner of the mandible.

Qubin (GB 7) 曲鬓 [qū bīn] A point of Gallbladder Meridian of Foot-*shaoyang*, the confluence of foot-*taiyang* and foot-*shaoyang* meridians. Location: Approx. 1 transverse crease fingerwidth, anterior to Jiaosun (TE, SJ 20), directly above the posterior edge of the temporal hair, anterior to the ear. Regional anatomy: There are the perietal branches of the superficial frontal artery and vein in the frontal muscle. The frontal branch of the auriculofrontal nerve is distributed. Indication: Migraine, swelling of the cheek and submental region, closejaw, vomiting, toothache, congestive and painful eyes, stiffness of the neck and nape. Puncture: 1—1.5 cm horizontally. Moxibustion: 1—3 moxa cones or 3—5

minutes with warming moxibustion.

Qugu 曲骨 [qū gǔ] 1. Referring to symphysis pubis. 2. Qugu (CV 2) the meridian point pertaining to CV, the confluence of CV and foot-*jueyin* meridian, also termed 屈骨. Location: At the midpoint of the superior edge of symphysis pubis. Regional Anatomy: At the white abdomininal line. There are the branches of the inferior hypogastric artery and the obturator artery. The branch of the iliohypogastric nerve is distributed. Indications: Fullness and pain in the lower abdomen, dribbling of urine, nocturnal emission, impotence, irregular menstruation, leukorrhea, enuresis, incontinence of urine, retention of urine, uteroptosis. Puncture: 3—4.5 cm perpendicularly. (cautiously used for the pregnant woman) Moxibustion: 2—7 moxa cones or 10—20 minutes with warming moxibustion. (Fig 104)

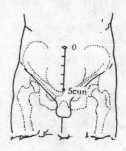

Fig 104

Ququan (LR 8) 曲泉 [qū quán] A point of Liver Meridian of Foot-*jueyin*, the sea-like (water) point of the meridian. Location: With the elbow flexed, in the depression superior to the end of the medial side of the transverse crease of the cubital fossa. Regional anatomy: Anterior to the semimembranous muscle and semitendinous muscle and at the posterior edge of the sartorius muscle. There is the great saphenous vein and the supreme genicular artery. The saphenous nerve is distributed.

Indications: Irregular menstruation, dismenorrhea, leukorrhea, prolapse of uterine, itch in the pubic region, postpartum abdominal pain, spermatorrhea, impotence, hernia, dysuria, headache, vertigo, mania, swelling and pain of the knees, atrophy of the lower abdomen. Puncture: 3—4.5 cm perpendicularly. Moxibustion: 3—5 moxa cones or 5—10 minutes with warming moxibustion.

R

Rangu(**KI 2**)然谷[rán gǔ]A point of Kidney Meridian of Foot-*shaoyin*. The stream-like point of the meridian, also termed Nongyan, Rangu. Location: Anteroinferior to the medial ankle, in the depression at the anteroinferior edge of the portubelance of the navicular bone. Regional anatomy: At the adductor muscle of toe. There is the terminal branch of the medial cutaneous nerve of leg. The medial lateral nerve distributed. Indications: Irregular menstruation, prolapse of uterus, itch of the pubic region, spermatorrhea, impotence, dysuria, diarrhea, distension and pain in the chest and hypochondrium, hemoptysis, infantile umbilical convulsion, lockjaw, emaciation-thirst disease, jaundice, atrophy of the lower limbs, pain in the dorsal foot. Puncture: 2.5—3.5 cm perpendicularly. Moxibustion: 3—5 moxa cones or 5—10 minutes with warming moxibustion.

rangu 然骨[rán gǔ]1. Referring to the protuberance of the medial ankle; 2. Referring to Rangu (KI 2).

Ranunculus sceleratus L. 石龙芮 [shí lóng ruì] One of drugs used to cause blistering by dressing it on a certain point. Fresh leaves of Ranun-applying culus japoincus Thunb.

rapid pulse 疾脉[jí mài]The pulse with a rate over 90 times per minute. It usually indicates the heat syndrome.

reinforcing the maternal viscus in a deficiency and reducing the oppspring in an excess 虚则补其母,实则泻其子[xū zhé bǔ qí mǔ shí zhé xiè qí zǐ]According to the five-element theory, there exists a relationship of deficiency, excess, reinforcement and reduction among the five storing viscera. In a deficiency syndrome, the maternal viscus is reinforced while in an excess one, the offspring one is reduced. For instance, in the case of the kidney and liver, the kidney pertains to water, the mother and the liver, wood, the son. In a deficiency of the liver, the kidney may be reinforced. This is 'In a deficiency, reinforce the mother.' In the case of the liver and heart, the liver pertains to wood, the mother and the heart, fire, the son. In the hepatic substantive fire syndrome the heart fire may be reduced. This is 'In an excess, reduce the son.'

residance of the kidneys 肾之府 [shèn zhī fǔ] Referring to the waist. It is therefore called because the kidneys dwell in it.

repeated moxibustion 报灸 [bào jiǔ] A term for moxibustion technique that is to repeat moxibustion treatment, used in moxibustion with multiple *zhuang* or the disease needling to be treated by repeated moxibustion. E. g., for the patient with deviated mouth and eye caused by apoplexy, the number of moxa cone on the head, face and four limbs would not exceed 30 (*zhuang*) but repeat moxibustion once every 3 days. Repeat moxibustion as the previous method 3 times for the mild case, 9 times for the severe.

reinforcing-reducing manipulations according to the direction of the tip of needle 针向补泻 [zhēn xiàng bǔ xiè] Referring to the reinforcing-reducing manipulations decided by the direction of the tip of the needle. "If reducing manipulation is required, the tip of the needle needs to be against the coming of the meridian, that is to be against the flourishing *qi* to deprive *qi*, that is so called against *qi*. If reinforcing manipulation is required, make the tip of the needle be along with the flow of *qi* in meridians. That is to go along with *qi*, that is to make the needle go along with the qi flow to reinforce *qi*, it is so called being along with. " (Eighty-one Difficult Classic with Illustrations)

reinforcing-reducing manipulations with the head of needle 针头补泻 [zhēn tóu bǔ xiè] Also termed *shou zhi bu xie*. Referring to accessary acupuncture manipulation by mainly using the left hand. (Fig 105)

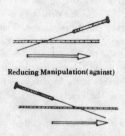

Reducing Manipulation(against)

Reinforcing Manipulation (along)

Fig 105

region of the kidneys and the liver 肾肝之部 [shèn gān zhī bù] The division of acupuncture. Referring to the deep stratum of muscles.

reinforcing and reducing manipulations 补泻手法 [bǔ xiè shǒu fǎ] The operation method of reinforcing and reducing by acupuncture. A variety of reinforcing and reducing manipulations are usually named with the manipulation, e.g., manipulation of "the dark-green dragon sways its tail", manipulation of "the red phoenix shakes its head", etc. It is not advisable to call them the manipulation that some of reinforcing and reducing methods do not pertain to the manipulative operation, e.g., off spring-maternal reinforcing and reducing, respiratory reinforcing and reducing, etc. In general it is termed acupuncture reinforcing and reducing methods.

reinforcing-reducing manipulation by finger 手指补泻法 [shǒu zhǐ bǔ xiè fǎ] Various manipulations used to promote *qi*, circulate *qi* and administer reinforcing-reducing manipulation in the course of acupuncture operation. In Difficult Classic the important role of the action of press by the left hand in acupuncture treatment has been empha-

sized. various auxiliary manipulations concerning acupuncture were generally called reinforcing-reducing manipulations by hand, which are 14 in total.

red phoenix extends its wings 赤凤迎源 [chì fèng yíng yuán] An acupuncture manipulation. Symetrical to 'The turtle explores the point' (cang gui tan xue). That is to insert the needle into the deep first, then thrust it to the superficial. After acquiring *qi* insert the needle into the middle and then to lift and thrust it left and right, up and down, and twirl it with the fingers twirling, and taking off the needle just like the phoenix extending its wings. It has the action of unobstructing collateral meridians. (Fig 106)

restlessness of cardiac *qi* 心气不宁 [xīn qì bù níng] Restlessness due to the decline of cardiac functions with the symptom of palpitation, restlessness, anxiety, insomnia, and irregular pulse, etc.

renal blockage 肾闭 [shèn bì] An osseous blockage syndrome, which is refractory to prolonged treatment, progresses to affect the kindey and thus, includes the symptoms of the curved waist and back, unable to extend, straight or the swollen joint, unable to flex, etc.

regurgitation of *qi* 气逆 [qì nì] The symptoms due to improper circulation and backing up of *qi*. Often referring to the upward spreading symptoms due to the functional disturbance of the lungs, stomach and liver, such as cough, dyspnea, vomiting, belching, hiccup as well as dizziness, vertigo, tinnitus, etc.

Renheng 人横 [rén héng] I.e., Daheng (SP 15).

residance of marrow 髓府 [suǐ fǔ] Referring to bones because the marrow is stored in them.

renal yang 肾阳 [shèn yáng] Also termed *yuan yang*, *zheng huo*, *shen huo*, *ming huo*, *mingmen zhi huo*, *xiantiang zhi huo*, Functional activities of the kidney are the very souce of heat of the human body. Patholo-

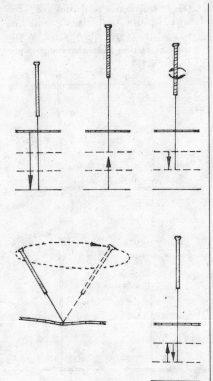

Fig 106

gically they are related to the ebb and flow of cold or heat. When they are hypofunctional and accompanied with cold manifestions, it is deficiency of renal yang. When they are hyperfuctional and accompanied with heat manifestations, it is excess of renal yang or 'exces of renal fire.'

repeated shallow puncture 赞刺 [zàn cì] One of the twelve needling techniques for treating carbuncle. It is repeatedly to insert and withdraw the needle vertically and superficially to cause little bleeding at the affected area.

refined *qi* 精气 [jīng qì] 1. Same as antipathogenic *qi* and usually referring to the essential materials and functions of life. 2.

Usually referring to essence from water and grain, which maintain the activities of life and metabolism.

retching and vomiting 呕吐 [ǒu tù] The symptoms as the result of the reflux of gastric *qi*. It is called 'ou' (retching). When the sound of straining is heard but nothing is brought up, while it is called ' *tu* ' (vomiting). When sound of the gastric contents are regurgiteated but no sound is heard. Since they are actually inseparable, they are collectively termed *'outu'* .

repeated left-right twirling 龙虎交战 [lóng hǔ jiāo zhàn] The acupuncture manipulation. The inserted needle is twirled left and right repeatedly. First mainly twirl it left, i. e. , twirl the needle more powerfully forwardly with the thumb in the number of nine, then mainly right, i. e. , twirl the needle more powerfully with the index finger, in the number of nine, repeat it. It can also be carried or according to the superficial, middle and deep strata. It is used for treating cancer.

Renzhong 人中 [rén zhōng] 1. In the depression at the middle of the upper lip; 2. Also called Shuigou, i. e. , Shuigou (GV 26).

reactive point 反应点 [fǎn yìng diǎn] A way of calling the *shu*-point in modern times, also called the reactive point of disease. It is therefore called because certain points have the action of reflecting certain disorder or disease.

reinforcing-reducing with moxibustion 艾灸补泻 [ài jiǔ bǔ xiè] Reinforcing and reducing are differentiated according to different power of fire while administering moxibustion.

regularly intermittent pulse 代脉 [dài mài] A rather slow and weak pulse with missing beats at regular intervals. It is often seen in deficiency of visceral *qi*, heart diseases, etc.

retention of placenta 胞衣不下 [bāo yī bú xià] The placenta is not delivered spontaneously, long after delivery of the infant.

residence of tendon 筋之府 [jīn zhī fǔ] Referring the knee. It is therefore called because the bigger tendons gather at it.

retain the needle in case of cold 寒则留之 [hán zé liú zhī] One of the principles of acupuncture treatment. Febrile diseases can be changed into cold by retaining the needle while cold diseases can be changed into heat by retaining the needle.

retention of lochia 恶露不下 [è lù bù xià] Little, if any of the fluids or decomposed blood in the uterus is discharged from the vagina during the pueperium.

residence of the chest 胸中之府 [xiōng zhōng zhī fǔ] Referring to back.

reinforcement of the spleen to help the lungs 培土生金 [péi tǔ shēng jīn] The method for treating deficiency of the lungs by reinforcing the spleen. It is indicated for such symptoms as chronic cough caused by deficiency of the lungs, copious watery phlegm, poor appetite, loose stools, whitish coating of the tongue, small and weak pulse, etc.

retarded pulse 迟脉 [chí mài] The pulse with a rate below 60 times per minute. It usually indicates the heat syndrome.

residence of intelligence 精明之府 [jīng míng zhī fǔ] Referring to the head because all the essence of the five storing viscera and six emptying viscera gathers in the head. Especially important are the eyes. Their appearance and luster usually reflect the functional state of these viscera.

reinforcing-reducing with the tip of needle being against and along the direction of *qi* 迎随补泻 [yíng suí bǔ xiè] One of acupuncture reinforcing and reducing manipulations, also called *zhen xiang bu xie*, which is to differentiate reinforcing and reducing manipulations according the puncturing along or against direction of meridian *qi*.

real intestine 真肠 [zhēn cháng] The wrong form of *zhichang* (rectum), an alternate term for Chengjin (BL 56).

reinforcing and reducing by the speed of inserting the needle 徐疾补泻 [xú jí bǔ xiè]

One of acupuncture reinforcing and reducing manipulations. Reinforcing or reducing manipulations are differentiated by the speed of inserting and withdrawing the needle. (Fig 107)

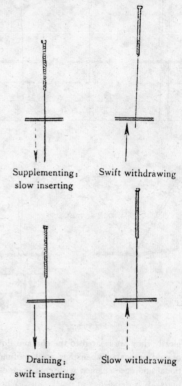

Supplementing: slow inserting   Swift withdrawing

Draining: swift inserting   Slow withdrawing

Fig 107

reinforcing and reducing by lifting and thrusting the needle 提插补泻 [tí chá bǔ xiè] One of acupuncture reinforcing and reducing manipulations. The reinforcing and reducing manipulations are differentiated according to the strength and speed of lifting and thrusting the needle while puncturing. In modern times it reinforcing manipulation the needle is usually thrusted swiftly and lifted slowly; In reducing manipulation the needle is usually lifted swiftly and thrusted slowly. (Fig 108)

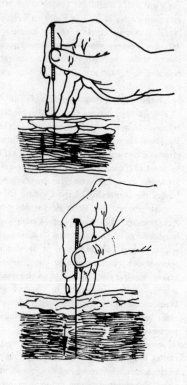

Fig 108

reinforce in case of deficiency 虚则补之 [xū zé bǔ zhī] The therapeutic principle of acupuncture, contrary to reduce in case of excess, also termed *"xu ze shi zhi"*. It implies that for deficiency syndrome it is advisable to use reinforcing manipulation to reinforce it, for cold syndrome of deficiency type warming moxibustion can be used.

Refu 热府 [rè fǔ] An alternate term for Fengmen (CV 16).

reduce in case of excess 盛则泻之 [shèn zé xiè zhī] The principle of acupuncture treatment, contrary to 'reinforce in case of excess', also called 'excrete it in case of full-

ness.' It implies that it is advisable to use reducing manipulation for excess syndrome to make it weakened.

renal yin 肾阳 [shèn yīn] Also termed *yuan yin*, *zheng yin*, *zhengshui*, *shenshui*. As a contrast of renal yang, it refers to the refined materials and fluids in the kidney.

reugulation between water and fire 水火相济 [shuǐ huǒ xiāng jì] Here, water refers to renal water while fire cardiac fire. They regulate each other so as to keep physiologic dynamics in equilibrium.

Riyue (GB 24) 日月 [rì yuè] A point of Gallbladder Meridian of Foot-*shaoyang*, the anterior referred point of the gallbladder, the confluence of foot-*taiyin*, foot-*shaoyin* meridian, also termed Shenfuang. Location: In the 7th intercostal space, directly below the nipple. Regional anatomy: There is the 7th and 8th intercostal artery and vein. The 7th or 8th intercostal nerve are distributed. Indications: Distension, swelling and pain in the hypochondrium, vomiting, acid regurgitation, hiccup, jaundice. Puncture: 1—2 cm obliquely, Moxibustion: 3—5 moxa cones or 5—10 minutes with warming moxibustion.

rolling spur sylinder 滚刺筒 [gǔn cì tóng] A kind of skin needle. It is composed of the two parts. One is the handle, the other is the rorlling sylinder on which the short needles are distributed over. While using it, hold the handle with one hand, and then roll it on the area where stimulation is needed. Suitable for superficial puncture on a larger area. (Fig 109)

round needle 员针 [yuán zhēn] A round needle.

round needle 圆针 [yuán zhēn] One of the nine ancient needles. It is called the needle with a round head. Since its head is oval-shape, it is used to do massage on the body surface to treat disorders and pain of tendens and muscles.

rotatory kneeding manipulation 搓法 [cuō fǎ] An accessary acupuncture manipulation. To take off the needle immediately after rotat-

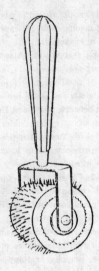

Fig 109

ing it with thumb, index finger. (plus the middle finger)

rough and large needle 絮针 [xù zhēn] An anciant needling instrument for daily life. The round needle and the sharp needle mentioned in Miraculous Prvot are derived from it.

Rouxi 肉郄 [ròu xī] An alternate term for Chengshan (BL 57).

roujiong 肉腘 [ròu jiǒng] I. e. , the assembled muscle.

root of gansui Euphorbia kanshui 甘遂 [gān suì] The drug for dressing and moxibustion.

Rongzhu 容主 [róng zhǔ] I. e. , Kezhu, an alternate term for Shangguan (GB 3).

reinforcing body resistance to elimilate pathogenic qi 扶正祛邪 [fú zhèng qù xié] *Fuzheng* refers to reinforcing the body resistance while *quxie* eliminating external pathogenic *qi* and internal pathologic products.

regular points 正穴 [zhèng xué] The *shu* points of the fourteen meridians contrary to the extra points.

regular meridians 正经 [zhèng jīng] 1. Referring to the twelve meridians, contrary to the eight extra meridians (vessels); 2. the meridian itself; 3. Yellow Emperor's Regular Classioc. It refers to Yellow Emperor's *Mintang* Points, which is preserved to be the book dealing with meridian points represented by Systematic Classic of Acupuncture.

Ren Zuotian 任作田 [rèn zuò tián] (1886—1950) An acupuncture specialist in modern times, born at Liaoyang, Liaoning Province. He took on acupuncture with rich clinical experiences. after '9. 18' (1931), he went to Yanan and took part in the anti-Japanese work for saving his motherland. Under the leadership of the Chinese Communist Party, he created Institute of Acupuncture Treatment at Yanan and handded over acupuncture techniques, which played a certain role in developing the people's health cause in the liberated areas. He was once honoured as the model worker of the integration of Chinese and Western medicine by the border government of Sha'anxi, Gansu and Ningxia provinces.

reinforcing and reducing according to respiration 呼吸补泻 [hū xī bǔ xiè] One of acupuncture reinforcing-reducing manipulations. The reinforcing and reducing manipulations are differentiated by inserting and withdrawing the needle in cooperation with the patient's exhalation and inhalation. (Fig 110)

Rhyt hmed Articles for Emergency 肘后歌 [zhǒu hòu gē] Written by an unknown person. In the article distal and proximsal combination of points for common diseases and symptoms were enumerated. It is of reference value in clinic.

rhinorrhea 鼻渊 [bí yuān] A disease of the nose mainfested by copious foul, prurulent discharge from the nose accompanied by obstruction of the nose, vertigo, dizziness, etc. Simlar to sinusitis.

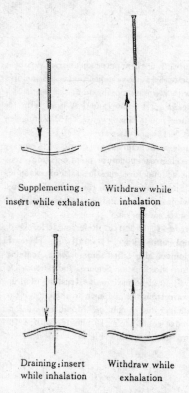

Supplementing:
insert while exhalation

Withdraw while
inhalation

Draining:insert
while inhalation

Withdraw while
exhalation

Fig 110

ring finger and fourth toe 小指次指 [xiǎo zhǐ cì zhǐ] Referring to the ring finger or 4th toe.

root of Japanese snakegourd fruit 土瓜根 [tǔ guā gēn] One of the interposing things used in moxibustion.

Ruxia 乳下 [rǔ xià] An extra point. Located 6 cm directly below the nipple. Indications: Abdominal pain and fullness, pains in the abdomen and hypochondrium, swollen

breast and insufficiency of lactation, chronic cough, regurgitation, dry vomiting, epigastric pain, amenorrhea. Moxibustion: 3—5 moxa cones or 5—10 minutes with warming moxibustion.

Rugen (ST 18) 乳根 [rǔ gēn] A point of Stomach Meridian of Foot-*yangming*. Location: Directly below the nipple, in the 5th intercostal space, 12 cm lateral to Zhongting (CV 16) of the thoracic midline. Regional anatomy: There is the greatest muscle of chest, the medial and lateral muscle of the 5th intercostal nerve and the branch of the intercostal artery and vein. The branch of the 5th intercostal nerve is diseributed. Indications: Cough, depressed chest and thoracalgia, breast carbancle, insufficient lactation, hiccup. Puncture: 1—1. 5 cm obliquely. Moxibustion: 5—10 minutes with warmmg monithustion.

ruizhong 锐中 [ruì zhōng] I. e. , Shengmen (HT 7).

Rushang 乳上 [rǔ shàng] A point, located 3 cm directly above the nipple, Indications: Mammarry trouble and thoracalgia. Moxibustion: 3—5 moxa cones or 5—10 minutes with warming moxibustion.

Ruzhong (ST 17) 乳中 [rǔ zhōng] A point of Stomach Meridian of Foot-*yangming*. Location: In the centre of the nipple. Regional anatomy: There is the greatest muscle of chest, the 4th intercostal medial and lateral muscles, and the lateral pectoral artery and vein. The anterior cutancous branch and the lateral cutaeneous branch of the 4th intercostal nerve are distributed. In contemprary times it is not used for puncture but for the mark of locating the point at the chest.

rush-fire moxibustion 灯草灸 [dēng cǎo jiǔ] I. e. , *deng hue jiu*.

S

Sanshang 三商 [sān shāng] An extra point. A collective term for Laoshang, Zhongshang and Shaoshang. Laoshang is located on the ulnar side of the great thumb, 0.3 cm lateral to the root of the fingernail; Zhongshang is located in the middle of the dorsal side of the thumb, 0.3 cm to the root of the fingernail; Shaoshang pertains to the well-like point of the Lung Meridian of Hand-*taiyin*, 0.3 cm lateral to the root of the corner of the fingernail on the radial side of the thumb. Puncture: Cause little bleeding with a triangular needle. (Fig 111)

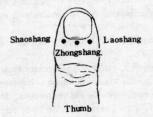

Fig 111

Sanjiaoshu (BL 22) 三焦俞 [sān jiāo shū] The back-*shu* point of the triple energizer. Location: 5 cm lateral to Xuanshu (GV, DU 5) between the spinal processes of the 1st and 2nd lumbar vertebrae. Reginal anatomy: In the illocostal muscle and the longest muscle, there is the posterior branch of the 1st lumber artery and vein. The lateral cutaneous branch of the posterior branch of the 10th thoracic nerve is distributed. The lateral branch of the posterior nerve of the 1st lumbar nerve is in the deeper. Indications: Abdominal distension, borborygmus, indigestion, vomiting, diarrhea, dysentery, edema, jaundice, nocturnal emission, aliguria, with short micturition, pains in the waist and back, gastritis, enteritis, nephritis, diabetes, insipidus neurasthenia. Punc-

ture: 1.5—3cm perpendicularly. Moxibustion: 5—7 moxa cones or 10—15 minutes with warming moxibustion.

sanguan 三管 [sān guǎn] A brief term for three points, Shangwan (CV 13), Zhongwan (CV 12) and Xiawan (CV 10).

simple acupuncture 干针 [gān zhēn] Contrary to electroacupuncture, point injection, etc., in acupuncture anesthesia. For example, "Simple acupuncture can make *qi* acquired while retention of the inserted needle can cause anesthesia."

sangda 颡大 [sǎng dà] Referring to forehead.

Sanqi points 疝气穴 [shàn qì xué] The extra points, also called *sanjiao jiu* in Acupuncture Moxibustion Science. Indications: Deviation of hernia, *bentun* (rushing of *qi* upward from the abdomen to the chest) cardialgia due to cold *qi*. Moxibustion: 3—5 moxa cones or 5—10 minutes with warming moxibustion. (Fig 112)

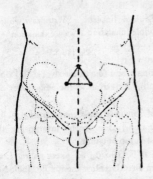

Fig 112

sanzonggu 三宗骨 [sān zōng gǔ] Referring to sacrum.

Sanjiejiao 三结交 [sān jié jiāo] Referring to Guanyuan (RN 4).

Sacral vertebra 骶椎 [dǐ zhuī] An ear point at the protruding spot of the starting part of the antihelix. Divide the interspace between Cervicle Vertebra and Sacral Vertebra into the two equivalent parts.

Sanxiao 散笑 [sān xiào] An extra point located lateroinfrerior to Yingxiang (LI 20) at the midpoint of the nasolabial groove. Indications: Stuffy nose, facial deep-rooted sore, deviated mouth and eyes. Puncture: 1—1. 5 cm horizontally.

Sancai points 三才穴 [sān cái xué] The points of Baihui (GV, DU 20), Xuanji (CV, RN 21) and Yongquan (KI 1). In ancient China, the heaven, man and earth were called three *cai* while the three points are distributed over the head, chest and foot.

Sanchi 三池 [sān chí] An extra point, located on the radial side of the elbow, 3 cm superior and inferior to Quchi (LI 11), 3 in total. Indications: Febrile diseases, rhinites, pain in the elbow and arm, paralysis of the upper limb. Puncture: 3—4 cm perpendicularly. Moxibustion : 3—5 moxa cones or 5—15 minutes with warming moxibustion.

Sanmen 三门 [sān mén] I. e. , Sanjian (LI 3).

sanshui 三水 [sān shuǐ] It means three yin, i. e. , *taiyin* (Yang Shangshan's Notes). *Sanshui* means three yin storing viscera… Three storing viscera refers to the liver, spleen and kidney. It is therefore called because they are located below the diaphragm. " (Wang Bin's Notes)

Sanmao 三毛 [sān máo] The area posteior to the toenail of the great toe, where hair grows.

sacral end 骶端 [dǐ duān] Referring the lower end of sacrum, i. e. , coccyx.

salt-interposing moxibustion 隔盐灸 [gé yán jiǔ] A kind of moxibustion . To fill in the umbilical fossa with stir-fried salt, then to do moxibustion with a big moxa cone. Change the cone when the patient feels scorching pain. Moxibustion can also be done by putting the moxa cone on the umbilicus that is filled with salt and circled with rinsed flour like a well. (Fig 113).

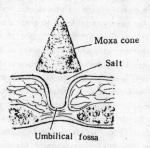

Moxa cone
Salt
Umbilical fossa

Fig 113

Sanli 三里 [sān lǐ] The name of the meridian points. One pertains to Large Intestine Meridian located at the forear; The other pertains to Stomak Meridian, located in front of the tibia. In order to differentiate them, the former is called Shousanli (LI 10), while the latter Zusanli (ST 36). In general, it refers to the latter.

Sanjiaojiu 三角灸 [sān jiǎo jiǔ] I. e. , Sanqi point.

Sanjian(LI 3) 三间 [sān jiān] A point of Large Intestine Meridian of Hand-*Yangming*. The stream-like point of the meridian it pertains to. Also named Shaogu. Location: On the radial side of the small head of the 2nd metacarpal bone in the depression posterior to the metacarpo-phalangeal bone at the dorso-palmar boundary. Select it by slightly forming a fist. Regional anatomy: The branch of the 1st dorsal artery of palm through the 1st interosseous dorsal muscle to reach the adductor muscle of thumb. Indications: Ocular pain, toothache, sore throat, toothache, pains in the fingers and dorsal hand, epistaxis, dry lips and mouth, lethargy, abdominal fullness, borborygmus and diarrhea. Puncture: 1. 5 cm perpendicularly. Moxibustion: 3—5 moxa cones or 5—10 minutes with warming moxa.

Sanyangwuhui 三阳五会 [sān yáng wǔ huì] An alternate term for Baihui (GV 20).

Sanyangluo (TE8) 三阳络 [sān yáng luò] Also termed Tongjian. Location: 12 cm above the transverse crease of the dorsal wrist between radius and ulna. Reginal anatomy: Between the common extensor muscle of finger and long abductor muscle of thumb. There is the dorsal interosseous artery and vein of forearm. The dorsal cutaneous nerve of forearm is distributed. The dorsal interosseous nerve of forearm is in the deeper. Indications: Headache, deafness, sudden aphohia, toothache, pain in the arm. Puncture: 3. 3 cm perpendicularly. Moxibustion: 3—5 moxa cones or 5—10 minutes with warming moxibustion.

Sanyinjiao (SP 6) 三阴交 [sān yīn jiāo] The confluence of foot-*taiyin*, foot-*jueyin* and foot-*shaoyin* meridians. Location: 1 dm directly above the tip of the medial ankle, in the depression of the posterior edge of the medial side of the tibia. Reginal anatomy: Between the posterior edge of fibula and soleus muscle, passing through long flexor muscle of toe, there is the greater saphenous vein, posterior artery and vein of tibia. The medial cutaneous nerve of the leg is distributed. The tibial nerve is in the deep. Indications: Weakness of spleen and stomach, borborygmus, abdominal distension, indigestion, irregular menstruation, metrorrhagia, amenorrhea, prolapse of genitalia, dystochia, postpartum retention of lochia, nocturnal emission, impotence, enuresis, hernia, atrophic foot, foot *qi*, insomnia, neurodermatites, urticaria, eczema, hypertension.

Sciatic 坐骨神经 [zuò gǔ shén jīng] An ear point located between Hip and Sympathetic.

scorching moxibustion 烧灼灸 [shāo zuó jiǔ] To directly scorch the skin of the point with direct moxibustion to make it blister or suppuration. It is divided into blistering moxibustion and suppurative moxibustion.

scrofula 瘰疬 [luǒ lì] Lymphadentitis scrofula of the neck. The smaller one is called *luo* and the larger, *li*.

sciatica 坐骨神经痛 [zuò gǔ shén jīng tòng] It belongs to the category of blockage syndrome, mainly manifested as the radiating pain at a segment or the whole path of the sciatic nerve. Treated by mainly selecting the points of foot-*taiyang* and foot-*shaoyang* meridians. The case with muscular atrophy, the points of foot-*yangming* and foot-*taiyin* meridians are selected in association. The common acupoints are Dachangshu (BL 25).

scratching manipulation 刮法 [guā fǎ] Referring to sratching the handle of the needle up and down so as to reinforcing needling sensation. (Fig 114)

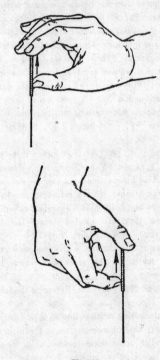

Fig 114

scalp needling 头针 [tóu zhēn] Also called *tou pi zhen*. A therapy to puncture the specific region at the scalp area. It was reported in 1972. In location of the point the function of the cerebral cortex is referred in combination with the location of disease, and its corresponding stimulation region is selected. While puncturing, No 26 filiform needle (6 cm in length) is usually used and puncture is horizontal with swift needle-rotation for a longer time, usually used for treating apoplexy with paralplegia, cerebral astheriosclerosis, aphagia, Parkinson's disease, etc. Their difference can be seen in the following table and figures. (Fig 115)

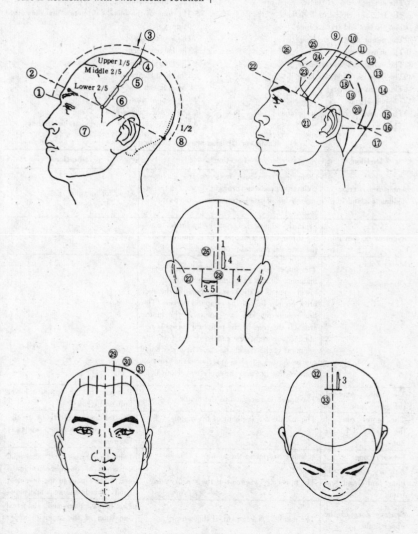

Fig 115

①Interspace between the two eyebrows
②The superior edge of the midpoint of the eyebrow
③The midpoint of the anteroposterior midline
④The motor zone of the lower limb and trunk
⑤The motor zone of the upper limb
⑥The motor zone of the face (language zone)
⑦The anterior edge of the temporal line
⑧The lateral occipital protuberance
⑨The cholera and tremor zone
⑩The motor zone
⑪The sensory zone
⑫The motor and sensory zone of foot
⑬The node of the vertex bone
⑭The language zone₂
⑮The visual zone
⑯The lateral occipital protuberance
⑰The balance zone

⑱The application zone
⑲The zone of motion sickness and listening
⑳The language zone₂
㉑The anterior edge of the temporal hair
㉒The superior edge of the midpoint of the eyebrow
㉓The genital zone
㉔The stomach zone
㉕The zone of the blood contraction and diastolization
㉖The visual zone
㉗The balance zone
㉘The lateral occipital protuberance
㉙The chest cavity zone
㉚The stomach zone
㉛The genital zone
㉜The motor zone of foot
㉝The midpoint of the anteroposterior midline

Table For Division of Scalp Needling

Division	Location	Indications
Anterior-posterior midline (sagital line)	From the interspace between the eyebrows (Yintant), passing through Vertex, to the interior edge of the external occipital protuberance	Used for locating
Eyebrow-occiput line	From the superior edge of the eyebrow, passing through the temporal area to the top end of the external occiptal protuberance	
Moter Zone	The upper point is 0.5 cm posterior to the midpoint of the anteroposterior midline, the lower point is at the crossing point of the eyebrow-occiput line of the temporal corner. The line connecting the two points is the motor area (If the edge of the temporal corner is not obtained, a right line can be drawn from the midpoint of the zygomatic arc. The lower point can be located . 0.5 cm anterior to the crossing point of this line and the eyebrow-occiput line)	
The motor zone of the upper zone	The upper 1/5 segmen of the motor	Paralysis of the opposite lower limb and trunk
The motor zone of the face (Motor Zone₁)	The middle 2/5 segment of the motor	Central facial paralysis of the opposite side, kinetic aphasia, lacrimation
Sensory Zone	1.5cm posterior to the motor	Pain, numbness and abnormal sensation of the opposite limbs and trunk, pain in the posterior head, pain in the neck and nape
Aensory Zone of the lower limb, head, and trunk	The upper 1/5 segment of the sensory sore	
Sensory Zone of the upper limb	The middle 2/5 segment of the sensory	Numbness, pain and abnormal sensation of the apposite upper limb

Continued

Division	Location	Indications
Sensory Zone of the face	The lower 2/5 segement of the sensory	Numbness, of the opposite side of face, migraine and triangular neuralgia
Motor-sensory Zone of foot	1 cm lateral to the midpoint of the anteroposterior midline, draw a line of 3 cm backwardly and straight line of 3 cm backward and that is parallel with the anteroposterior midline	Paralysis, numbness, pain and abnormal sensation of the opposite foot and lower abdomen, acute lumbar sprain, cortical profuse urine, night urination
Korea-tremor-central Zone	1.5 cm forwardly removed from the motor	Child cholera, paralysis agitans
Vasomotion Zone	3 cm removed forwardly from the Motor	Cortical puffiness, hypertension, angiitis
Syncope-hearing Zone	Draw a straight line of 4 cm from the place 1 cm lateral to the external occipital protuberance in parallel with the anteroposterior midline	Vertigo, tinnitus, reduced hearing
Visual Zone	Draw a straight line of 4 cm from the place 1 cm lateral to the external occipital protuberance upwardly in parallel with the midline	Cortical visual disturbance, myopia
Balance Zone	Draw a straight line of 4 cm from the place 3.3 cm lateral to the external occipital protuberance drawn in parallel with the anteroposterior midline	Balance disturbance caused by cerebellum
Language Zone$_2$	Draw a straight line of 3 cm from the place 2 cm below the motch of the parietal bone backward in parallel with the anteroposterial midline	Nominal aphasia
Language Zone$_3$	Draw a straight line of 4 cm from the midpoint of the Syncope-hearing Zone backwardly	Sensory aphasia
Application Zone	Draw a straight line of 3 cm respectively from the node of the parietal bone vertically downwardly, anteriorly downward, posteriorly downward that form a 40° angle	Apraxia
Stomach Zone	Draw a straight line of 2 cm from the hairline the pupil directly ascends to respectively in parallel with the anteroposterior midline	Stomachache, discomfort at the epigastrium
Chest Cavity Zone	Draw a straight line of 2 cm above and below the hairline between stomach Zone and the anteroposterior hairline	Discomfort of chest, asthma, palpitation
Genital Zone	Draw a straight line of 2 cm backward in parallel with the anteroposterior midline at the corner of the hair	Dysfunctional metrorrhagia, profuse leukorrhea, nocturnal emission, treating prolapse of uterus in cooperation with foot-motor-sensory Zone

sequential points 步穴 [bù xué] Referring to introduction to the needling techniques according certain sequence.

Selecting the meridian for the disease neither excess nor deficiency 不盛不虚以经取之 [bù shèn bù xū yǐ jīng qǔ zhī] The principle of acupuncture treatment. For the disease that is not obviously caused by deficiency or excess is just treated by selecting the point according to the meridian but not necessarily differentiate reinforcing and reducing manipulations.

selection of the upper point for treating the lower diseases 下病上取 [xià bìng shàng qǔ] One of the principles of selecting the point in Internal Classic. The points at the upper part of the body are selected for treating the diseases at the upper.

Setting the mountain on fire 烧山火 [shāo shān huǒ] An acupuncture manipulation symetrical to cool at a clear sky night, a synthetical application of acupuncture reinforcing manipulation. After the needle is inserted subcutaneously, it is repeatedly thrusted thrice according to the sequence of the superficial, medial and deep strata, and lifted once so as to make the patient feel warm. It suits cold syndrome. (Fig 116)

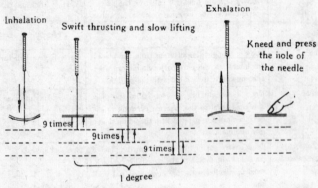

Fig 116

second lateral line of abdomen 腹第二侧线 [fù dì èr chè xiàn] The line for locating the meridian points, 6 cm to the abdominal midline, where Stomach Meridian of Foot-*yangming* passes through. Distributed are Burong(ST 19), Chengman(ST 20), Liangmen (ST 21), Guanmen (ST 22), Taiyi (ST 23), Huaroumen (ST 24), Tianshu (ST 25), Wailing (ST 26), Daju (ST 27), Shuidao (ST 28), Guilai (ST 29), Qichong (ST 30).

selection of points from other meridians 异经取穴 [yì jīng qǔ xué] The point-selected method, contrary to selection of the points from the meridian. Also termed *ta jing gu xue*. It refers to selection of the point or the other meridians concerning the diseased meridian, including the external-internal meridians, the meridain with the same name. etc. For stomach trouble, Gongsun (SP 4) of foot-*taiyin* meridian is selected, for hemorrhoids, Kongzui (LU 6) of Lung Meridian of Hand-*taiying* is selected, etc.

sea of qi 气海 [qì hǎi] 1. The reservoir of *qi*, referring to the part of the chest between the two breasts or that of the abdomen below the umbilicus; 2. The name of the acupuncture point, Qihai (CV 6).

seventh vertebra 第七椎 [dì qī zhuī] Referring to the 7th thoracic vertebra.

second lateral line of back 背第二侧线 [bèi dì èr chè xiàn] A line locating the meridian point. The area 6 cm distal to the midline of the back is where Bladder Meridian of Foot-*taiyang* passes throuogh, the points such as Fufen (BL 41), Naohu (GV, DU 17), Gaohuang (BL 43), Shentang (BL 44), Yixi (BL 45), Geguan (BL 46), Hunmen (BL 47), Yanggang (SI 5), Yishe (BL 49), Weiicang (BL 50), Huangmen (BL 51), Zhishi (BL 52), Baohuang (BL 53) and Zhibian (BL 54) are distributed over.

sea of meridians 经脉之海 [jīng mài zhī hǎi] Referring to *chogmai* (Vital Vessel).

selecting the points of the same meridian 接经取穴 [jié jīng qǔ xué] One of the point-selected methods, also called *tong ming jing qu xue*. In the twelve meridians, the meridians of the hand and foot with the same name are connected from upper to lower. According to this relationship, the pathological change of certain meridian can be treated by it. So, the disorders of the hand-*taiyin* and hand-*yangming* meridians can be treated by selecting the points on the foot-*taiyin* and foot-*yangming* meridians and the disorders of foot-*taiyin* and foot-*yangming* meridians can be treated by selecting the points on hand-*taiyin* and hand-*yangming* meridians.

selecting the points along the meridians 循经取穴 [xún jīng qǔ xué] One of the point-selected methods. To select the point concerned according to the scale of the meridian connects with. In clinic it mainly refers that the diseases or symptoms in the aspect of the viscera are treated by selecting the distal points of the four limbs distal of the meridians concerned, as well as the proximal meridian points where the diseases or sympstoms are located. So it can be classified into distal selection of the point along the meridian and proximal selection of the point along the meridian.

searching for the basic cause of the ailment in treatment 治病求本 [zhì bìng qiú běn] In treating a disease its primary cause should

be ascertained by grasping the meaning of its manifestations.

sea of medulla 髓海 [sui hǎi] One of the 'four seas', referring to brain.

selection of the surrounding points for the middle disease 中病旁取 [zhōng bìng páng qǔ] One of the principles of selection the point in Internal Classic. The disease at the middle part of the body is treated by selecting its surrounding points.

serpiginous-belt erysipelas 蛇丹 [shé dān] A serpiginous vesicular eruption of the skin around the waist, which is red in color, like a snake encircling the waist, similar to herpes zoster.

sea of water and grain 水谷之海 [shuǐ gǔ zhī hǎi] One of the 'four seas'. Referring to stomach.

selection of the point from the other meridian 他经取穴 [tā jīng qǔ xué] I. e., *yu jing qu xue*.

second lateral line of head 头第二侧线 [tóu dì èr chè xiàn] The line to locate the meridian point, which connects Toulinqi (GB 15) and Fengchi (GB 20) where Gallbladder Meridian of Foot-*taiyang* passes through. Toulinqi (GB 15), Muchuang (GB 16), Zhengying (GB 17), Chengling (GB 18), Naokong (GB 19) and Fengchi (GB 20) are distributed over.

selecting the point from the distal segement 远节段取穴 [yuǎn jié duàn qǔ xué] A classification of point-selected method. It referes that the point selected in clinical treatment or acupuncture anesthesia and the painful or operated location are not controlled by the same or proximal segment of the spinal cord. E. g., for head trouble, the cranial opertation the patient of the lower limb is selected, for trouble of the waist and leg, the point on the upper limb is selected.

selection of the point from the point-located meridian 本经取穴 [běn jīng qǔ xué] One of point-selected methods. Referring to selection of the point from the merifian the disease pertains to. Usually the point distal to the affected area is selected. For instance, for cougha Chize (LR 3) of the foot-*jueyin* meridians is selected. It also includes selection of the point proximal to the affected area, e. g., hypochondriac pain due to disorder of liver *qi*, Zhangmen (LR 13) of Liver Meridian of Foot-*jueyin* is selected. For toothache due to flaring up of stomach fire, Xiaguan (ST 7) of Stomach Meridian of foot-*yangming* is selected. Refer selection of the point along the meridian.

sea of the five storing viscera and six emptying viscera 五脏六腑之海 [wǔ zàng liù fǔ zhī hǎi]Referring to stomach, also referring to Vital Vessel.

seven emotions 七情 [qī qíng] Seven kinds of emotional reactions, namely joy, anger, anxiety, worry, grief, apprehension and fright.

sea of the twelve meridians 十二经之海 [shí èr jīng zhī hǎi] Referring to the vital Vessel, also termed the sea of blood.

severe-pain syndrome 急痛证 [jí tòng zhèng] The severe pain occurring at different portions of the human body. 1. Severe cardiac pain: Danzhong (CV 17), Neiguan (PC 6), Xinshu (BL 15), Zusanli (ST 36); 2. Severe biliary pain: Riyue (GB 24), Zhongwan (CV12); Yanglingquan (GB 34), Zusanli (ST 36), Taichong (GB 9); 3. Severe stomachache: Zhongwan (CV 12), Zusanli (ST 36).

second lateral line of chest 胸第二侧线 [xiōng dì èr chè xiàn] A line for locating the meridian point, i. e., the line connecting the middle of the supraclavicular bone and that of the nipple, 12 cm to the midline of chest, where Stomach Meridian of Foot-*yangming* passes through. Quepeng (ST 12), Qihu (ST 13), Kufang (ST 14), Wuyi (ST 15), Yingchuang (ST 16), Ruzhong (ST 17), and Rugen (ST 18) are distributed.

seven-time vessels 七次脉 [qī cì mài]CV and GV that run over the neck, three yang meridiands and three yin meridians of hands and feet have a main point each.

They are sequentially Renying (ST 9) — CV, Futu (LI8) —Hand-*yangming* Meridian; Tianchuang (SI16) —Hand-*taiyang*; Tianrong (TE, SJ16) —Foot-*shayang*; Tianzhu (BL10) —Foot-*shoyang*; Fengfu (GV16) —GV.

Seven-star needle 七星针 [qī xīng zhēn] A kind of cutaneous needle, shaped as a small hammer, formed with seven thready needles, used to tapping the skin to puncture the skin superficially. (Fig 117)

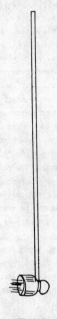

Fig 117

seven important portals 七冲门 [qī chōng mén] The seven portals of the digestive system, viz, lips, teeth, epiglottis, cardia, pylorus ilicecal valve, and anus.

seasonal variation of pulse 脉合四时 [mài hé sì shí] The pathologic changes of the pulse according to the changes of four seasons. For example, the pulse in spring is somewhat taut; in summer, somewhat full; in autumn, somewhat floating; in winter, somewhat deep. All of these changes are normal.

Secret Handed-down Moxibustion Techniques 灸法秘传［jiǔ fǎ mì chuán］A book compiled by Jinye Tianchuan and Lei Shaoyi in Qing Dynasty (1644—1911), one volume. It contains the illustration of the anterior side, the illustration of the posterior side, the illustration of the finger joints, the illustration of moxibustion with moxibustion lamp, miraculous prescriptions of drugs for moxibustion, prohibitions of moxibustion techniques 70 symptoms, indications of moxibution, etc. Of them a technique that a kind of specially-prepared medicinal mugwort is put into a silver moxibustion bowl to carry on moxibustion treatment was introduced, which is of certain characteristics. At the end of the book "Prescriptions of *Taiyi* Miraculous Acupuncture" were appended into it by Liu Guoguang. It is a special book of moxibustion techniques and was published in 1883.

selecting the point from the couple meridians 偶经取穴［ǒu jīng qǔ xué］One of the point-selected methods, also called selecting the points from the externally-internally related meridians. According to the external-internal relationship between the meridians, select the point of on the meridian which is externally-internally related to another meridian. E. g., for common cold that pertains to the disorder of Lung Meridian of Hand-*taiyin*, Hegu(LI 4) of Large Intestine Meridian of Hand-*yangming* is selected; For stomach trouble that pertains to Stomach Meridian of Foot-*yangming*, Gongsun (SP 4) of Spleen Meridian of Foot-*taiyin* is selected.

seven apoplexy points 中风七穴 ［zhòng fēng qī xué］Seven empirical effective points for treating apoplexy. They are as follows: Baihui GV 20), Erqianfaji, Jianjing (GB 21), Fengshi (GB 31), Zusanli (ST 36), Juegu point, Quchi (LI 11). (Prescriptions of Peaceful Holy Benevolence.)

Secret Moxibustion Classic for Carbuncles and Furuncles 痈疽神秘灸经［yōng zǔ shén mì jiǔ jīng］An acupuncture book, also inscribed as Moxibustion Classic of Carbuncles and Furuncles written by Hu Yuanqing in Yuan Dynasty (1271—1386). It contains treatment of surgical carbuncles and furuncles with moxibustion, and respectively describes the major *shu* points of the fourteen meridians, which are used for treating carbuncles and furuncles, appended with illustrations. In the book a number of secret points were collected, which can not be seen in other acupuncture books. It is a special book to explore the pathogenesis and moxibustion treatment of carbuncles and furuncles, completed in 1354.

seven important portals 七冲门［qī chōng mén］The seven portals of the digestive system, viz, lips, teeth, epiglottis, cardia, pylorus, ileocecal valve, and anus.

shaking of needle 针摇［zhēn yáo］A manipulation, i. e., shaking manipulation, enumerated as one of the twelve manipulations in Compendium of Acupuncture.

shaking manipulations 动法［dòng fǎ］The acupuncture manipulation. Enumerated as one of the fourteen manipulations in Key to Acupuncture Classic. It is that if *qi* does not move, the needle may be lifted, if *qi* does not flow, the needle may be shaked like shaking a ball, moving and shaking…"

sharp-round needle 圆利针［yuán lì zhēn］One of the nine ancient needles. Clinically used for treating carbuncle, swelling and blockage syndrome.

sharp needle 锐针［ruì zhēn］Referring to the sharp needle.

shaking manipulation 摇法［yáo fǎ］Referring to the acupuncture manipulation of shaking the body of needle. Used in withdrawing the needle in reducing manipulation.

Shangmen 上门 ［shàng mén］An alternate term for Younen (KI 21).

Shangjuxu (ST 37) 上巨虚［shàng jù xū］A point of Stomach Meridian of Foot-*yang-*

ming, called Juxushang, the lower joining point of the large intestine. Location: 1.8 dm directly below Dubi (ST 35) on the lateral side of the patellar ligament below Zusanli (ST 36). Regional Anatomy: In the anterior muscle of tibia, they are the anterior artery and vein of tibia. The branches of the lateral cutaneous nerve of calf and of the proper nerve are distributed. The deep femoral nerve is in the deeper. Indications: Pain in the intestine, diarrhea, dysentery, constipation, intestinal carbuncle, foot *qi*, paralysis due to apoplexy, abdominal distension. Puncture: 3—5 cm perpendicularly. Moxibustion: 3—7 moxa cones or 5—15 minutes with warming moxibustion.

Shangqihai 上气海 [shàng qì hǎi] An alternate term for Danzhong (CV 17), contrary to Xiaqihai.

Shangguan (GB 3) 上关[shàng guān] A point of Gallbladder Meridian of Foot-*shaoyang*, also called Kezhuren, the confluence of hand-*shaoyang*, foot-*shaoyang* and foot-*yangming* meridians. Location: On the superior edge of the zygomatic arc, 3 cm at the anterior edge of auricle directly opposite to Xiaguan (ST 7). Regional anatomy: Below the temporal muscle. There are the temporal orbital artery and vein. The temporal branch of the facial nerve and the zygomatic-facial nerve are distributed. Indications: Headache, tinnitus, deafness, toothache, deviated mouth and eyes, epilepsy due to fright, clonic convulsion, neural deafness, otitis, media. Puncture: 1—2 cm perpendicularly. Moxibustion: 2—5 minutes with warming moxibustion.

Shanglian 上廉 [shàng lián] 1. A point of Large Intestine Meridian of Hand-*Yangming*. Location: On the radial side of the dorsal forearm, on the line connecting Yangxi (LI 5) and Quchi (LI 11), 1 dm below Quchi (LI). Regional anatomy: In the long extensor muscle of the wrist and the supinator muscle. There are the muscular branches of the radial artery and cephic

vein. The dorsal cutanous nerve of forearm and the deep branch of the radial nerve are distributed. Indications: Headache, paraplegia, soreness and pain in the elbow and arm, abdominal pain, borborygmus, diarrhea. Puncture: 1.5—3 cm perpendicularly. Moxibustion: 3—5 moxa comes or 5—10 minutes with warming moxibustion. 2. Referring to Shangjuxu (ST 37).

Shangshan 伤山 [shāng shān] The wrong form of Changshan, another name of Changshan (BL 57).

Shaoyangwei 少阳维 [shào yáng wéi] An extra point. Located at the midpoint, at the line connecting Taixi (KI 3) and Futu (KI 7). Indications: Foot *qi*, chronic eczema, lumps, paralysis of the lower limbs. Puncture: 1—2 cm perpendicularly. Moxibustion: 3—5 moxa cones or 5—10 minutes with warming moxibustion.

shaoyin **meridian** 少阴脉 [shào yīn mài] The name of the meridian during the early period. Referring to foot-*shaoyin* meridian.

shaogu 少谷 [shào gǔ] Another the name of Sanjian (LI3).

Shaofu (HT 8) 少府[shào fǔ]A point of Heart Meridian of Hand-*shaoyin*, the spring-like point (fire) of the meridian. Location: Between the 4th and 5th metacarpal bones at the level with Laogong (PC 8) when the fingers are flexed. To form a fist, the point is where the tip of the small finger touches. Regional anatomy: Passing through the 4th lumbricoid muscle and the superficial deep flexor muscle of the 4th and 5th fingers, reaching the interosseous muscle. There is the common artery and vein on the metacarpo-phalangeal side. The 4th palmar common nerve is distributed. Indications: Palpitation, thoracalgia, intestinal carbuncle, itch of the pubic region, prolapse of uterus, pubic pain, dysuria, anuresis, contracture of the small finger, feverish sensation in the palms. Puncture: 1—2 cm perpendicularly. Moxibustion: 1—3 moxa cone or 3—5 minutes with warming moxibustion.

Shaoze (ST 1) 少泽 [shào zé] A point of Small Intestine Meridian of Hand -*taiyang*, the well-like (metal) point of the meridian. Also termed Xiaoji. Location: Approx. 3 cm lateral to the corner of the fingernail, on the ulnar side of the small finger, sore throat, nebula, enroachment of pterugium to the corner, swelling breast, insufficient secretion of lactation, debility of the small fingers, first aid in coma. Puncture: 0.3—0.6 cm obliquely, or cause little bleeding with a triangular needle. Moxibustion: 1—3 moxa cones or 3—5 minutes with warming moxibustion.

shaoyang **meridian is selected for flaccidity and looseness of joint** 骨繇者取之少阳 [gǔ yáo zhě qǔ zhī shào yáng] As for the treatment of the flaccidity and looseness of the joint *shaoyang* meridian may be first considered.

Shangen 山根 [shān gēn] Referring to the root of the nose, approx. at the level with the inner canthus of the eyes.

Shaoguan 少关 [shào guān] An alternate term for Yinjial (CV 7).

shaoyang **meridian** 少阳脉 [shào yáng mài] The name of the meridian during the early period, referring to foot-*shaoyang* meridian.

Shaoyinxi 少阴郄 [shào yīn xī] I. e., Yinxi (HT 6).

Shaoyinshu 少阴俞 [shào yīn shū] Referring to Shenshu (BL 23).

shaofu 少腹 [shào fù] 1. Same as *xiao fu* (the lower abdomen); 2. The bilateral lower part of the abdomen.

Shaoji 少吉 [shào jí] I. e., Xiaoji, an alternate term for Shaoze (ST 1).

sharp round needle 员利针 [yuán lì zhēn] I. e., 圆利针.

Shao hai (HT 3) 少海 [shào hǎi] A point of Heart Meridian of Hand-*shaoyin*, the sealike (water) point of the meridian. Also termed Qujie. Location: Between the end of the transverse crease of the medial side of

elbow and the mediosuperior condyle of the humur. Regional anatomy: There is the round pronator muscle and brachial muscle, the basilic vein, the infroulnar accessory artery and vern, the ulnar artery and vein. The medial cutaneaus nerve of forearm is distributed. Indications: Febrile diseases, coma due to apoplexy, insufficiency of lactation, headache, stiff neck, hypochondriac pain, numb arm, tremor of elbow, breast carbuncle, sore throat, nebula, malaria, headache, deafness, tinnitus, pain in the lateroposterior aspect of the shoulder and arm. Puncture: 1.5—3 cm perpendicularly. Moxibustion: 3—5 moxa cones or 5—10 minuts with warming moxibustion.

Shangqiu (SP 5) 商丘 [shāng qiū] A point of Spleren Meridian of Foot-*taiyin*, the stream-like (metal) point of the meridian. Location: In the depression anterior to the medial ankle of foot. Regional anatomy: There is the medial artery of the dorsal foot and the greater saphenous vein. The branch of the medial cutaneous nerve of the medial side of leg is distributed. Indications: Abdominal pain, abdominal distension, nausea and vomiting, stiffness and pain in the tongue proper, borborygmus, diarrhea, vomiting, mental fatigue, tremor of the body, pain in the chest and hypochondrium, jaunidice, abdominal masses, infantile malnutrition, pain in the lumbar spine. Puncture: 1.5—2.5 cm perpendicularly. Moxibustion: 1—3 moxa cones or 5—10 minutes with warming moxibustion.

Shangcigang 上慈宫 [shàng cí gōng] An alternate term for Chongmen (SP12).

Shangying li 上龈里 [shàng yíng lǐ] An extra point located in the centre of the mucoid membrane of the upper lip, externally opposite to Shuigou (GV 26). Puncture: 0.3—0.6 cm perpendicularly or prick to cause little bleeding with a triangular needle. (Fig 118)

Shangguan 上管 [shàng guǎn] I. e., Shangwan (CV 13).

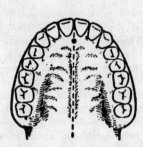

Fig 118

Shangliao 上髎 [shàng liáo] A point of Bladder Meridian of Foot-*taiyang*, the connecting point of foot-*taiyang* and foot-*yangming* meridians. Location: At the lateral aspect of the sacral crest, in the posterior forearm of the 1st sacrum, or select it in the depression between the posterosuperior iliac spine and the pseudospinous process. Regional anatomy: There is the posterior branch of the lateral artery and vein of sacrum. The posterior branch of the 1st sacral nerve is distributed. Indications: Lumbago, irregular menstruation, prolape of uterus, leukorrhea, spermatorrhea, impotence, difficulty in micturation and defecation. Puncture: 3—4 cm perpendicularly. Moxibustion: 3—7 moxa cones or 5—15 minutes with warming moxibustion.

Shangkunlun 上昆仑 [shàng kūn lún] I.e., Kun lun (BL 60).

Shanglin 上林 [shàng lín] I.e., Shangjuxu (ST 37).

Shangzhu 上杼 [shàng zhù] Alternate name of Dazhui (GV 14).

Shangyinxiang 上迎香 [shàng yíng xiāng] An extra point. Location: In the depression of the nasal bone at the end of the upper end of the nasolabial groove. Indications: Prolonged shedding of cold tear, redness and ulceration of lid margin, rhinitis, nasosinusitis. Puncture: 1.5 cm horiontally.

Shanggai 商盖 [shāng gài] I. e., Gsaogai. an alternate term for Dushu (Bl 16).

Shaochong (HT 9) 少冲 [shào chōng] A point of Heart Meridian of Hand-*shaoyin*, the well-like (wood) point of the meridian, also termed Jingshi. Location: 0.3 cm lateral to the corner of the fingernail on the radial side of the small finger. Regional anatomy: There is the network of the artery and vein formed by the proper artery and vein at the digito-palmar side. The proper nerve at the digiial-pains in the chest and hypochondrium, mania, febrile disesses, coma due to apoplexy, stools with purulent blood, spitting blood. Puncture: 0.3—0.6 cm obliquely or cause bleeding with a triang ular needle. Moxibustion: 3—5 moxa cones or 5—10 minutes with warming moxibustion.

Shangxing (GV 23) 上星 [shàng xīng] A point of Governor Vessel, also called Shentang. Location: On the midline of the anterior head, congestive, swelling and painful eyes, rhinorrhea, nasal polyp, epistaxis, infantile convulsion, malaria, febrile diseade, mania, rhinitis, epilepsy. Puncture: 1—2 cm horizontally. Moxibustion: 3—5 moxa cones or 5—10 minutes with warming moxibustion.

Shanggu 上骨 [shàng gǔ] Referring to radius.

Shangdu 上都 [shàng dū] An extra point. One of Baxie (EX-VE 9).

Shangwan (CV 13) 上脘 [shàng wǎn] A point of Conception Vessel, the confluence of CV, foot-*yangming* and hand-*taiyang* meridians. Location: On the abdominal midline, 1.5 dm above the umbilicus. Regional anatomy: In the white abdominal line. There are the superior epigastric artery and vein. The branch of the 7th intercostal nerve is distributed. Indications: Epigastric pain, abdominal distension, vomiting, hiccup, indigestion, jaundice, diarrhea, cough with profuse phlegm, epilepsy, spitting blood due to consumptíve disease. Puncture: 3—4 cm perpendicularly. Moxibustion: 3—7 moxa cones or 5—15 minutes with warming moxibustion.

Shangexue 上腭穴 [shàng é xué] An extra point, located at the midpoint of the superior edge of the upper gum. Puncture: 0. 3—0. 6 cm obliquely or prick to cause little bleeding. Indication: jaundice. (Fig 119)

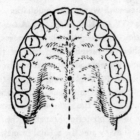

Fig 119

Shangyang (LI 1) 商阳 [shāng yáng] A point of Large Intestine Meridian of Hand-*yangming*, the well-like (metal) point of the meridian, also termed Jueyang. Location: Approx. 0. 3 cm lateral to the corner of the fingernail at the radial aspect of the index finger. Indications: Sore throat, swollen cheek, pain in the lower teeth, deafness, tinnitus, glaucoma, syncope, coma, asthmatic breath, shoulder, pain referring to the supraclavicular fossa. Puncture: 0. 3 cm obliquely or to prick to cause little bleeding with a triangular needle. Moxibustion: 1—3 moxa cones or 5—10 minutes with warming moxibustion.

Shanggu 尚骨 [shàng gǔ] An alterante term for Jianyu (LI 15).

sharp primatic needle 锋针 [fēng zhēn] One of the nine ancient needles, termed a triangular needle in latter generations. In clinic it is mainly used in surgery for piercing abscess and carbuncle to discharge pus and treatment of febrile dieases.

Shangqu (KI 17) 商曲 [shāng qū] A point of Kidney Meridian of Foot-*shaoyin*, the confluence of Vital Vessel and foot-*shaoyin* meiridian, also termed Gaoqu. Location: 1. 4 cm lateral to Xiawan (CV 10), and 6 cm above the umbilicus. Regional anatomy: At the medial edge of the straight muscle of abdomen. There is the superior and inferior artery and vein. The 9th intercostal nerve is distributed. Indications: Abdominal pain, diarrhea, constipation, something accumulating in the abdomen. Puncture: 3—4. 5 cm perpendicularly. Moxibustion: 5—7 moxa cones or 10—15 minutes with warming moxibution.

Shaoshang (LU 11) 少商 [shào shāng] A point of Lung meridian of Hand-*taiyin*, the well-like (wood) point of the meridian. Location: Approx. 3 cm lateral to the corner of the fingernail. Regional anatomy: There is the network of artery and vein formed by the digital-palmar proper artery and vein. The mixed branch of the lateral cutaneous nerve of the forearm and the superficial branch of the radial nerve and the network of the nerve endings formed by the central nerve and the digiatl-palmer proper nerve are distributed. Indications: Sore throat, cough, asthmatic breath, epigastric epistaxis, fullness in the epigastrum, coma due to apoplxy, cough and anxiety, swelling neck, throat blockge, febrile diseases, mania, vomiting due to heatstroke, infantile convulsion, spasm of the fingers and wrists. Puncture: 0. 3—0. 6 cm obliquely or cause little bleeding. Moxibustion: 4—7 moxa cones or 5—10 minutes with warming moxibustion.

shenmai (BL 62) 申脉 [shēn mài] A point of Bladder Meridian of Foot-*taiyang*, produced by Motility Vessel of Yang. One of the eight confluential points, communicated with Motility Vessel of Yang. Locations: At the centre of the depression below the lateral ankle. Regional anatomy: Epilepsy, mania, headache, vertigo, insomnia, lumbness, cold feet, inability to sit long, congestion and pain in the eyes, stiff neck. Regional anatomy: Between the cruciate ligament of leg and short peroneal muscle. The short extensor muscle of toe is in the deeper. There is the arterial network at the lateral ankle, and the gastracnemius muscle is distributed. Puncture: 1—2 cm perpendicularly. Moxibustion: 3—5 moxa cones or 5—10 minutes with warming moxibustion.

Shexia 舌下 [shé xià] An extra point located at the lateral side of the tongue, just opposite to the corner of the mouth when the tongue is fully extended. Puncture: 0. 3—0. 6 cm perpendicularly.

She zhu 舌柱 [shé zhù] Referring to trenulum of tongue. (Fig 120)

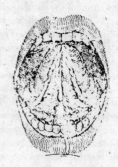

Fig 120

Sheben 舌本 [shé běn] 1. The root of the tongue; 2. Another name of Fengfu (GV 16); 3. An alternate term for Yamen (GV 15).

Sheyan 舌厌 [shé yàn] Another name of Yamen (GV 15).

Shenshu (BL 23) 肾俞 [shèn shū] A point of Bladder Meridian of Foot-*taiyang*, the back *shu* point of the kidneys. Location: 4. 5 cm lateral to Mingmen (GV, DU 4) between the spinal processes of the 2nd and 3rd lumbar vertebrae. Regional anatomy: Between the longest muscle and the iliocostal muscle. There is the posterior branch of the 2nd artery and vein. The lateral cutaneous branch of the posterior branch of the 1st lumbar vertebra is distributed. The lateral branch of the posterior branch of the 1st lumbar nerve is in the deeper. Indications: spermatarrhea, impotence, enuresis, frequent urination, irregular menstruation, leukorrhea, pains in the waist and knees,

blurred vision, tinnitus, deafness, dysuria, edema, diarrhia, cough and short breath. Puncture: 1. 5—3. 5 cm perpendicularly. Moxibustion: 5—7 moxa cones or 5—15 minutes with warming moxibustion.

Shenzhu (GV 12) 身柱 [shēn zhù] A GV point. Location: Between the spinal process of the 3rd thoracic vertebra and that of the 4th thoracic vertebra at the posterior midline. Reginal anatomy: Passing through the fasciae of the waist and back, the supraspinal ligament, and the interspinal ligaments. There is the posterior branch of the 3rd intercostal artey and the medial branch of the posterior branch of the 3rd thoracic vertebra. The spinal cord is in the deeper. Indications: General fever, headache, cough, asthmatic breath, mania, epilepsy, stiffness and pain in the lumbar spine, deep-rooted sore. Puncture: 1. 5—3 cm obliquely. Moxibustion: 3—5 moxa cones or 5—10 minutes with warming moxibustion.

shen 神 [shén] Referring to the human body's (antipathogenic) *qi* (body resistance).

Shemen （HT 7） 神门 [shén mén] A point of Heart meridian of Hand-*shaoyin*, the stream-like (earth) and source point of the meridian, also termed Duichong, Zhongdu, Ruizhong. Location: At the end of the ulnar end of the transverse crease of the posterior palm. In the depression at the radial edge of the ulnar flexor muscle of wrist. Regional anatomy: Between the ulnar flexor muscle of wrist and the superifical flexor muscle of finger. There is the ulnar artery that passsess through. The medial cutaneous nerve of forearm is distributed. The ulnar nerve is in the deeper. Indications: Cardialgia, anxiety, trance, insomnia, amnesia, palpitation with fright, idiocy, mania, epilepsy, yellow eyes, hypochondriac pain, feverish sensation in the palms, hemoptysis, spitting blood, stools with purulent blood, headache, vertigo, dry throat, poor appetite, aphonia, asthmatic breath.

Shenguang 神光 [shén guāng] An alternate

term for Riyue (GB 24).

Shenxi 肾系 [shèn xì] An extra point, located 3 cm below Futu (SY 32). According to Prescriptions Worth a Thousand Gold, it is used for emaciation-thirst disease with frequent urination.

Shenshou 神授 [shén shòu] An extra point. Located on Large Intestine Meridian of Hand-*yangming*.

Shentang (BL 44) 神堂 [shén táng] 1. A point of Bladder Meridian of Foot-*taiyang*. Location: 9 cm lateral to Shendao (GV, DU 11) between the spinal processes of the 5th and 6th thoracic vertebrae. Regional anatomy: In the trapezius muscle and the rhomboid muscle. There are the posterior branches of the 5th intercostal artery and vein and the descending branch of the cervical transverse artery. The medial cutaneous branch of the posterior branch of the 4th and 5th thoracic nerve is distributed. The lateral branch of the posterior branch of the 4th and 5th thoracic nerves and the dorsal scarpular nerve are in the deeper. Indications: Cough and asthmatic breath, fullness in the chest and abdomen. Puncture: 1.5—2.5 cm obliquely. (It is not advisable to puncture.) Moxibustion: 3—5 moxa cones or 5—15 minutes with warming moxibustion. An alternate term for Shangxing (EV 23).

Shenfu 神府 [shén fǔ] An extra point, located 1 cm below Zhongting (CV 16). Indication: Cardialgia. Puncture: 1—1.5 cm horizontally. Moxibustion: 3—5 moxa cones or 5—10 minutes with warming moxibustion.

Shenfeng (KI 23) 神封 [shén fēng] A point of Kidney Meridian of Foot-*shaoyin*. Location: 6 cm lateral to Danzong (CV 17) on the midline of chest, in the 4th intercostal space. Regional anatomy: In the broadest pectoral muscle. There is the 4th intercostal artery and vein, and the anterior cutanous branch of the 4th intercostal artery and vein. The anterior cutanous branch of the 4th intercostal nerve is distributed. The 4th intercostal nerve is in the deeper. Indications: Cough, asthmatic breath, fullness in the chest and hypochondrium, vomiting, anorexia, breast carbuncle. Puncture: 1—1.5 cm obliquely. (It is not advisable to puncture deep). Moxibustion: 3—5 moxa cones or 5—10 minutes with warming moxibustion.

Shenting (GV 24) 神庭 [shén tíng] A GV point, the confluence of GV, foot-*taiyang* meridian and foot-*yangming* meridians, also termed Faji. Location: At the midline of the forontal head, 1.5 cm into the anterior hairline. Regional anatomy: At the crossing point of the left and right frontal muscles. There are the branches of the frontal artery and vein and the branches of the superficial temporal artery and vein. The branch of the temporal nerve is distributed. Indications: Headache, vertigo, congestion, swelling and pain in the eyes, lacrimation, nebula, night blindness, rhinitis, epistaxis, epilepsy, opithotonos. Puncture: 1—1.5 cm horizontally. Moxibustion: 3—5 moxa cones or 5—10 minutes with warming moxibustion.

Shenjiao 身交 [shēn jiāo] An extra point. Located 9 cm below the umbilicus, same with Guangyuan (CV 4) in location. (Fig 121)

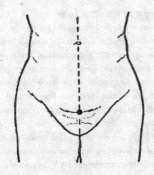

Fig 121

Shendao (GV 11) 神道 [shén dào] A GV point, also termed Zanshu. Location: At the midline of the back, between the spinal processes of the 5th and 6th thoracic verte-brae. Regional anatomy: There is the poste-rior branch of the 5th intercostal artery. The medial branch of the posterior branch of the 5th thoraic nerve is distributed. Indications: Cardialgia, palpitation with fright, insomnia, amnesia, appoplexy, aphasia, epilepsy, stiffness of the lumbar spine, pains in the shoulder and back. Puncture: 1.5—3 cm obliquely. Moxibustion: 3—5 moxa cones or 5—10 minutes with war-ming moxibustion.

she manipulation 摄法 [shè fǎ] An accessary acupuncture manipulation. Referring to pressing, pinching and scratching the meridianal location with the fingernail. (Fig 122)

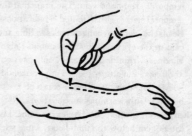

Fig 122

Shenque (CV 8) 神阙 [shén què] A CV point, also termed Jizhong, alternately termed Qishe, Weihui, Qihe, Huangu. Location: In the centre of the umbilical fossa. Region-al anatomy: There is the inferior epigastric artery and vein. The anterior cutaneous branch of the intercostal nerve is distribu-ted. Indications: Collapse, symptom of apoplexy, clammy cold of four limbs, epilepsy, pain in the surrounding umbili-cus, edema, tympanlite, prolapse of anus, diarrhea, constipation, incontinence of urine, infertility. Puncture is prohibited. Moxibustion: 5—15 moxa cones with salt-interposed moxibustion or 15—30 minutes with warming moxibustion.

Shencong 神聪 [shén cōng] An extra point,

also termed Sishencong. One proportional *cun* to Baihui (GV 20) from the four direc-tions. Indications: Apoplexy, headache, ver-tigo, eplilepsy, mania and neural asthenia. Puncture: 1—1.5 cm horizontally. Moxi-bustion: 1—3 moxa cones or 3—5 minutes with warming moxibustion. (Fig 123)

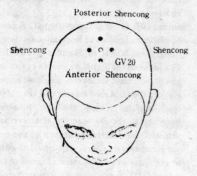

Fig   123

Shenmen 神门 [shén mén] An ear point near 1/2—1/3 of the upper foot of the antithe-lix.

Shenqi 肾气 [shèn qì] An alternate term for Daheng (SP 15).

Sheheng 舌横 [shè héng] An alternate term for Yamen (GV 15).

Shencang (KI 25) 神藏 [shén cáng] A point of Kidney Meridian of Foot-*shaoyin*. Loca-tion: 6 cm lateral to Zigong (CV 19) at the midline of chest, in the 2nd intercostal space. Regional anatomy: In the greater pectoral muscle. There is the 2nd inter-costal artery and vein. The anterior branch of the 2nd intercostal nerve is distributed. The 2nd intercostal nerve is in the deeper. Indications: Cough, asthmatic breath, tho-racalgia, anxiety, vomiting, anorexia. Punc-ture: 1—1.5 cm obliquely. (It is not advis-able to puncture deep.) Moxibustion: 3—5 moxa cones or 5—10 minutes with war-ming moxibustion.

shen 胂 [shèn] 1. The muscles below crista iliaca; 2. Generally referring to paravertebral musculature.

Shetou 蛇头 ［shé tóu］ An alternate term for Wenliu (LI 7).

Shimian point 失眠穴［shī mián xué］An extra point, located at the heel, at the crossing point of the line connecting the midline of the sole and the line connecting the medial and lateral ankle. Indications: Insomnia, pain in the sole. Puncture: 1—2 cm perpendicularly or 5—15 minutes with warming moxibustion.

Shizhitou 十指头［shí zhǐ tóu］I. e., Guicheng (Shixuan, EX-UE 11).

Shitou 势头 ［shì tóu］ An alternate term for penis.

Shixuan (EX-UE 11) 十宣［shí xuān］An extra point. Located 0.3 cm to the tip of the fingesnail, 10 in total. Indication: Tonsilitis. Treatment: To cause little bleeding with a friangalar needle.

Shiqizhui (EX-B 8) 十七椎 ［shí qī zhuī］ Shiqizhui (EX-B 8) An extra point, located at the posterior midline below the spinal process of the 5th lumbovertebra. There is locally the suraspinal ligament, interspinal ligament, the branch of the medial branch of the posterior branch of the 5th lumbar nerve, and its accompanying branches of the artery and vein; There is the intervertebral ligament (the yellow ligament), the spinal duranater, arochnoid, subarochnoid cavity and cauda equina. Indications: Lumbago, pain in the leg, paralysis of the lower limb, dysuria due to pressure of the fetus, dysmenorrhea, anal trouble, sciatica, metrorrhagia. Puncture: 1.5—3 cm perpendicularly. Moxibustion: 3—7 moxa cones or 10—16 minutes with warming moxibustion. Also referring to the 5th lumbar verterbra. (Fig 124)

Shiguan (KI 18) 石关 ［shí guān］ 1. A point of Kindney Meridian of Foot-*shaoyin*, the confluence of Vital Vessel and foot-*shaoyin* meridian. Also termed Shigque. Location: 1.5 cm lateral to Jianli (CV 11), 1.2 dm above the umbilicus. Regional anatomy: At

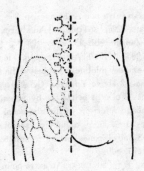

Fig 124

the medial edge of the straight muscle of abdomen. There are the branches of the hypogastric artery and vein. The 8th intercostal nerve is distributed. Indications: Vomiting, abdominal pain, constipation, postpartum abdominal pain, infertility. Puncture: 3—4 cm perpendicularly. Moxibustion: 5—7 moxa cones or 10—15 minutes with warming moxibustion; 2. The extra point, located 9 cm lateral to Juque (CV 14).

Shigong 石宫［shí gōng］An alternate term for Yindu (KI 19).

Shique 石阙 ［shí què］ An alternate term for Shiguan (KI 19).

Shigong 食宫［shí gōng］An alternate term for Yindu (KI 19)

Shidou 食窦 ［shí dòu］ 1. A point of Spleen Meridian of Foot-*taiyin*. Location: 18 cm lateral to Zhongting (CV 16) on the line of chest, at the 5th intercostal space. Regional anatomy: At the serratus anterior muscle. There is the lateral artery and chest and the thoracico-abdominal vein. The lateral cutaneous branch of the 5th intercostal nerve is distributed. Indications: Distansion and pain in the chest and hypochondrium, abdominal distension and borborygmus, regurgitation, belching, edema. Puncture: 1—1.5 cm obliquely. (deep puncture is prohibitted.)Moxibustion: 3—5 moxa cones or 5—10 minutes with warming moxibustion;

2. An extra point, Mingguan.

Shiguang 始光 [shǐ guāng] An alternate term for Zanzhu (BL 2).

Shisu 始素 [shǐ sù] An extra point, located at the axillary midline, 6 cm below the axillary fossa, 3 above Yuanye (GB 22). Indications: Fullness below the hypochondrium, lumbago referring to the abdomen. Puncture: 1—1.5 cm obliquely. Moxibustion: 1—3 moxa cones or 3—5 minutes with warm needling.

Shicang 食仓 [shí cāng] An extra point, located 9 cm lateral to Zhongwan (CV, RN 12) or 1.5 cm bilateral to Jianli (CV 11). Indication: Gastritis, enteritis, indigestion. Puncture: 3—4.5 perpendicularly. Moxibustion: 5—7 moxa cones or 10—15 minutes with warming moxibustion.

Shimen (CV 5) 石门 [shí mén] A CV point. the anterior-referred point of the triple energizer. Also termed Liji, Jinglou, Dantian, Mingmen. Location: 6 cm below the umbilicus, on the abdominal midline. Regional anatomy: In the white line of abdomen, there are the branches of the superficial artery and vein of the abdominal wall and the branches of the inferior artery and vein of the abdominal wall. The anterial cutaneous branch of the 11th intercostal nerve is distributed.

Shiwang 十王 [shí wáng] An extra point, located on the dorsal site of the ten fingers, approx. 0.3 cm to the skin toward the midpoint of the root of the fingernail. Indications: Coma, high fever, sunstroke, cholera, infantile convulsion. Prick to cause a little bleeding with a triangular needle.

Shouzhanghoubijian point 手掌后臂间穴 [shǒu zhǎng hòu bì jiān xué] An extra point, located on the flexor side of the forearm, 5 transverse finger-widths above the transverse crease of wrist between the long palmar muscle and the radial flexor muscle of wrist. Puncture: 1.5—3 cm perpendicularly. Moxibustion: 3—5 moxa cones or 5—10 minuts with warming moxibustion.

Shouhuaigu 手踝骨 [shǒu huái gǔ] An extra point, located on the dorsal side of wrist at the highest point of the node of radius. Indications: Spasm of the ten fingers, pain in the upper and lower teeth. Moxibustion: 3—7 moxa cones or 5—15 minutes with warming moxibustion.

Shousuikong 手髓孔 [shǒu suí kǒng] I.e., Shouzusuikong, the extra point.

Shoulder joint 肩关节 [jiān guān jié] An ear point in the first equally divided zone (Divide the scaphoid fossa between Clavicle and into the four equivalent zones).

Shoulder 肩 [jiān] An ear point located in the equivalent zone superior to Clavicle.

Shoushaoyinxi 手少阴郄 [shǒu shào jīn xī] I.e., Yinxi (HT 6).

Shouxin 手心 [shǒu xīn] An extra point located on the line connecting the midpoint of the transverse crease of the metacarpophalangeal joint of the middle finger and Daling (PC 7)

Shouzhanghoubairouji point 手掌后白肉际穴 [shǒu zhǎng hòu bái ròu jì xué] An extra point, located at the dorsopalmar boundary of the midpoint of the transverse crease posterior to the palm. Indications: Cramp in cholerammorbus. Puncture: 1.5—3 cm perpendicularly. Moxibustion: 3—5 moxa cones or 5—10 minutes with warming moxibustion.

Shounizhu 手逆注 [shǒu nì zhù] An extra point, located 1.8 dm above the transverse crease of the wrist, on the flexor side of the forearm, between the long palmar muscle and the flexor radial muscle. Indications: Hysteria, pain, spasm and numbness of the forearm. Puncture: 1.5—3 cm perpendicularly. Moxibustion: 3—7 moxa cones or 5—10 minutes with warming moxibustion.

short needling 短刺 [duǎn cì] An needling technique to insert the needle deep to the proximal bone and shake the body of the needle in association with gentle kneading, so as to treat disorder and pain in the deeper part of the body.

shouyu 手鱼 [shǒu yú] The protrusion formed by the ball muscle of thumb. Also called *yu*.

Shouqiaoyin 首窍阴 [shǒu qiào yīn] I. e., Touqianyin (GB 11).

shoulder meridian 肩脉 [jiān mài] A name of meridian during early period, similar to hand-*taiyang* meridian.

Shouzhongzhidiyijie-point 手中指第一节穴 [shǒu zhōng zhǐ dì yī jié xué] An alternate term for Zhongzhiji, the extra point.

Shoudazhijiahou 手大指甲后 [shǒu dà zhǐ jiǎ hòu] An extra point, located at the dorsopalmar boundary of the head of the transverse crease of the metacarpal joint, on the edge of the ulnar side of the thumb. Indications: Infantile intestinal disorder, conjunctivites, corneal macula, nyctalopia. Puncture: 0. 3—0. 6 cm perpendicularly or prick to cause little bleeding with triangular needle. Moxibustion: 3—5 moxa cones or 5—10 minutes with warming moxibustion.

short pulse 短脉 [duǎn mài] The pulse that is shorter than its normal one. It usually indicates stagnation or deficiency of *qi*.

Shousanli (LI 10) 手三里 [shǒu sān lǐ] A point of Large Intestine Meridian of Hand-*yangming*. Location: 6 cm below Quchi (LI 11), on the line connecting Yangxi (LI 5) and Quchi (LI 11), on the radial side of the dorsal forearm. Regional anatomy: Passing through the long extensor muscle of the wrist, reaching the spinator. There are the branches of the radial artery and vein. The dorsal cutaneous nerve of forearm and the deep branch of the radial nerve are distributed. Indications: Febrile disease, sore throat, swelling and pain of the arm, paralysis of the upper limbs, weakness of the elbow, irregular menstruation and diarrhea, scaby erysepilas, abdominal pain and diarrhea, dysentery, toothache, redness and pain of the eyes, hyepertension, mania, malaria. Puncture: 3 cm perpendicularly. Moxibution: 3—5 moxa cones or 5—10 minutes with warming moxibustion.

Shouzudazhizaojia 手足大指爪甲 [shǒu zú dà zhǐ zǎo jiǎ] I. e., the extra point, Guiyan.

Shouzusuikong point 手足髓孔 [shǒu zú suí kǒng] The extra point. "In administering moxibustion for treating hemiplegia, first do it on Tianchuang (SI 16), then Damen··· and then Shousuikong located at the sharp bone posterior to the wrist ··· finally Zusuikong 3 cm psterior to the lateral ankle. "

Shoushanglian 手上廉 [shǒu shàng lián] I. e., Shanglian (LI 9).

Shouwuli (LI 13) 手五里 [shǒu wǔ lǐ] A point of Large Intestine Meridian of hand-*yangming*. Location: 1 dm above Quchi (LI 11) on the line connecting Quchi (LI 11) and Jianyu (LI 15). Regional anatomy: At the starting point of the brachio-radial muscle and the anterior edge of brachial triceps muscle. There is the radial artery and vein. The dorsal cutaneous nerve of forearm is distributed. The radial nerve is in the deeper. Indications: Spasm and pain in the elbow and arm, scrofula, cough and spitting blood, malaria, scrofula. Puncture: 1. 5—3 cm perpendicularly. Moxibustion: 3—5 moxa cones with warming moxibustion.

Shuaigu (GB 8) 率谷 [shuài gǔ] A point of Gallbladder Meridian of Foot-*shaoyang*, the confluence of foot-*taiyang* meridian and foot-*shaoyang* meridian, an alternate term for Erjian (LI 2). Location: Directly above the tip of ear, 4. 5 cm into the hairline. Regional anatomy: At the temporal muscle. There is the parietal branch of the superficial tempopral artey and vein. The anastomotical branch of the aurotemporal nerve and the greater occipital nerve are distributed. Indications: Headache, vertigo, vomiting, infantile convulsion. Puncture: 1—1. 5 cm horizontally. Moxibustion: 1—3 moxa cones or 3—5 minutes with warming moxibustion.

Shuishuwushiqi points 水俞五十七穴 [shuǐ shū wǔ shí qī xué] Also called Shuishuwushiqichu. For details, see Shenshuwushiqi point.

Shuwei 鼠尾 [shǔ wěi] An extra point located at the midline of the heel at the superior edge of Achilles.

Shulei 属累 [shǔ lèi] An alternate term for Mingmen (GV 4).

***shu* points** 腧穴 [shū xué] Referring to the area where *qi* in the viscera and meridians is transported, irrigated, goes out and comes in. They are the stimulation point in acupuncture treatment, also the certain reactive points of certain diseases and pains. They are communicated with the meridians and the viscera, and can reflect the physiopathological changes of various viscera, and are suitable for external treatments, such as acupuncture, moxibustion, and massage. The reconginiton in the succeeding dynasties of the *shu* points has been enriched. They are generally classified into three main categories: Those pertaining to certian meridians are called the *shu* points of the fourteen meridians (meridianal points), those that were added to the original meridian points are called extra points, those that have no fixed loations but are located along with the affected area or tenderness are called Ahshi points.

***shu-mu* points combined method** 俞募配穴法 [shū mù pèi xué fǎ] One of the point-combined methods. Referring to the combination and application of the back-*shu* points and anterior referred points that pertain to the pathological viscera. E. g., for stomach trouble Weishu (BL 21) and Zhongwan (CV 12) are selected, for bladder trouble Pangguangshu (BL 28) and Zhongji (CV 3) are selected.

***shu* point of viscera** 脏俞 [zàng shū] Referring to the points of the well-like, spring-like, stream-like and sea-like points of yin meridians of the five storing viscera. There are 25 points of the meridians of the five storing viscera unilaterally, 50 bilaterally.

Shuaigu 率骨 [shuài gǔ] I. e., Shuaigu (GB 8).

shu 输 [shū] 1. Referring to the *shu* point, also specially referring to the *shu* point among the five *shu* points; 2. Referring to communication and irrigation.

***shu* meridian** 输脉 [shū mài] Also termed *shu zhi mai*, referring to the meridian connecting with the viscera at the back.

Shuigou (GV 26) 水沟 [shuǐ gōu] A GV point. The confluence of GV, hand-*yangming* and foot-*yangming* meridians, also termed Renzhong. Location: At the crossing point of the upper 1/3 and middle 1/3 of the philtrum. Regional anatomy: In the orbicular muscle of mouth, there are the artery and vein of the upper lip, the buccal branch of the facial nerve and the branch of the facial nerve and the branch of the infraorbital nerve are distributed. Indications: Coma, syncope, summer-heat disease, mania, epilepsy, acute/chronic convulsion, stuffy nose, epilepsy, puffy face, epistaxis, toothache, close jaw, jaundice, emaciation, thirst disease, cholera, pest, stiffness and pain in the spine, strain and lumbago. Puncture: 1 cm upwardly obliquely.

Shuimen 水门 [shuǐ mén] An alternate term for Shuitu (ST 10).

Shuifen (CV 9) 水分 [shuǐ fēn] A CV point. An alternate term for Zhongshou. Location: 3 cm above the umbilicus on the abdominal midline. Regional anatomy: In the white abdominal line. There are the hypogastric artery and vein. The anterior cutaneous branch of the 8th and 9th intercostal nerve are distributed. Indications: Borborygmus, diarhea, abdominal pain, abdominal distension, edema, infantile sunken fontanel, stiffness of the lumbar spine. Puncture: 3—4 cm perpendicularly. (For the pregnant woman it should be used cautiously.) Moxibustion: 3—7 moxa cones or 5—15 minutes with warming moxibustion.

Shuixue 水穴 [shuǐ xué] An alternate term for Futu (ST 32).

Shuiquan (KI 5) 水泉 [shuǐ quán] A point of Kidney Meridian of Foot-*shaoyin*, the gap-like point of the meridian. Located 3 cm directly below Taixi (KI 3) at the midpoint of the line connecting the medial ankle and the level of Achilles tendon. Regional anatomy: The medial branch of the calcaneus of the posterior tibial artery. The medial cutaneous branch of leg and the mediala branch of the tibial nerve of leg are distributed. Indication: Irregular menstruation, dysmenorrhea, prolapse of uterus, dyspnea, blurred vision, abdominal pain. Puncture: 1 cm perpendicularly. Moxibustion: 3—5 moxa cones or 5—10 minutes with warming moxibustion.

Shugu (BL 65) 束骨 [shù gǔ] A point of Bladder Meridian of Foot-*taiyang*, the streamlike (wood) point of the meridian. Regional anatomy: There is the common planter artery and vein of the 4th toe. The common planter nerve of the 4th toe and the lateral cutaneous nerve of the dorsal foot are distributed. Location: In the depression posterior to the small head of the 5th metatarsal bone on the edge of the lateral side of foot at the dorso-planter border. Indications: Mania, headache, stiff neck, vertigo, pain in the waist and back, pain the posterior aspect of the lower limb. Puncture: 1—1.5 cm perpendicularly. Moxibustion: 3—5 moxa cones or 5—10 minutes with moxibustion.

shu **puncture** 输刺 [shū cì] 1. One of the nine needling techniques. It refers to the needling technique of selecting the well-like, spring-like, stream-like, river-like and sea-like points (the five *shu* points) and back *shu* points of the viscera; 2. One of the twelve needling techniques. It refers to treatment of excess syndrome by applying lifting-thrusting manipulation of directly inserting and withdrawing the needle with less needlings by deep puncture; 3. One of the five needling techniques. It refers to deep pucture for treating bone blockage including the deep diseases and symtoms, similar to *shu* puncture of the twelve

needling techniques but different from classification. *Shu* puncture said in modern clinic usually refers to this.

Shuitu (ST 10) 水突 [shuǐ tū] A point of Stomach Meridian of Foot-*yangming*. Also termed Shuimen. Location: At the midpoint of the line connecting Renying (ST 90) and Qishe (ST 11), on the anterior edge of the sternocleidomastoidous muscle on the anterolateral neck. Regional anatomy: Passing through the broader muscle of neck to reach the crossing point of sternocleidomastoidous muscle and the upper edge of the omohyoid muscle. There are the branches of the common artery of neck and lateral artery of neck. The cutaneous nerve of neck is distributed. The descending branch of the infralingual nerve is in the deeper. Indications: Cough, asthmatic breath, sore throat, swelling of the shoulder, hiccup, goiter, scrofula. Puncture: 1 cm perpendicularly. Moxibustion: 1—3 moxa cones or 5—10 minutes with warming moxibustion.

Shuiyuan 水原 [shuǐ yuán] I. e., Shuiquan (KI 5)

Shuidao (ST 28) 水道 [shuǐ dào] A point of Stomach Meridian of Foot-*yangming*. Location: 6 cm latral to Guanyuan (RN 4), 1 dm below the umbilicus. Regional Anatomy: At the straight muscle of abdomen, there are the branches of the infrocostal artery and vein. The hypogastric artery and vein are at its lateral aspect. The branch of the infrocostal nerve is distributed. Indications: Distension and pain in the lower abdomen, hernia, dysmenorrhea, dysuria. Puncture: 3—4 cm perpendicularly. Moxibustion: 5—7 moxa cones or 10—20 minutes with warming moxibustion.

Shuaigu 蟀骨 [shuài gǔ] I. e., Shuaigu (GB 8).

shu **points** 俞穴 [shū xué] General referring to all *shu* points. Also specially referring to back-*shu* points.

Shuqiao 俞窍 [shū qiào] Referring to the *shu*

point between the bone and the tendon.

Shufu (**KI 27**) 俞府 [shū fǔ] A point of Kidney Meridian of Foot-*shaoyin*. Location: Below the clavicular bone, 6 cm lateral to Xuanji (CV 21) on the midline of chest. Regional anatomy: Above the greater pectoral muscle. There are the perforating branches of the inframammary artery and vein. The anterior branch of the supraclavicular nerve is distributed. Indications: Cough, asthmatic breath, thoracalgia, vomitting, anorexia. Puncture: 0. 9—1. 5 cm obliquely. Moxibustion: 3—5 moxa cones or 5—10 minutes with warming moxibustion.

Sibai (**ST 2**) 四白 [sì bái] A point of Stomach Meridian of Foot-*yangming*. Location: In the inferior orbital foramen of the maxillary bone. Regional anatomy: Between the obicular muscle of the eye and the quadrate muscle of the upper lip, to reach the infraorbital foramen. There are the branches of the facial artery and vein and the infraorbital artery and vein. The branch of the facial nerve is distributed, just at the infraorbital nerve. Indications: Congestion, swelling, itch and pain in the head and face, lacrimation. Puncture: 1—2 cm perpendicularly.

Sihua 四华 [sì huá] I. e., Sihua point.

Siguan 四关 [sì guān] 1. The two elbows and knees; 2. The name of grouped point, Hegu (LI 4) and Taichong (LI 3).

Sihua 四花 [sì huā] An extra point, 1. 4 cm lateral to the inferior of the 7th and 10th thoracic vertebral spines, i. e., Feshu (BL 17)and Dashu(BL 19); 2. Take the distence from Dazhui (GV, DU 14) to Jiuwei (CV 15) as the length, measure from Adam's Apple (via Dazhui) downward to the midpoint of the back spine, 0. 5 mouth *cun* to its upper, lower, left and right points, 4 in total. Indications: Consumptive disease, cough, asthma, weak and thin. Moxibustion with moxa cone 3—7 moxa cones.   (Fig 125)

single point 孤穴 [gū xué] Referring to the single point on the midline.

side-lying postiion 侧卧位 [cè wò wèi] See lying position.

side-sitting position 侧倚位 [cè yǐ wèi] See sitting position.

silver needle 银针 [yín zhēn] The needling instrument mainly made of silver. It is favourable in conducting heat and in electric conduction. Usually used for warming needling.

Six Collections of Acupuncture Prescriptions 针方六集 [zhēn fāng liù jí] A book written by Wu Kun in Ming Dynasty (1368—1644). The whole book is divided into six collections. 1. The first one introduces meridians, *shu* points, bone measurement, etc., appended with illustrations; The 2nd one notes Biaoyou Fu and describes the five and eight methods and 66 points; The 3rd cites the original of Internal Medicine, minutely describes the nine needles, the acupuncture manipulations such as waiting for *qi*, seeing *qi*, taking *qi*, maintaining *qi*, etc.; The 4th describes the comparison of the effects between acupuncture and drugs, appended with a commentary on Gold Needle; The 5th describes the indication and operation of *shu* points; The 6th compiles and records various schools' rhythmed articles and moxibustion techniques, accompanied with the author's commentar and viewpoints. It was completed in 1618.

superficial pulse 浮脉 [fú mài] The pulse which can be easily felt with a gentle touch, but easily obliterated by a heavy press. It usually indicates the exterior syndrome.

six excesses 六淫 [liù yín] As a contrast to six *qi* it refers to six abnomarl climates, viz., wind, cold, summer heat, dampness, dryness and fire (intense heat).

sitting position 坐位 [zuò wèi] One of the body positions for acupuncture, also divided into the supine-sitting position (for puncturing the face and nape), lateral-sitting position (for puncturing one side of the face

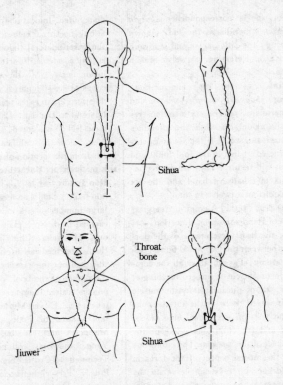

Fig 125

and temple), the head-supported position (for puncturing the vertex), prone-sitting position (for puncturing the flexor side of the upper limb), the elbow-flexed and palm-prone position (for puncturing the extensor side of the forearm), the elbow-flexed and hand-held position (for puncturing the radial side of the upper limb), and the sitting position. (for puncturing the anterior medial and lateral aspects of the lower limb)

Six-point moxibustion 六之灸 [liù zhī jiǔ] To administer moxibustion on the six points, Gechu (BL 17), Ganshu (BL 18), and Pishu (BL 20) for treating gastric expansion, gastric spasm, stomach cancer, enteritis, reduced appetite, indigestion, spasm of the diaphragm, asthmatic breath, pleurasy.

sixty-six points 六十六穴 [liù shí liù xué] A collective term for the well-like, spring-like, stream-like, river-like and sea-like points of the twelve meridians, i.e., the well-like, spring-like, stream-like, river-like and sea-like points of each yin meridian, 30 in total; The well-like, spring-like, stream-like, source, river-like and sea-like points of each yang meridian, 36 in total. The total number is 66. The needlings in midnight-noon ebb-flow of *qi* are based on them.

six correspondences 六合 [liù hé] 1. The six correspondences between the heaven and earth, upper and lower and four directions; 2. The external-internal correspondence of the twelve meridians. According to Miraculous Pivot, the 1st correspondence is *taiyin* and *yangming* meridians, the 2nd, *shaoyin* and *taiyang*, the 3rd, *jueyin* and *shaoyang* meridians; 3. Referring to twelve branch meridians.

six meridians 六经 [liù jīng] The *taiyang*, *yangming*, *shaoyang*, *taiyin*, *shaoyin* and *jueyin* meridians. "The six meridians resemble the mountains while the intestines and stomach the sea." If the six meridians are obstructed, pains in the four limbs and stiff waist will result." They are divided into the six meridians of hand and the six meridians of foot, twelve in total.

Sidu (TE 9) 四渎 [sì dú] A point of Energizer Meridian of Hand-*shaoyang*. Location: 2. 1 cm above the transverse crease of the dorsal wrist, between the two radial bones. Regional anatomy: Passing through the common extensor muscle of finger, reaching at the ulnar side of the long extensor muscle of thumb where there is the interosseous artery and vein on the dorsal side of the forearm, and the cutaneous nerve of the dorsal aspect of the forearm. The cutaneous nerve of the medial aspect of the forearm and the deeper interosseous nerve on the dorsal aspect of the forearm are distributed. Indications: Sudden deafness, toothache, short breath, sudden blindness, obstruction of the throat, pain in the forearm. Puncture: 1. 5—3 cm perpendicularly. Moxibustion: 3—5 moxa cones with 5—10 minutes with warming moxibustion.

Siman (KI 14) 四满 [sì mǎn] 1. A point of Kidney Meridian of Foot-*shaoyin* the confluence of Vital Vessel and foot-*shaoyin* meridian. Also termed Suifu, Danzhong. Location: 1. 5 cm lateral to Shimen (RN 5) below the umilicus. Regional anatomy: Passing through the anterial sheath of the straight muscle of abdomen and the straight muscle of abdomen. Reaching at the transverse fascia. There is the muscular branch of the artery and vein below the abdominal wall. The 11th intercostal nerve is

distributed. Indications: Irregular menstruation, nocturnal emission, hernia, pain in the lower bilateral abdomen, enuresis, constipation, edema. Puncture: 3—4. 5 cm perpendicularly. Moxibustion: 3—5 moxa cones or 5—10 minutes with warming moxibustion; 2. An extra point. Located 4. 5 cm bilateral to Dantian. Dantian is where Shimen (RN 5) is located, 5 cm bilateral to and 6 cm below the umbilicus, which is different from the location of the meridian point.

silk manuscripts Unearthed from Mawangdui Han Tombs 马王堆汉墓帛书 [mǎ wáng duī hàn mù bó shū] The medical literatures. A large number of silk manuscripts were unearthed from No 3 Han tomb at Mawangdui, Changsha, China in 1973. Many of them are medical literatures. Originally they had not the names of the chapters and the names of the book. The systematizers nomenclatured them according to their contents, i. e., Eleven Meridians and Moxibustion Classic of Foot and Arm, Eleven Meridians and Moxibustion of Yin and Yang (the first volume), Pulse-feeling Techniques, Critical Sign of Yin and Yang Pulse, Prescriptions for Fifty-two Diseases. The above ones were combined as one volume of silk manuscripts, *Quegu Shiqi*, Eleven Meridians Classic of Yin-yang for Moxibustion, Illustration of *Daoyin*. The above three were combined as one volume of silk manuscripts. Prescriptions for Health Preservation, Miscellaeous Prescriptions and Obstetric Book, each of which was one volume of the silk manuscript. Eleven Meridians and Moxibustion Classic is the earliest literature concerning meridians, or called Silk Manuscripts on Meridians, which can verify with meridians, a chapter of Miraculous Pivot.

sign of excess in extreme deficiency 至虚有盛候 [zhì xū yǒu shèng hòu] The pseudo-excess symptoms appear at the critical stage of the deficiency syndrome.

six emptying viscera aim at transmission 六腑以通为用 [liù fǔ yǐ tōng wéi yòng] The function of these organs is to keep on being unobstructed. Otherwise, pathologic changes will occur.

six emptying viscera 六腑 [liù fǔ] A collective term for the gallbladder, stomach, small intestine, large intestine, bladder and triple energizer. Traditional Chinese medicine regards the six emptying vescera in a more of less similar manner as Western medicine because a *zang* (storing) viscus and a *fu* (emptying) one are interrelated superficially and internally. Each of them has its own intrinsic characteristics.

six *qi* 六气 [liù qì] Referring to six kinds of normal climate, viz., wind, cold, summerheat, dampness and fire (intense heat).

sixteen gap-like points 十六郄穴 [shí liù xī xué] See gap-like points.

sixteen collateral meridians 十六络脉 [shí liù luò mài] It is collectively termed the sixteen collateral meridians that the fifteen collateral meridians are added with the big collateral meridian of stomach.

simultaneous selection of *shu* (stream-like) **and source points** 返本还原 [fǎn běn huán yuán] A term of needling technique of midnight-noon ebb-flow. When the steam-like point is selected according to certain time, the source point that pertains to the same meridian the open well-like point pertains to must be selected.

SI diseases 手太阳小肠经病 [shǒu tài yáng xiǎo cháng jīng bìng] The main diseases and symptoms are: Sore throat, swelling cheek, deafness, yellow eyes, stiff neck, pains in the scapula and posterolateral side of the upper limb, pain in the lower abdomen that refers to the lumbar spine, dearrhea, distension and difficulty in defecation.

sifeng 四缝 [sì fèng] An extra point located on the midpoint of the transverse crease of the proximal finger, at the lateral side of the 2nd, 3rd, 4th and 5th metacarphalangeal bones. Regional anatomey: There is the filliform fibrous sheath of finger, the synovial sheath of finger, and the deeper flexor muscle of finger. The articular cavity of finger is in the deeper. There is the proper nerve on the metacarpophalangeal side and the branches of the artery and vein. There are four in each hand, 8 in total. Indications: Infantile malnutrition, infantile indigestion, pertusis, ascadriasis, arthralgia of finger. Prick to cause little bleeding with a triangular needle, and soueeze out yellow-white mucoid liquid. (Fig 126)

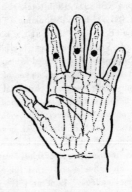

Fig 126

Sihengwen 四横纹 [sì héng wén] See *zhi gen*.

simple needling 白针 [bái zhēn] Referring to simple acupuncture technique. Contrary to warming acupuncture, also called cold acupuncture.

giant typhonium tuber 白附子 [bái fù zǐ] One of interposing things used in moxibustion, the dried root of Aconitum Corenuum (Lev1.) Raipaics.

Sishencong (EX-HT 1) 四神聪 [sì shén cōng] Another name of Shencong.

six emptying viscera 六腑 [liù fǔ] A general term for the gallbladder, stomach, large intestine, small intestine, bladder and triple energizer. Their actions are transporting and digesting food and acuqueous matter.

sitting prone position 伏案位 [fú àn wèi] The

name of the body position of acupuncture. See sitting position.

SI points 手太阳小肠经穴[shǒu tài yáng xiǎo cháng jīng xúe] They are Shaoze (SI 1) (well), Qiangu (SI 2) (spring), Houxi (SI 3) (stream), Wangu (SI 4) (source), Yingu (KI 10) (river), Yanglao (SI 6) (gap), Zhizheng (SI 7) (connecting), Xiaohai (SI 8) (sea), Jianzheng (SI 9), Naoshu (SI 10), Tianzong (SI 11), Bingfeng (SI 12), Quyuan (SI 13), Jianwaishu (SI 14), Jianzhongshu (SI 15), Tianchuang (SI 16), Tianrong (SI 17), Quanliao (SI 18), Tinggong (SI 19), 19 in total.

Sizu 丝竹 [sī zú] I.e., Sizhukong (TE 23).

Sizukong (TE 23) 丝竹空 [sī zhú kōng] A point of Triple Energizer Meridian of Hand-*Shaoyang*. Also termed Mulao. Location: In the depression on the end of the lateral side of the eyebrow. Regional anatomy: There are the frontal branches of the superficial temporal artery and vein. The zygomatic branch of the facial nerve and that of the auricular temporal nerve are distributed. Indications: Headache, blurred vision, congestive and painful eyes, toothache, epilepsy. Puncture: 1.5—3 cm horizontally.

skin-touched moxibustion 着肤灸 [zháo fū jiǔ] I.e., direct moxibustion.

skin puncture 毛刺 [máo cì] To puncture the skin of the disease or symptom at the superficial part of the body. Plum needle applied in modern times is developed from this, and the scale of treatment has been enlarged. Superficial puncture in five needlings is similar to this.

slow insertion and swift withdrawal resulting in reinforcing 徐而急则实 [xú ér jí zé shí] A key point of acupuncture reinforcing manipulation, parallel to swift inserting and slow withdrawing resulting in reducing. It implies that the techniques of slowly inserting the needle and swiftly withdrawing the needle in latter generations. Three times of insertion and one time of withdrawal or two

insertions and one withdrawal originate from this. Refer reinforcing and reducing manipulations by inserting the needle swiftly and withdrawing the needle slowly.

slow lifting and swift thrusting 慢提急按 [màn tí jí àn] See *jin ti man an*.

slow-down pulse 缓脉 [huǎn mài] 1. The moderate forceful and even pulse with a rate of 60 times per minute, seen in a healthy person; 2. The pulse that is loose and slow. It usually indicates the damp syndrome or weakness of the spleen and the stomach.

small head of fibula 外辅[wài fǔ] Contrary to internal *fu*, collectively called fibula.

small intestine 小肠 [xiǎo cháng] One of six emptying viscera. Its action is to transport and digest food and excrete residues. Small Intestine Meridian of Hand-*taiyang* pertains to the small intestine and Heart Meridian of Hand-*shaoyin* connects with the small intestine. Its back-*shu* point is Xiaochangshu (BL 27), its anterior referred point is Guanyuan (CV 4), and its lower joining point is Xiaojuxu (ST 39).

small intestine meridian of hand-*taiyang* 小肠手太阳之脉 [xiǎo cháng shǒu tài yáng zhī mài] The original name of small Intestine Meridian of Hand-*taiyang*.

small pulse 细脉 [xì mài] The pulse which is small, soft and forceless as thread but can still be obviously felt. It usually indicates deficiency an dampness.

slippery pulse 滑脉 [huá mài] The pulse which feels even and smooth like pearls rolling on a dish. It usually indicates the substantive heat syndrome, phlegm, dyspepsia, pregancy, etc.

small and large depressions 溪谷 [xī gǔ] A term of location. '*Gu*' modifies the large depression appearing at the muscle while '*xi*' the small depression.

smashed garlic 蒜泥 [suàn ní] One of drugs for application. To smash the head of garlic into very small pieces, then apply them on the point. If they are applied on Yuji (LU

10), sore throat can be cured. If on the sole, fast dysentery can be cured. One to two hours after external application blisters will be caused on the skin. If blistering is not needed, a layer of vasilin may be dressed on the skin so as to protect the skin.

small eyebrow knife 小眉刀 [xiǎo méi dāo] An acupuncture instrument, used for cutting, pricking and discharging blood, also called *shadao*. It is made of steel, 3—6 cm in length and its deviated edge likes an eyebrow.

Small Intestine 小肠 [xiǎo cháng] An ear point at the upper edge of the crus of helix, opposite to pylorus.

small needle 小针 [xiǎo zhēn] Also called tiny needle.

Small Intestine Meridian of Hand-*taiyang* (SI) 手太阳小肠经 [shǒu tài yáng xiǎo cháng jīng] One of the twelve meridians. The course: Starts from the end of the small intestine, ascends to the wrist along the ulna side of the palm, emerges from the styloid process of the ulna, directly asscends along the ulnar side, emerges between the superomedial condyle of the medial side of the elbow and acromion, ascends along the posterrolateral side of the upper arm, emerges from the scapular joint, winds the scapula, crosses at the shoulder, enters into the supraclavicular fossa, connects with the heart, runs along the pharynx and passes through the diaphragm, goes over the stomach, and finally joins the small intestine. The branch: Starts from the supraclavicular fossa, ascends to the cheek along the lateral neck, reaches at the outer canthus, turns back and enters into the ear. One branch splits from the cheek ascends to the place below the eye , goes near the lateral nose and reaches at the inner canthus. (connects with Bladder Meridian of Foot-*taiyang*).

sore throat 咽喉肿痛 [yān hóu zhǒng tòng] A common symptom in the throat trouble.

soft pulse 濡脉 [rú mài] The pulse, which is small, soft and superficial, can be felt by gentle touch, but becomes indistinct on a heavy press. It indicates dampness and deficiency.

source-connecting point combined method 原络配穴法 [yuán luò pèi xué fǎ] One of the point-combined methods. To select the source points of the mainly diseased meridian as the main, and the connecting point of the externaly-internally related meridian as the accessary.

'shaking off dusts' 振埃 [zhèn āi] One of the five needling techniques. For full chest, asthmatic breath, etc. , caused by adverse flow of yang *qi*, Tianrong (SI 17) and Lianquan (CV, RN 23) are selected for checking its adverse flow; Its effect is just like shaking off dusts.

source point selected method 拔原法 [bá yuán fǎ] One of point-selected methods. It refers to treatment of diseases of varities of miridians with the source points of their own.

'solving the puzzling problem' 解惑 [jiě huò] A needling technique in Internal Classic. According to Miraculous Pivot, solving the puzzling problem implies that one should know well how to regulate yinyang, reinforce the deficiency and reduce the exeess. In the work, the big wind disease should be treated by reducing the excess and reinforcing the deficiency as blood is comparatively insuficieney, so as to balance yin-yang. If one masters this principle, the diseases can be treated just like solving the puzzling problem.

something-interposing moxibustion 隔物灸 [gé wù jiǔ] A kind of indirect moxibustion, i. e. , including ginger-interposing moxibustion, garlic interposing moxibustion, medicinal paste-interposing moxibustion, etc.

source points 原穴 [yuán xué] The *shu* points where primordial *qi* of the viscera passes through or retains. The twelve meridians have one source point each. The source points of yin meridians are the same with stream-like points of the five *shu* points, the source points relate to primordial *qi* while primordial *qi* spreads over various source points through the triple energizer. So they can be used for treating troubles of the viscera. In modern times it is also used for examination of meridians and is taken as a representative points of a meridian. (Fig 127)

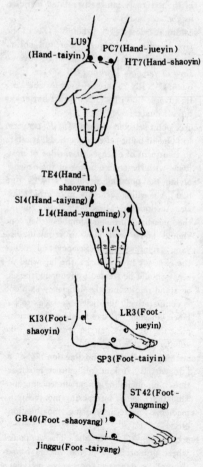

Fig 127

The names of the source points are tableted as follows:

Lungs	Taiyauan (LU9)
Larege Intestine	Hegu (LI 4)
Stomach	Chongyang (ST 42)
Spleen	Taibai (SP 3)
Heart	Shenmen (GB 12)
Small Intestine	Wangu (GB 12)
Bladder	Jinggu (BL 3)
Kidneys	Taixi (KI 3)
Pericardium	Daling (PC 7)
Triple Energizer	Yangchi (YE, SJ 4)
Gallbladder	Qiuxu (GB 40)
Liver	Taichong (LR 3)

sparrow-pecking moxibustion 雀啄灸 ［què zuó jiǔ］ One of moxibustions with moxa stick. To appoint the point with the burning ignited end of the moxa stick and move it up and down, so as to give it continuous stronger stimulation. (Fig 128)

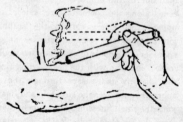

Fig 128

sparrow-pecking method 雀啄法［què zuó fǎ］ After inserting the needle carry on vertical spotting puncture superficially and frequently.

springing manipulation 弹法［táng fǎ］ An accessary acupuncture manipulation. Two explanations: One refers to springing the skin with a finger before acupuncture, the other refers to springing the handle of the needle after acupuncture. (Fig 129)

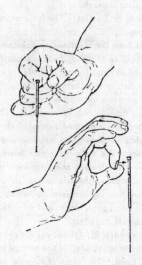

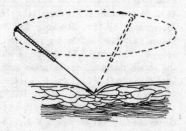

Fig 130

Fig 129

sprain 扭伤[niǔ shāng] The injury of the soft tissue around the joint due to violent traction and twist.

Spleen 脾 [pí] A point located lateroinferior to the Stomach Zone Point.

spermatorrhea 遗精[yí jīng] The emission of seminal fluid during sleep or even involuntarily in day time. It is called dreamy spermatorrhea that the seminal fluids escapes in dream, it is called slippery spermatorrhea when the seminal fluid is involuntarily excreted without dream.

spleen meridian of foot-*taiyin* 脾足太阴之脉 [pí zú tài yīn zhī mài] The original name of Spleen Meridian of Foot-*taiyin*.

spiralling manipulation 盘法 [pán fǎ] After inserting the needle superficially into the subcutaneous region, make the body of the needle deviated and make it spiral in a circle. Mainly used at the abdomen. The left spiralling with the needle pressed is reinforcing (tonifying) manipulation while the right spiraling with the needle lifted is re-

ducing (purging) manipulation. (Fig 130)

Spleen Meridian of Foot-*taiyin* (SP) 足太阴脾经 [zú tài yīn pí jīng] One of the twelve meridians. Called *pi zu tai yin zhi mai*. The course: Starting from the end of the great toe, running along the dorso-planter boundary at the medial side of the 1st metatarsal bone, ascending to the anterior aspect of the medial ankle, ascends along the medial aspect of leg, and the posterior tibia, crossing and emerging from the foot-*jueyin*-meridian, ascending to the knee in front of the medial thigh, entering into the abdomen, pertaining to the spleen, connecting with the stomach, passing through the diaphragm, running by the esophagus, connecting with the root of tongue, and distributing itself over the inferior tongue. One branch splits from the stomach, passes through the diaphragm, and runs into the heart (connecting with Heart Meridian of Hand-*shaoyin*). And the big collateral of spleen is termed Dabao, which emerges from the chest and hypochondrium.

SP points 足太阴脾经穴 [zú tài yīn pí jīng xué] According to Systematic Classic of Acupuncture they are Yinbai (SP 1) (well-like), Dadun (SP 2) (spring-like), Taibai (SP 3) (seam-like and source), Gongsun (SP 4) (connecting), Shangqiu (SP 5) (river-like), Sanyinjiao(SP 6)(foot-*shaoyin* and foot-*jueyin* meridians), Lougu (SP 7), Diji (SP 8) (gap-like), Yinlingquan (SP 9) (sea-like), Xuehai (SP 10), Jimen (SP

11), Chongmen (SP 12), Fushe (SP 13), Fujie (SP 14), Daheng (SP 15), Fuai (SP 16), Shidou (SP 17), Tianxi (SP 18), Xiongxiang (SP 19), Zhourong (SP 20), Dabao (SP 21) (the big collateral of spleen), 21 in total. The points of which the spleen meridian crosses other meridians: Zhong fu (LU 1) (foot-*taiyin*); Qimen (LR 14) (foot-*jueyin*); Riyue (GB 24) (foot-*shaoyang*); Xiawan (CV 10); Guanyuan (CV 4); Zhongji (CV 3). There is also Pishu (BL 20) pertaining to foot-*taiyang* meridian; the anterior-referred point, Zhangmen (LR 3) pertaining to foot-*shaoyang* meridian.

SP diseases 足太阴脾经病 [zú tài yīn pí jīng bìng] The main diseases and symptoms are vomiting, jaundice, abdominal mass, loose stool.

splenic yin 脾阴 [pí yīn] As a contrast to splenic yang, it refers to the yin essence of the spleen itself.

spleen, the foundation of life 脾为后天之本 [pí wéi hòu tiān zhī běn] After a man is born, the needs for growth and development can be met, depending mainly upon the health and integraty of the functioning of the stomach and pariculary the spleen. Thus , the spleen is regarded as the foundation of life.

splenic blockage 脾闭 [pí bì] A blockage syndrome which is refractory to prolonged treatment, progresses to affect the spleen and this includes the symptoms of weak limbs, sene of suppression in the chest, cough, vomiting watery salivation, etc.

spring-like point 荥穴 [yíng xué] One of the five *shu* points. The *qi* in the meridian flows here just like spring that has formed a small stream. It is often used for treating febrile diseases.

spring-like and river-like points treating external meridians 荥俞治外经 [yíng shū zhì wài jīng] One of point-selected principles in Internal Classic. The spring-like and river-like points of various meridians are used for treating the diseases and symptoms where the externally running meridians pass through.

splenic *qi* 脾气 [pí qì] The functioning of the spleen.

Special Book for Moxibustion Treatment 采艾篇 [cǎi ài piān] A book compiled by Ye Guang in Qing Dynasty (1644—1911). It was divided into the four volumes. The 1st one contains general introduction, meridians, moxibustion treatment; The 2nd records the explained names of the twelve meridians, indications and diagnostic techniques; The 3rd records moxibustion techniques for diseases and symptoms of internal medicine, the 4th records moxibustion techniques for diseases and symptoms of pediatrics, gynecology, and surgery. It was published in 1668.

Spinal Cord₁ 脊髓₁ [jǐ suǐ yī] An ear point at the most upper edge of the root of ear.

Spinal Cord₂ 脊髓₂ [jǐ suí èr] An ear point anterior to the mastoid process at the lower edge of the root of ear.

spasmotic blockage 挛痹 [luán bì] A blockage syndrome with spasm, numbness and pain of the tendons, muscles and skin, and limitations of the movement of joints.

splenic yang 脾阳 [pí yáng] Referring to the functioning of the spleen, especially its transmitted and digestive capabilities and the thermal energy generated in the process of such activities. If the spleen does not function sufficiently and cold symptoms appear, it is regarded as deficieincy of splenic yang.

spleen 脾 [pí] One of the five striong viscera, located at the abdomen, governing transportation and digestion (dietary food), the origin of producing nutrition and blood. It can control blood, transport equeous fluid and govern the nutrition of the four limbs and muscles. Spleen Meridian of Foot-*taiyin* pertains to the spleen, stomach Meridian of Foot-*yangming* connects with the spleen and its *shu* point is Pishu (BL

20) and its anterior referred point is Zhang-men(LR 13).

spleen, the resource of growth and development 脾为升化之源 [pí wéi shēng huà zhī yuán] The spleen is compared to Earth that is the resource from which everything grows and flourishes. It is an important viscus which digests food, absorbs nourishment, and manufacture *qi* and blood to support and nourish all the internal organs, tissues and structures.

squint 斜视 [xié shì] It denotes that the two eyes can not look straight foreward.

storage with no excretion 藏而不泻 [cáng ér bú xiè] Referring to the physiologic functions of the five storing viscera. In general, these organs are abundent in tissues and have the functions of storing, secreting and producing the refined *qi*, but most of them do not open directly to the exterior and the refined materials which are stored in them cannot be excreted freely to the outside of the body.

stagnation of *qi* 气滞 [qì zhì] *Qi* does not circulate freely, becomes stagnant and causes distension, distress and pain.

stimulation strength 刺激强度 [cì jí qiáng dù] A term of needling techniques. Referring to the degree of the strength of acupuncture. It is divided into strong stimulation, moderate stimulation and weak stimulation. It is formed appropriately by the strength of manipulation, depth of puncture, diameter of needle, number of needles, speed of stimulation frequency and duration of stimulation. The strong stimulation is formed by powerful manipulation, deep insertion of stimulation; While the lighter, smaller, less, slower and shorter consist of weak stimulation; It is called moderate stimulation that it is between the two. Different stimulation strengths generate different effects to the body and the reaction of different patients to the same strong acupuncture stimulation. So, one should accord with the principple of syn-drome differentiation to master the proper strength of stimulation flexibly while carrying on acupuncture treatment.

stringy pulse 弦脉 [xuán mài] The pulse that is taut and long, giving the feeling of string of a violin. It usually indicates diseases of the liver and gallbladder, the pain syndrome, phlegm, hypertension, arteriosclerosis, etc.

stomach 胃 [wèi] One of the six emptying viscera, also called the "sea of water and cereals" and "the sea of the five storing and six emptying viscera." Its action is to receive diets so as to nourish the whole body. A-mong the meridians Stomach Meridian of Foot-*yangming*, Spleen Meridian of Foot-*taiyin*, Lung Meridian of Hand-*taiyin*, Small Intestine Meridian of Hand-*shaoyang*, Liver Meridian of Foot-*taiyin*, Small Intestine Meridian of Hand-*shaoyang* and Liver Meridian of Foot-*jueyin* all are connected with the stomach. Its back *shu* point is Weishu (BL 21), its anterior referred point is Zhongwan (CV 12) and its sea-like point is Zusanli (ST 36).

stuck needle 滞针 [zhì zhēn] After needle insertion the body of the needle is stagnant and can not be rotated and further inserted and withdrawn. An abnormal condition during acupuncture that the needle after being inserted into the body is stuck and firmly held.

stomachache 胃痛 [wèi tòng] Also termed epigastric pain. Since the ache occurs at the epigastrum and its surrounding area, it is generally termed 'cardiac ache' in ancient China.

Stomach 胃 [wèi] An ear point at the area where the crus of antihelix disappears.

stomach, spirit and root 胃神根 [xèi shén gēn] The three qualities necessary for normal pulse. That the pulse is moderate, un-hurried and regular is said to have 'gastric *qi*', that the pulse is storing is said to have 'spirit'; that the pulse can be taken on deep palpation is said to have 'root'.

stimulation point 刺激点 [cì jí diǎn] A kind of calling to the *shu* point of acupuncture in contemporary times, or it is called the stimulation point of acupuncture treatment. It is so called because all the points have the action of treating diseases.

stimulation region 刺激区 [cì jí qū] Comparatively speaking to the stimulative spot. The location stimulated is a region but not a spot. E. g., for the needling technique of plum needling the human body is divided into several stimulation regions.

stimulation parameter 刺激参数 [cì jí cān shù] Various data in the aspect of adding the stimulation condition to the point and stimulation volume during acupuncture. The stimulation parameter of the manipulative needling includes thrusting and lifting and the amplitude of twirling, frequencies and duration in the course of the manipulative operation. The parameter of electroacupuncture generally includes strength (current and voltage), frequency, wave-type, wave width and stimulation duration of the pulse current. The clinical effects vary because of different stimulation parameters. There is the interaction among various items, and it is also related to the length of stimulation time to certain extent. It is of important significance to research the acupuncture mechanism, improve clinical therapeutic effects and exchange experiences by recording and accumulating stimulation parameters and analysing them.

storying viscera troubles treated by selecting stream-like points 治脏者治其俞 [zhì zàng zhě zhì qí shù] One of the point-selected principles in Internal Classic. It implies that for treating disorders of the five storing viscera the stream-like point of the five *shu* points of the meridian should be selected.

stomach meridian of foot-*yangming* 胃足阳明之脉 [wèi zú yáng míng zhī mài] The original name of Stomach Meridian of Foot-*yangming*.

stiff neck 落枕 [luò zhěn] Referring to simple stiffness and pain of the neck, which is limited in movement.

straight and side puncture 傍针刺 [páng zhēn cì] One of the twelve needling techniques for treating carbuncles. It is repeatedly to insert and withdraw the needle vertically and superficially to cause little bleeding at the affected area.

style 针眼 [zhēn yǎn] The little furuncle at the margin of the eyelid, i. e., hordeolum externum.

stasis revoved by puncturing bleeding 宛陈则除之 [yàn chén zé chú zhī] It imphies that it is advisable to use the method of pricking to cause slight bleeding for certain diseases, stasis of *qi* and blood, and pathogenic *qi* at blood phase.

stainless steel needle 不锈钢针 [bù xiù gāng zhēn] An acupuncture instrument. The medical acupuncture instrument is made of stainless steel in contemporary times. In general, it is made of stainless chome-nickle steel, which is hard, elastic and hardly to be stained, and is commonly used in clinic.

Stomach Meridian of Foot-*yangming* (ST) 足阳明胃经 [zú yáng míng wèi jīng] One of the twelve meridians. The course: It starts by the nose, crosses in the root of nose, meets foot-*taiyang* meridian by the nose, descends along the lateral side of nose, enters into the upper tooth, emerges and runs by the mouth, and winds the lips. Its lower part crosses Chengjiang (CV, RV 24), then, withdraws and runs along the mandible and emerges from Daying (ST 5) and runs along Jiache (KI 8), ascends in front of the ear, passes through Shangguan (GB 3), runs along the hairline to the middle of the forehead, the cranial region. One branch descends from the anterior Daying (ST 9), runs along the throat and enters into the supraclavicular fossa, passes through the diaphragm, pertains to the stomach and connects with the spleen. The one running externally descends from the supracalvicular fossa, passes through the breast, again descends by the umbilicus, enters into the inguinal artery. One branch descends from the opening of the stomach along the inner abdomen to join the previous one at the inguinal artery, descends and passes through the anterior hip joint to the protuberance of the tibial muscle of thigh, descends to the inner, and then descends along the guadraceps of tibia to the dorsal foot, enters into the medial side of the middle toe (emerges from the end of the middle toe). The branch splits from the place 3 cm below the knee, descends and enters into the lateral side of the middle toe (merges from the end of the second toe.) One branch splits from the dorsal foot, enters into the great toe, and emerges from its end. (connects with Spleen Merdian of Foot-*taiyin*)

ST points 足阳明胃经穴 [zú yáng míng wèi jīng xué] They are Chengqi (ST 1), Sibai (ST 2), Juliao (ST 3), Dicang (ST 4), Daying (ST 5), Jiache (ST 6), Xiaguan (ST 7), Touwei (SY 8), Renying (SY 9), Shuitu (ST 10), Qishe (ST 11), Quepeng (ST 12), Qihu (SY 13), Kufang (ST 14), Wuyi (ST 15), Yingchuang (ST 16), Ruzhong (ST 17), Rugen (ST 18), Burong (ST 19), Chengman (ST 20), Liangmen (ST 21), Guanmen (ST 22), Taiyi (ST 23), Huarumen (ST 24), Tianshu (ST 25), Wailing (ST 26), Daju (ST 27), Shuidao (ST 28), Guilai (ST 29), Qichong (ST 30), Piguan (ST 31), Futu (ST 32), Yinshi (ST 33), Liangqiu (ST 34) (gap), Dubi (ST 35), Zusanli (ST 36) (correspondence of stomach), Shangjuxu (ST 37) (correcpondence of large intestine), Tiaokou (ST 38), Xiajuxu (ST 39) (corresondence of small intestine), Fenglong (ST 40) (connecting), Jiexi (ST 41) (river), Chongyang (ST 42) (source), Xiangu (ST 43) (stream), Neiting (ST 44) (spring), Lidui (ST 45) (well), 45 in total. The points where the meridian crosses other meridians are: Yingxiang (LI 20) (hand-*yangming*), Jingming (BL 1) (foot-*taiyang*), Hanyan (GB 4), Xuanli (GB 6), Shangguan (GB 3) (foot-*shaoyang*), Shuigou (GV 26), Shenting (GV 24), Dazhui (GV 14), Chengjiang (CV 14), Shangwan (CV 13), Zhongwan (CV 12). There are also Weishu (BL 21) that pertains to foot-*taiyang*, the anterior referred point, Zhongwan (CV 12) that pertains to CV.

ST diseases 足阳明胃经病 [zú yáng míng wèi jīng bìng] They are chiefly chills and fever, malaria, mania, stuffy nose, epistaxis, deviated mouth, swelling neck, sore throat, distension and fullness of the abdomen, pain in the epigastrum, nausea, vomiting, indigestion.

Suizhong 髓中 [suǐ zhōng] I. e., Suifu, an alternate term for Siman (KI 14).

sunlight moxibustion 日光灸 [rì guāng jiǔ] A kind of moxibustion. Cover the abdomen with a layer of mugwort floss and expose the abdomen in sun.

shugu 束骨 [shù gú] 1. The portion of the 5th metatarsophalangeal joint on the lateral aspect of the foot; 2. Sugu, the name of the acupuncture point, located in the depression posterosuperior to the 5th metatar sophalangeal joint.

superficial puncture 半刺 [bàn cì] One of five needlings. The needling that the skin is punctured superficially and the inserted needle is swiftly withdrawn, similar to shallow puncture in nine needlings. The plum needle applied in modern times developed from it.

Supplement of Miraculous Pivot and Meridians 灵枢经脉翼 [líng shū jīng mài yì] A book written by Xia Ying in Ming Dynasty (1368—1644). Its contents are the notes to Meridians, a chapter of Miraculous Pivot on the basis of the Expounding of Fourteen Meridians.

subcutaneous needle 皮内针 [pí nèi zhēn] Specially made for subcutuaneous embedding of the needle, varied in the granual type and thumb-tag type. (Fig) The first one is 1.5 cm or 3 cm in length, like the filiform needle in diameter. Its tail is granual like. While using it, pinch its body with a forceps, gently and slowly puncture the skin with it horizontally 1—2 cm deep. Then slowly puncture the skin with it horizontally 1—2 cm deep, and then slowly puncture the skin with it horizontally and fix it with rubberized cloth. The body is winded into a circle, its tip is exposed and appoints to the point. After slightly rotating it, press it into the point, then fix it with rubberized cloth. The duration of retaining the needle is decided by the concrete condition. (Fig 131)

Fig 131

swift lifting and slow inserting 急提慢按 [jí tí màn àn] See *jin ti man an*.

superficial-deep point-combined method 表里配穴法 [biǎo lǐ pèi xué fǎ] One of point-composed methods. Referring to combination of the points according to the superficeal-deep relationship between the yang and yin meridians of the twelve meridians. E. g. , for stomach trouble, select Zusanli (ST 36) of Stomach Meridian of Foot-*yangming* and Gongsun (SP 4) of Spleen Meridian of Foot-taiyin; For sore throat select Hegu(LI 4)of Large Intestine Meridian of Hand-*yangming* and Yuji (LU 10) of Lung Meridian of Hand-*shaoyin*. The source-connection points-combined method recorded in ancient literatures pertains to this category.

Supplementary Illustrations of Classified Classic 类经图翼 [lèi jīng tú yì] A book written by Zhang Jiebing. The continuous compilation of Classified Classic, 11 volumes. The part dealing with meridians and

acupuncture all has the appending illustrations and is of important reference value. At the end of the book Appended Supplements is appended.

supine position 仰卧位 [yǎng wò wèi] The name of the body position of acupuncture. See lying position.

supine-sitting position 仰靠位 [yǎng kào wèi] The name of the body position of acupuncture. See sitting position.

superficial puncture and swift insertion for febrile syndromes 热则疾之 [rè zé jí zhī] One of the therapeutical principles of acupuncture. As for febrile diseases pathogenic heat can be reduced by superficial puncture and swift insertion of the needle. Refer retain the needle for cold syndromes.

Supplementary Notes to Illustrated Classic of the Bronze Fi-gure with *Shu* Points 补注铜人腧穴针灸图经 [bǔ zhù tóng rén shū xué zhēn jiǔ tú jīng] A book written by an unknown person. It is based on Illustrated Classic of Acupuncture of the Bronze Figure with *Shu* Points (3 volumes). The 1st and 2nd volumes record the points of the twelve meridians, (arranged from the four limbs to the trunk) the points of GV and those of CV (arranged from the upper part to the lower); The 3rd, 4th, and 5th were divided into the twelve parts, introducing the indications of various points and acupuncture and moxibustion treatment of various points. It aids in the systematization of the meridians and points. As compared with Systematic Classic of Acupuncture, it adds Yaoyangguan (GV 3), Lingtai (GV 10), Jueyinshu(BL 14), Gaohuangshu (BL 43), and Qingling (HT 2).

Sun Simiao 孙思邈 [sūn sī miǎo] (581—682) An eminent medial specialist in Tang Dynasty (618-907 A. D.)born at Yao County, Shanxi Province. During childhood, he learned medicine due to his illness, and he researched medicine very conscientiously and was very familia to theories of various schools and Budhist Classics. He summed up clinical experiences and drugs and acupuncture knowledge and wrote the books. Prescriptions with A Thousand Gold and Supplementary Prescriptions With A Thousand Gold, both of which contain the special chapter of acupuncture.

Suikong 髓孔 [suǐ kǒng] 1. An alternate term for Daying (ST 5); 2. I. e. , Suikong, an alternate term for Yaoshu (GV 2).

Suihui 髓会 [suǐ huì] One of the eight confuentical points. Generally explained as Xuanzhong (GB 39), also as Yangfu (GB 38), both of which pertain to Gallbladder Meridian of Foot-*shaoyang*, located at the fibular region.

Suikong 髓空 [suǐ kōng] An alternate term for Yaoshu (GV 2).

Suifu 髓府 [suǐ fǔ] An alternate term for Siman (KI 14).

Suishu 髓俞 [suǐ shū] An alternate term for Yaoshu (KI 14).

superficial collateral meridians 浮络 [fú luò] Referring to the collateral meridians at the body surface.

substantial gallbladder 胆实 [dǎn shí] The syndrome due to stagnation of biliary *qi*. The main symptoms are distension and pain of the hypochondrium, bitter taste in the dry mouth, aching of the temporal regions, headache, pain in the eyes, etc.

substantial heat in the liver and gallbladder 肝胆湿热 [gān dǎn shī rè] The pathologic changes due to stagnation of pathogenic dampness and heat in the liver and the gallbladder. The main symptoms are jaundice, fever, bitter taste, pain in the hypochondrium, nausea and vomiting, anorexia, aversion to fatty food, abdominal distension and pain, yellowish urine, loose stools, yellowish glossy coating of tongue, stringy rapid pulse, etc.

substantial pulse 实脉 [shí mài] 1. A general term for various kinds of forceful pulses; 2. The large, forceful and substantive pulses, indicating the excess syndrome.

superficial puncture 浮刺 [fú cì] To puncture obliquely the muscle to treat coldness and contricture of the muscle. Similar to oblique puncture alpplied in modern clinic.

suppurative moxibustion 化脓灸 [huà nóng jiǔ] A kind of moxibustion with moxa cone, also termed scarring moxibustion. To administer moxibustion directly on the point on the skin with moxa cone, so as to gradually cause suppuration, leaving scar at last. After 5—9 moxa cones of moxibustion on each point, plaster of moxibustion scar (mild plaster) is used to seal the point and change it once a day. After 4—7 days, the point where moxibustion is administered becomes suppurative, forming moxibustion scar. Usually used for asthma, chronic gastroenteritis.

Supplementary Prescriptions Worth a Thousand Gold 千金翼方 [qiān jīn yì fāng] A medical book written by Sun Simiao in Tang Dynasty (618—907A. D.), 30 volumes, the continuous compilation of Prescreptions Worth a Thousand Gold. In the 26th—28th volumes, three chapters of acupuncture were added, which recorded and described way of selecting the points, acupuncture-moxibustion techniques for various diseases, as well as "miscellaneous methods", "acupuncture prohibitions" etc.

Suliao (GV 25) 素髎 [sù liáo] A CV point also termed Mianwany. Location: In the centre of the tip of nose. Regional anatomy: There is the doral nasal branch of the faicial artery and vein. The lateral nasal branch of the anterior ethemoidal nerve is distributed. The cartilage of the tip of nose is below. Indications: Stuffy nose, epistaxis, thin nasal discharge, nasal polyp, rhinitis, brandy nose, coma. Puncture: 1—1. 5 cm obliquely or prick to cause little bleeding with a triangular needle. Moxibustion is prohibited.

sui **point** 隧穴 [suì xué] '*Sui*' means the meridian tunnel, while '*xue*' means *shu* points. Here it generally refers to the meridians points of the whole body.

sudden blindness 暴盲 [bào máng] Originally the patient did not suffer from any ocular disease but suddenly becomes blind in one or both eyes. Similar to embolism of the central retinal artery.

sudden *jue* symptom complex 暴厥 [bào jué] Sudden fainting with abrupt, rapid pulse.

sudden collapse 暴脱 [bào tuō] Collapse occurring suddenly.

swift lifting and slow thrusting 紧提慢按 [jǐn tí màn àn] Contrary to swift thrusting and slow lifting. Usually used in cool to a clear sky night.

swift needle insertion 快插进针 [kuài chā jìn zhēn] See injection-like needle insertion.

sword-like needle 披针 [pī zhēn] I. e., sword-like needle.

sword-head needle 箭头针 [jiàn tóu zhēn] I. e., the arrowhead needle.

sword-like needle 剑针 [jiàn zhēn] Called *pizhen* in ancient China.

swift insertion and slow withdrawal lead to reducing 急而徐则虚 [jí ér xú zé xū] An acupuncture reducing manipulation, parallel to slowing and swifting leading to reinforcing. It implies that swiftly inserting the needle and slowing withdrawing the needle can weaken pathogenic *qi*, i. e., reducing. That in needling techniques in latter generations one insertion and three withdrawals or one insertion and two withdrawals are used for reducing originates from this.

swift thrusting and slow lifting 紧按慢提 [jǐn àn màn tí] Contrary to swift lifting and slow thrusting. Referring to the action of reinforcing manipulation by lifting and thrusting the needle. Usually used in Setting the mountain on fire.

syndrome of emptying viscera 腑证 [fǔ zhèng] The manifestations of the disease of the three yang meridians with involvement of their related emplying viscera.

symptoms of the upper energizer 上焦病证 [shàng jiāo bìng zhèng] Those of the early stage of an acute febrile disease, includ-

ing manifestations of the invasion of the large intestine meridian and pericardium meridian by pathogenic *qi*.

symptoms of the middle energizer 中焦病证 [zhōng jiāo bìng zhèng] Those of the late stage of an acute febrile disease, including manifestations of the invasion of the liver and kidney by pathogenic *qi*.

syndrome differentiation in accordance with the triple energizer 三焦辨证 [sān jiāo biàn zhèng] The method to identify the location, nature and characteristics of the three different stages of the clinical course of an acute feabrile disease due to external affection, as well as the ebb and flow of pathogeni *qi* and anti-pathogenic *qi*, which are used by the experts of acute febrile diseases by borrowing the terms of the upper, middle and lower energizers.

syndrome differentiation in accordacne with the etiology 病因辨证 [bìng yīn biàn zhèng] The procedure to analyse and sum up the symptoms and signs, so as to identify the causes of disease.

syndrome differentiation in accordance with *qi* and blood 气血辨证 [qì xuè biàn zhèng] The procedure to analyze and sum up the symptoms and signs according to the pricniples of *qi* and blood.

syndrome differentiation in accordance with body fluids 津液辨证 [jīn yè biàn zhèng] The procedure to analyse, sum up and judge the condition of the disease according to the signs of body fluids.

Systematic Classic of Acupuncture 针灸甲乙经 [zhēn jiǔ jiá yǐ jīng] A book compiled by Huangfu Mi during Wei and Jin Periods (951—1115), originally called Huangdi San-bu Zhenjiu Jia Yi Jing, also called Huangdi Jia Yi Jing, Huangdi Sanbu Zhenjing, briefly called Jai Yi Jing. Basing on Plain Questions. Acupuncture Classic and Essential Treatment of *Mingtang* Points and Acupuncture-Moxibustion(lost), it collects the contents concerning acupuncture and systematized them. The edition that is handed down contains 10 volumes, in which the theories such as storing-emptying viscera, meridians and treatment are briefly described and minutely records the locations of 649 point of the whole body and their indications, depth of puncture, number of moxa cone, etc. It is the earliest famous and systematical acupuncture book and exerts agreat influence upon the development of acupuncture science at home and abroad. It was completed in 256—259 A. D.

syndrome differentiation in accordance with the principles of *wei*-defence, *qi*-vital energy *ying*-nutrition and *xue*-blood 卫气营血辨证 [wèi qì yíng xuè biàn zhèng] The method to identify the location, nature and variation of the four phases of the clinical course of an acute febrile disease due to external affection as well as the ebb and flow of pathogenic *qi* and of anti-pathogenic *qi*.

syndrome differentiation with the names of six meridians 六经辨证 [liù jīng biàn zhèng] The names of the six meridians are used to identify the location and the nature of the disease, characteristics of pathologic changes, and the ebb and flow of the pathogenic *qi* during the different stages of onset and development of the infectious desease of external causes in On Febrile Diseases written by Zhang Zhongjing in Han Dynasty (206 B. C. — 220A. D.)

synthetical manipulation 综合手法 [zōng hé shǒu fǎ] Contrary to basic accessary manipulations. Referring to the comparatively complex manipulation formed by some single manipulations. E. g. , setting the mountain on fire, cool to a clear sky night, yin hiding in yang, yang hiding in yin, etc. Some pertain to reinforcing manipulation, some other pertain to reducing manipulation, some pertain to reinforcing-reducing manipulation, still some other pertain to the method of promoting *qi* flow.

Sympathetic 交感 [jiāo gǎn] An ear point at the end of the lower foot of the antihelix.

Taiyuan (LU 9) 太渊 [tài yuān] A point of Lung Meridian of Hand-*tatyin*, the stream-like (earth) and source point of the meridian, the confluence of meridian of eight confluent points. Location: On the end of the radial side of the transverse crease of the wrist of the posterior palm , at the pulsation of the radial artery. Regional anatomy: Between the radial flexor muscle of wrist and the long abductor muscle of thumb. There are the radial artery and vein. The lateral cutaneous nerve of forearm and the superficial branch of the radial nerve are distributed. Indications: Headache, ocular pain, sore throat, toothache, deafness, tinnitus, asthmatic breath, cough, thoracalgia and hemoptysis, emaciation-thirst disease, insomnia, nocturnal emission, impotence, frequent urination, pain in the lumbar spine, irregular menstruation, pain in the medial ankle. Puncture: 1.5—3 cm perpendicularly. Moxibustion: 3—5 moxa cones or 5—10 minutes with warming moxibustion.

Taixi (KI 3) 太溪 [tài xī] A point of Kidney Meridian of Foot-*shaoyin*, the stream (eartn) and source point of the meridian it pertains to. Also termed Lidui, Neikunlun, Location: In the depression between the medial ankle and the tendon sheath. Select it at the level with and opposite to the tip of the medial ankle. Regional anatomy: Sore throat, toothache, deafness, coughing up blood, asthmatic breath, full chest and thoracalgia, emaciation-thirst disease, insomnia, nocturnal emission, impotence, spermatorrhea, frequent urination, soreness and pain in the lumbar spine, foot *qi*, irregular menstruation, pain in the sole, urethral infection, neuroasthenia, auditory vertigo, brachial asthma. Puncture: 1.5—3 cm perpendicularly. Moxibustion: 3—5 moxa cones, or 5—10 minutes with warming

moxibustion.

taking off the needle 拔针 [bá zhēn] I.e., withdrawing the needle.

tassel meridian 缨脉 [yīng mài] I.e., Foot-*yangming* meridian by the neck.

Taiyang 太阳 [tài yáng] An ear point at the edge of the cartillege of the antitragus between Occiput and Forehead.

Tan Zhiguang (1852—1930) 谭志光 [tán zhì guāng] A contemporary acupuncture expert, born at Changsha, Hunan Province. At his early age, he learned acupuncture from Liu Yunjie in Shanghai. Later he came back to Hunan to establish an acupuncture research institute in 1923, handed down acupuncture techniques and wrote the book Questions and Answers on Acupuncture.

Taodao (CV 13) 陶道 [táo dào] A GV point, the confluence of GV and foot-*taiyang* meridian. Location: At the midline of the back. Between the spinal processes of the 1st and 2nd thoracic vertebrae. Regional anatomy: Passing through the fascia of the waist and back, reaching at the supraspinal ligament and interspinal ligament. There is the posterior branch of the 1st intercostal artery, and the medial branch of the posterior branch of the 1st intercostal artery. The medial branch of the posterior branch of the 1st intercostal nerve is distributed. Indications: headache, stiffness in the neck, aversion to cold and fever, malaria, common cold, stiff neck, cough, asthmatic breath, steaming of bones, thoracalgia, pain in the spine, malaria, mania, opisthotonos. Puncture: 1.5—3 cm obliquely. Moxibustion: 3—5 moxa cones or 5—10 minutes with warming moxibustion.

Taicang 太仓 [tài cāng] 1. stomach; 2. An alternate term for Zhongwan (CV 12).

Taibai (SP 3) 太白 [tài bái] A point of Spleen Meridian of Foot-*taiyin*, the stream-like (earth) and source point of the meridian. Location: At the posterior edge of the small head of the 1st metatarsal bone on the medial side of the foot, at the dorso-ventral boundary. Regional anatomy: At the abductor muscle of the great toe: There is the dorsal venous network of foot and the medial vein of the sole and the branch of the medial artery. The branches of the proper nerve and the suerficial peroneal nerve are distributed. Indications: Stomachache, abdominal distension. abdominal pain, borborygmus, vomiting, diarrhea, dysentery, constipation, hemorrhoids, foot *qi*, poor appetite, indigestion, cardiac pain with slow pulse, distension and pain in the chest and hypochondrium, heavy sensation of the body and arthralgia, atrophy syndrome. Puncture: 1—2 cm perpendicularly. Moxibustion: 3—5 moxa cones or 5—10 minutes with warming moxibustion.

Taichong (LR 3) 太冲 [tài chōng] A point of Liver Meridian of Foot-*jueyin*, the stream-like (earth) and source point of the meridian. Location: In the depression anterior to the joining part of the 1st and 2nd metatarsal bones. Regional anatomy: At the lateral edge of the short extensor muscle of the great toe and the interosseous dorsal muscle. There is the dorsal venous network and the dorsal artery of the 1st metatarsal bone. The branches of the superficial and deep perroneal nerves are distributed. Indications: Enuresis, infantile convulsion, mania, epilepsy, hypochondriac pain, abdominal distension, jaundice, vomiting, sore throat, congestion and pain in the eyes, pains in the interior aspect of the knee and thigh, puffiness of the dorsal foot, atrophy of the lower limbs. Puncture: 1.5—3 cm perpendicularly. Moxibustion: 3—5 moxa cones or 5—10 minutes with warming moxibustion.

taichong mai 太冲脉 [tài chōng mài] Referring to Chongmai (Vital Vessel).

Taiyin 太阴 [tài yīn] 1. An extra point, Location: On the posterior edge of the medial side of tibia, 2.4 dm directly above the tip of the medial ankle. Indication: Foot *qi*. Moxibustion: 3—7 moxa cones; 2. The *taiyin* meridians, one of the three yin meridians, divided into hand-*taiyin* meridian foot-*taiyin* meridian.

Taiyang (EX-HN5) 太阳 [tài yáng] 1. An extra point, also called Qianguan, Dangyang. Location: Approx. 3 cm lateral to the midpoint of the line connecting the end of the eyebrow and the external corner of eye. Indications: Headache, migraine, common cold, vertigo, toothache, congestion and swelling and pain in the eyes, triangular neuralgia, facial paralysis, acute conjunctivitis, stye, retinal hemorrhage, keratitis. Puncture: 1.5 cm perpendicularly or 1.5 cm horizontally or cause little bleeding with traingular needle. 1. An alternate term for Tongziliao (GB 1); 2. The taiyang meridian, one of the three yang meridians, divided into the hand-*taiyang* meridian and foot-*taiyang* meridian. (Fig 132)

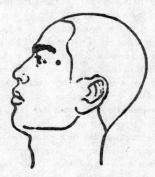

Fig 132

Taiyinyang 太阴阳 [tài yīn yáng] An alternate term for Yemen (TE 2).

Taiyinluo 太阴络 [tài yīn luò] Referring to Lougu (SP7).

Taiyinqiao 太阴跷 [tài yī qiào] I. e., Yinqiao, referring to Zhaohai (KI 6).

Taichong 太冲 [tài chōng] I. e. , Dazhong (KI 4).

Taiquan 太泉 [tài quán] I. e. , Taiyuan (EX-HN 5).

Taizhu 太祖 [tài zhǔ] Another name of Conggu.

Taisu 太素 [tài sù] A medical book. For details see Comprehensive Notes to Yellow Emperor's Internal Classic.

Tailing 太陵 [tài líng] I. e. , Daling (PC 7).

Taiyi (ST 23) 太乙 [tài yǐ] A point of Stomach Meridian of Foot-*yangming*. Location: 6 cm lateral to Xiawan (CV 10), 6 cm below the umbilicus. Regional anatomy: In the straight muscle of abdomen. There are the branches of 8th and 9th intercostal artery and vein and the branches of the hypogastric artery and vein. The branches of the 8th and 9th intercostal nerves are distributed. Indications: Stomachache, abdominal distension, diarrhea, mania, foot *qi*, anxiety, acute enteritis, indigestion, adhesion of the intestine. Puncture: 3—4 cm perpendicularly. Moxibustion: 3—5 moxa cones or 5—10 minutes with warming moxibustion.

Taiyi moxa stick 太乙神针 [tài yí shén zhēn] 1. A kind of moxibustion with moxa stick. Ignite one end of the moxa stick added with drug powder, then wrapp it with seven strata of cloth and press it on the ping, then change it after it becomes cold. Do moxibustion 5—7 times on each point. The drugs added in the moxa cone vary. In modern times the moxa cone is made by mixing mugwort floss with sandalwood, resurrection lilyrkizoma, motopterygium root, cinnamon twig, auklandis root realagar, dachurian angelica root, eagle wood, pubescent angelica root, wuplphur, spikenard, nutgrass flatsedge rhizome, red sage root, asarum herb.

Taiyi 太一 [tài yí] I. e. , Taiyi (ST 23).

Textral Study on Eight Extra Vessels 奇经八脉考 [qí jīng bā mài kǎo] A book written by Li Shizhen in Ming Dynasty (1368—1644). It had a textual study on the course of the eight extra vessels, their indications and the points pertaining to them and explored in combination with data in the aspect of *qigong*, and thought that "the meridians within the body can be observed only by". Its description about the eight extra vessels is more detailed than that of The Expounding of the Fourteen Meridians, but the points enumerated in it are somewhat different from those by Systematic Classic of Acupuncture. It was completed in 1577.

Textual Study on Meridians 经络考 [jīng luò kǎo] A book compiled by Zhang Sanxi in Ming Dynasty (1368—1644). One of Six Essentials of Medicine written by himself, only one volume. It was completed in 1609.

Textual Study on Illustrations of Meridian Points of Acupuncture 针灸经穴图考 [zhēn jiǔ jīng xué tú kǎo] A book written by Huang Zhuzai. It mainly contains Internal Classic and systematic Classic of Acupuncture, refers over sixty kinds of literatures, and systematically introduces the location, indication of the meridian points and techniques of acupuncture and moxibustion. It also supplements the meridian points to 365 points, and somewhat changes of tropism of a few points. In the last volume it checks and corrects the mistakes in Textual Study on Eight Extra Vessels. It was published in 1935.

terminal bone 穷骨 [qióng gǔ] Referring to sacrum and coccyx. In ancient China the sacrum and coccyx were often termed in a mixed way. .

technique of feeling pulse 操纵 [cāo zòng] The method of applying digital pressure in palpating pulse. Essentially the finger should first press gently and then harder or alternate, gentle and heavy pressures repeatedly so as to recognize different qualities of the pulse.

ten changes 十变 [shí biàn] 1. The name of the ancient literature; 2. The relationship of the change of the ten stems in cooperation.

tendinous blockage 筋闭 [jīn bì] A blockage syndrome characterized mainly with the symptoms of tendons. The chief manifestations are spasm of the tendons and pain and stiffness of the joints.

tense pulse 紧脉 [jǐn mài] The pulse that feels tense, forceful, and tight like rolling a rope to the finger. It usually indicates the pain syndrome and the cold syndrome.

tender point 压痛点 [yā tòng diǎn] The sensitive and painful spot discovered by pressing or pinching the body surface with the fingers. As to selection of the point in acupuncture a stress has been made on induction, as was said in Internal Classic, "feeling comfortable while pressing it, feeling responsible and painful while pressing it." According to the reaction of tenderness it is regarded as the chief reason for locating the point. Refer as hi point.

Textual Study on Illustrations of Meridians 经脉图考 [jīng mài tú kǎo] A book compiled by Chen Huichou in Qing Dynasty (1644—1911), four volumes, the 1st volume generally describes the 'internal scence', bone measurement, courses of meridians and important points; The 2nd and 3rd indications of the courses of the twelve meridians, illustrations and rhythmed articles. The 4th describes the courses of the eight extra vessels, indications and 'invention of the courses of variour meridians'. It mainly refers to Supplementary Illustrations of Classified Classic and Synopsis of Golden Chamber, and textually studied them. The illustrations are comparatively carefully and neatly down, published in 1878.

Testicle 睾丸 [gāo wán] An ear point located apporx. 0.2 mm posteroinferior to the parotid gland.

TE points 手少阳三焦经穴 [shǒu shào yáng sān jiāo jīng xué] According to Systematic Classic of Acupuncture, they are Guanchong (TE, SJ 10) (well-like), Yemen (TE, SJ 2) (spring-like), Zhongzhu (TE, SJ 3)

(stream-like), Yangchi (TE 4) (source), Waiguan (TE 5) (connecting), Zhigou (TE 6) (river-like), Tianjing (TE 7) (sea-like), Qinglengyuan (TE 11), Xiaole (TE 12), Naohui (TE 13), Jianliao (TE 14), Tianliao (TE 15), Tianyong (TE, SJ 16), Yifeng (TE, SJ 17), Chimai (TE, SJ 18), Luxi (TE, SJ 19), Jiaosun (TE 20), Ermen (TE 21), Heliao (TE 22), Sizukong (TE 23), 23 in total. The crossing points with other meridians are Binfeng (SI 12), Quanliao (SI 18), Tinggong (SI 19) (hand-*taiyang* meridian); Tongziliao (GB 1), Shangguan (GB 3), Hanyan (GB 4), Xuanli (GB 6), Jianjing (GB 21) (foot-*shaoyang* meridian), Dazhui (GV 1) and Sanjiaoshu (BL 22) pertaining to foot-*taiyang* meridian; The anterior-referred point of Triple Energizer Meridian, Shimen (CV 5) pertaining to CV; The lower joining points of Triple Energizer Meridian, Weiyang (BL 39) pertaining to foot-*taiyang* meridian.

TE diseases 手少阳三焦经病 [shǒu shào yáng sān jiāo jīng bìng] They are mainly deafness, tinnitus, swelling throat, sore throat, pain in the outer canthus, pain in the cheek, pain in the posterior ear and the region where the meridian runs over, firmness and fullness of the lower abdomen, tympanites, difficulty in micturition, enuresis.

third lateral line of chest 胸第三测线 [xiōng dì sān chè xiàn] A line locating the meridian point, i. e., descending from the supraclavicular fossa, 18 cm to the midline of chest, where Lung Meridian of Hand-*taiyin* and Spleen Meridian of Foot-*taiyin* pass through. Yunmen (LU 2), Zhongfu (LU 1), Zhourong (SP 20), Xiongxiang (SP 19), Tianxi (SP 18), and Shidou (SP 17) are distributed.

thoracic midline 胸正中线 [xiōng zhèng zhōng xiàn] The line for locating the meridian point, also called the midline of stern, where CV passes through and Tiantu (CV 22), Xuanji (CV 21), Huagai (KC 20), Zigong (CV 19), Yutang (CV 18),

Danzhong(CV 17), and Zhongting (CV 15) are distributed.

thoracic *shu* points 胸俞 [xiōng shū] Referring to the points at the 1st lateral line of chest. They are Shufu (KI 27), Yuzhong (KI 26), Shencang (CV 18), Lingxu (KI 24), Shenfeng (KI 23), Bulang (KI 22), twelve on the bilateral lines.

thoracic blockage 胸闭 [xiōng bì] The symptom-complex due to interference with flow of yang *qi* and stagnation of the phlegm and damp pathogen in the chest, chiefly manifested as upper back pain, feeling of suffocation in the chest, shortage of breath, cough with copious phlegm etc.

Thoracic vertebra 胸椎 [xiōng zhuī] An ear point in the 1st equivalent zone above Cervical Vertebra.

three yin meridians of foot 足三阴经 [zú sān yīn jīng] A general term for Spleen Meridian of Foot-*taiyin*, Kidney Meridian of Foot-*shaoyin* and Liver Meridian of Foot-*jueyin*. Distributing themselves over the medial side of the lower limb, ascending to reach the internal organs in the abdomen and chest. "Three yin meridians of foot run from foot to abdomen." (Miraculous Pivot)

three yang meridians of foot 足三阳经 [zú sān yáng jīng] A general term for Stomach Meridian of Foot-*yangming*, Bladder Meridian of Foot-*shaoyang*. Starting from the head and face, distributed over the trunk and the anterior, posterior and lateral aspect of the lateral side of the lower limb. "Three yang meridians of foot run from head to foot." (Miraculous Pivot)

three regions and nine modes 三部九候 [sān bù jiǔ hòu] The divisons for pulse diagnosis. "The heaven mode of the region is called the heaven region, that is the arteries at the bildteral forehead, the earth mode of the upper region is the arteries of the cheeks. The man mode of the middle region is hand-*taiyin*, the earth mode of middle region is hand-*yangming*, the man mode of the upper region is the heaven mode of the lower region is foot-*jueyin*, the earth mode of the lower region is foot-*shaoyin*, the man mode of the lower region is foot-*taiyin*." (Plain questions) The flourishing and decline of *qi* and blood of the internal organs concerned can be dignosed from the arteries of the various portions.

	Division	Artery	Point Concerned	Indication
upper	Heaven	Two forehead	Foot-*shaoyang*, Hanyan (G134)	*qi* at the corner of the head
	Earth	Two cheecks	Foot-*Yangming*, Daying (ST5)	*qi* at the mouth and eyes
	Man	In front of ears	Hand-shaoyang. Heliao (SJ 22)	*qi* at the ear and eyes
Middle	Heaven	Hand-*taiyin*	Lingqi (LU 8)	Lung
	Earth	Hand-*yangming*	Hegu(LI 4)	*qi* in the chest
	Man	Hand-*shaoyin*	Shnmen(HT 7)	heart
Lower	Heaven	Foot-*jueyin*	Wuli, Taichong (LR 3) (LI 13)	Liver
	Earth	Foot-*shaoyin*	Taixi(KI 3)	Kidney
	Man	Foot-*taiyin*	Jimen(SP 11)	spleen, stomach

Throat tooth 喉牙 [hóu yá] An ear point anteroinferior to Brain Stem.

Thyroid gland 甲状腺 [jiǎ zhuàng xiàn] An ear point located at the lateral 1/3 of the boundary line between Zone$_3$ and Zone$_6$.

third lateral line of abdomen 腹第三侧线 [fù dì sān chè xiàn] The line for locating the meridian points, 10 cm to the abdominal midline where Spleen Meridian of Foot-*taiyin*, Liver Meridian of Foot-*jueyin* and Gallbladder Meridian of Foot-*shaoyang* pass through. Distributed over are Qimem (LR 14), Riyue(GB 24), fuai(SP 16), Dahneg(SP 15), Fujie (SP 14), Fushe(SP 13), Chongmen(SP 12).

thready collateral meridians 丝络 [sī luò] The name of the collateral meridian.

three strata 三部 [sān bù] Referring superficial, middle and deep strata of the point. The superficial stratum is called the heaven stratum, the middle the man one, and the deep the earth one. Also called collectively *sancai*, which is divided into *tiancai*, *rencai* and *dicai*. (Fig 133)

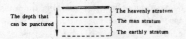

The depth that can be punctured

The heavenly stratum
The man stratum
The earthly stratum

Fig 133

three yang 三阳 [sān yáng] 1. 1) The name of the meridians, a collective term for *taiyang*, *yangming* and *shaoyang* meridians; 2) referring to *taiyang* meridian; 2. *Sanyang*, an alternate term for Baihui (GV, DU).

three yang and three yin 三阳三阴 [sā yáng sān yīn] Nomenclature of the meridians. Yang is divided into *taiyang*, *yangming* and *shaoyang*, collectively called three yang; Yin is divided into *taiyin*, *shaoyin* and *jueyin*, collectively called three yin. *Taiyang* can also be termed the 3rd yang, *yangming* the 2nd, and *shaoyang* the 1st; *taiyin* can also be termed the 3rd yin, *shaoyin* the 2nd, *jueyin* the 1st. *Tai* and *shao* refer to

the volume of *qi* of yin and yang. *Yangming* refer to the most flourishing of yang *qi*. *Jueyin* refers to the least of yin *qi*. That they are classified into the 1st, 2nd and 3rd refers to the sequence of six *qi*.

three strata 三才 [sān cái] Originally referring to heaven, man and earth. In acupuncture it refers to the upper, middle and lower strata or the superficial, middle and deep strata.

three transverse width *cun* 横三间寸 [héng sān jiān cùn] A term of moxibustion technique. Make three moxa cones with 0.9 cm transverse width, added with their interspaces. The distance of the two ends is totally 3 cm. It also implies that the diameter of the base of the moxa cone is standardized as 0.9 cm. It is usually used for suppurative moxibustion in clinic.

three insertions and one withdrawal 三进一退 [sān jìn yī tuì] An acupuncture technique in reinforcing manipulation, used in "Setting the mountain on fire." Contrary to one insertion and three withdrawals. It denotes that the needle is inserted according to the three strata gradually from the superficial

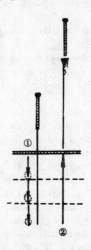

①

②

Fig 134

stratum to the middle, then to the deep, and withdraw once directly to the deep stratum, then to the superficial. It can be repeated. (Fig 134)

three yang meridians of hand 手三阳经 [shǒu sān yáng jīng] A collective term for Large Intestine Meridian of Hand-*yangming*, Small Intestine Meridian of Hand-*taiyang*, and Triple Energizer Meridian of Hand-*shaoyang*, distributed over the lateral (extending) side of the upper limb, and upwardly reaching at the head and face.

three yin meridians of hand 手三阴经 [shǒu sān yīn jīng] A collective term for Lung Meridian of Hand-*taiyin*, Heart Meridian of Hand-*shaoyin* and Pericardium Meridian of Hand-*jueyin*. Starting from the viscera in the chest, distributed over the medial (flexing) side of the upper limb.

three hundred and sixty five locations 三百六十五节 [sān bái liù shí wǔ jié] The locations where *qi* and blood of the meridians come and go.

three hundred and sixty-five points 三百六十五穴 [sān bái liù shí wǔ xué] The approximate number of the meridianal points of the whole body. (on the lateral side of the body)

three hundred and sixty-five collateral meridians 三百六十五络 [sān bái liù shí wǔ luò] Three hundred and sixty-five is the approximate number, which was used to call the collaterals and points and explain the connection between the points of the whole body and collateral meridians.

three strategic passes 三关 [sān guān] A collective term for the wind strategic pass, the *qi* strategic pass and the life strategic pass.

three varied punctures 三变刺 [sān biàn cì] The three acupuncture techniques, to cause little bleeding, coming out of *qi* and warming the meridian after acupuncture.

Throat 咽喉 [yān hóu] An ear point located 1/2 above the medial side of the tragus.

thirteen points 十三穴 [shí sān xué] The thirteen empirical points used to treat ma-

nia, etc., in ancient China. It was held that the diseases were caused by the ghost (gui). So, they were named with the ghost. They are Renzhong (GV 26), Shaoshang (LU 11), Fengfu (GV 16), Yinbai (SP 1), Daling (PC 7), Shenmen (BL 62), Jiache (ST 6), Chengjiang (CV 24), Laogong (PC 8), Shangxing (GV 23), Guicang (For the males it refers to Yinxiafeng, for the females it refers to Yumentou), Guicheng, Quchi (LI 11), and Guifeng referring to Shixiazhongfeng.

thumb *cun* 拇指法 [mǔ zhǐ fǎ] One of proportional *cun* in selecting the point. The length between the two ends of the transverse crease of the flexor side of the thumb is taken as 3 cm, often used for locating the points at the four limbs.

Tianding (LI 17) 天鼎 [tiān dǐng] A point of Large Intestine Meridian of Hand-*yangming*. Location: On the lateral side of the neck between Futu (LI 18) and Quepen (ST), at the posterior edge of the sternocleidomastoidous muscle. Regional anatomy: At the posterior edge of the sternocleidomasto-idous muscle, reaching the interspace of the anterior and middle scalene muscle. The external superficial vein of neck is in the shallow. The supraclavicular nerve is distributed. At the place where the cervical cutaneous nerve penetrates at the posterior edge of the sternocleudomastodous muscle. Indications: Sore throat, sudden aphonia, obstructed *qi*, goiter, scrofula. Puncture: 1.5—3 cm perpendicularly. Moxibustion: 3—5 moxa cones or 5—10 minutes with warming moxibustion.

tip of the small elbow 小肘尖 [xiǎo zhǒu jiān] The mediosuperior condyle of humerus.

Tianwen 天温 [tiān wēn] An alternate term for Tianquan (PC 2).

Tianshi 天湿 [tiān shī] The wrong form of Tianwen.

Tianchuang (SI 16) 天窗 [tiān chuāng] A point of Small Intestine Meridian of Hand-

taiyang. Also termed Chuanglong. Location: On the lateral side of the neck, below the corner of the mandible, 1 dm lateral to Adamp's Apple, i. e. , 1. 5 cm posterior to Futu (LI 18). Regional anatomy: Passing through the anterior edge of trapezius muscle and the posterior edge of the levator muscle of scapula. There are the branches of posteroauricular artery and vein and the occipital artery and vein. The cervical cutaneouso nerve, greater auricular nerve and lesser occipital nerve are distributed. Indications: Deafness, tinnitus, sore throat, stiffness and pain of the neck, sudden aphasia, pain in the cheek, cervical goiter, mania, apoplexy. Puncture: 1. 5—3 cm perpendicularly. Moxibustion: 3—5 moxa cones or 5—10 minutes with warming moxibustion.

Tiaokou (ST 38) 条口 [tiáo kǒu] A point of Stomach Meridian of Foot-*Yangming*. Location: 24 cm directly below Dubi (ST 35) at the lateral side of the patellar ligament, approx. in the centre of the anterolateral leg or 6 cm above Shangjuxu(ST 37). Reginal anatomy: In the anterior muscle of tibia. There is the tibial artery and vein. The lateral cutaneous nerve of calf and the branch of the saphennous nerve are distributed. The deep peroneal nerve is in the deeper. Indications: Cold, numbness and pain in the legs, hypogastric pain, swollen dorsal foot, pains in the shoulder and arm, charley horse. Puncture: 3—4. 5 cm perpendicularly. Moxibustion: 3—5 moxa cones or 5—10 minutes with warming moxibustion.

Tianrong (SI 17) 天容 [tiān róng] A point of Gallbladder meridian of Foot-*shaoyang*. Location: At the corner posterior to the nandible, in the depression at the anteror edge of the sternocleidoumastoidous muscle. Regional anatomy: The external cervical vein is in the front, there are the internal cervical artery and vein in the deeper. The anterior branch of the greater auricular nerve, the cervical branch of the facial nerve and the accessory nerve are distribut-

ed. The supracervical ganglion of the sympathetic nerve stem is in the deeper. Indications: Deafness, tinnitus, sore throat, obstruction of throat, swelling and pain in the shoulder. Puncture: 1. 5—3 cm perpendicularly. Moxibustion: 3—5 moxa cones or 5—10 minutes with warming moxibustion.

Tianlong 天笼 [tiān lóng] An alternate term for Tianchuang (SI 16).

Tiangai 天盖 [tiān gài] An alternate term for Quepen (ST 13).

tiankui 天癸 [tiān kuí] 1. A substance to induce sexual maturity and fertinity; 2. Another term of menstruation.

Tianying point 天应穴 [tiān yìng xué] Same with Ashi point.

Tianshu (ST 25) 天枢 [tiān shū] A point of Stomach Meridian of Foot-*yangming*, the anterior-referred point of the large intestine. Also termed Changqi, Gumen, Xuanyuan, Buyuan. Location: 6 cm lateral to Shenque (CV 8) in the umbilicus. Regional anatomy: In the straight muscle of abdomen. There are the branches of the 10th intercostal artery and vein and the branches of the inferior artery and vein of the abdominal wall. The branch of the 10th intercostal nerve is distributed. Indications: Pain in the surrounding umbilicus, abdominal distension, borborygmux, diarrhea, dysentery, edema, constipation, irregular menstruation, leukorrhea, amenorrhea, abdominal pain, abdominal mass, acute/chronic enteritis, bacterial dysentery, appendicitis, intestinal round-worms, obstruction of intestine, intestinal adhesion, intestinal paralysis. Puncture: 3—5 cm perpendicularly. Moxibustion: 5—7 moxa cones or 10—20 minutes with warming moxibustion.

Tianfu (LU 3) 天府 [tiān fǔ] A point of Lung Meridian of Hand-*taiyin*. Location: On the superficial side of the upper arm, 9 cm below the horizontal line at the upper end of the anterior fold of axilla, on the radial side of musculus biceps. Regional anatomy: At the radial aspect of biceps. There are the muscular branches of the cephacious vein and the artery and vein of arm. The lateral cutaneous nerve of arm and muscular cutaneous nerve are distributed. Indications: Pain in the surrounding umbilicus, vomiting, abdominal distension, borborygmus, dysentery, diarrhea, constipation, intestinal carbuncle, dysmenorrhea, irregular menstruation, hernia, edema. Puncture: 1.5—3 cm perpendicularly. Moxibustion: 3—5 moxa cones or 5—10 minutes with warming moxibustion.

Tianjin 天泾 [tiān jìn] An alternate term for Tianquan (PC 2).

Tianzong (SI 11) 天宗 [tiān zōng] A point of Small Intestine Meridian of Hand-*taiyang*. Location: at the depression in the centre of the depression of the lower fossa of the spine of scapula, directly upward opposite to Bingfeng. Regional anatomy: In the infraspinous muscle. There is the muscular branch of circumflex artery and vein of scapula. The suprascapular nerve is distributed. Indications: Pain in the scapular region, pain in the posterior aspect of the elbow and arm, swelling and pain in the cheek, asthmatic breath, breast carbuncle. Puncture: 1.5—3 cm perpendicularly or obliquely. Moxibustion: 3—5 moxa cones or 3—5 minutes with warming moxibustion.

Tianwuhui 天五会 [tiān wǔ huì] An alternate term for Renying (ST 9).

Tianjiu 天臼 [tiān jiú] An alternate term for Tongtian (BL 7).

Tianchong 天冲 [tiān chōng] A point of Gallbladder Meridian of Foot-*shaoyang*. Location: 6 cm in the hairline directly above the posterior edge of the root of ear. Regional anatomy: At the temporal muscle. There are the posteroauricular artery and vein. The branch of the greater occipital nerve is distributed. Indications: Headache, gingivites, epilepsy, fright and palpitation, goiter. Puncture: 1—3 cm horizontally. Moxibustion: 1—3 moxa cones or 3—5 minutes with warming moxibustion.

Tianqu 天衢 [tiān qú] I. e., Tianchong (GB 9).

Tianquan (PC 2) 天泉 [tiān quán] A point of Pericardium Meridian of Hand-*jueyin*. Also termed Tianwen. Location: 6 cm below the horizontal line of the head of the anterior axillary crease, anterrior to the upper arm, between the long head and the short head of biceps muscle of aim. Regional anatomy: Between two heads of biceps muscle of aim. There are the muscular branches of the artery and vein of arm. The medial cutaneous nerve of arm and the muscular cutanous nerve are distributed. Puncture: 1.5—3 cm perpendicularly. Moxibustion: 3—5 moxa cones or 5—10 minutes with warming moxibustion.

Tianjing (TE 10) 天井 [tiān jǐng] A point of Triple Energizer Meridian of Hand-*shaoyang*, the sea-like point (earth) of the meridian. Location: With the elbow flexed, in the depression 3 cm directly above the tip of the elbow (plecranon) in the fossa of olecranon at the lower end of humerus. Regional anatomy: At the tendon sheath. There are the network of artery and vein of the elbow joint. The dorsal cutaneous nerve of arm and the muscular branch of the radial nerve are distributed. Indications: Micraine, pains in the hypochondrium, neck, soulder and arm, deafness, scrofula, mania, epilepsy. Puncture: 1.5—3 cm perpendicularly. Moxibustion: 3—7 moxa cones or 5—15 minutes with warming moxibustion.

Tianyou (TE 16) 天牖 [tiān yǒu] A point of Triple Energizer Meridian of Hand-*shaoyang*. Location: Posteroinferior to the styloid process of the zygomatic bone, at the posterior edge of the sternocleidomastoidous muscle, at the level with the corner of the mandible or between Tianrong (SI 17) and Tianzhu (BL 10). Regional anatomy: At the posterior edge of the sternocleidomastoidous muscle, passing through the splenius muscle of head, reaching the longest muscle. There is the posteroauricular artery. The lesser occipital nerve is distributed. Indications: Headache, dizziness, swelling face, blurred vision, sudden deafness, stiff neck. Puncture: 1. 5— 3 cm perpendicularly. Moxibustion: 1—3 moxa cones or 3—5 minutes with warming moxibustion.

Tianchi 天池 [tiān chí] 1. A point of Pericardium Meridian of Hand-*jueyin*, the confluence of hand-*shaoyang* meridians, also termed Tianhui. Location: 3 cm lateral to the nipple in the 4th intercostal space. Regional anatomy: In the greater muscle of chest and thoracic muscle of chest. There is the vein of the thoracic and abdominal walls and the branches of the external artery and vein of chest. The muscular branch of the anterothoracic nerve and the 4th intercostal nerve are distributed. Indications: Depressed chest, anxiety, cough, profuse sptum, asthmatic breath, thoracalgia, pain below the axilla, scrofula, malaria, breast carbuncle. Puncture: 1—1. 5 cm obliquely with the tip of the needle outward. Moxibustion: 1—3 moxa cones of warming moxibustion; 2. An alternate term for Chengjiang (CV 24).

tian **moxibustion** 天灸 [tiān jiǔ] The technique of painting the point with drugs such as cinnbar, etc.

Tianman 天满 [tiān mǎn] An alternate term for Baihui (GV, DU 20).

Tianxi (SP 18) 天溪 [tiān xī] A point of Spleen Meridian of Foot-*taiyin*. Location: 18 cm lateral to Dazhong (CV, RN 17) on the thoracic midline, in the 4th intercostal space. Regional anatomy: At the serratus anterior muscle. There are the branches of the lateral artery and vein of chest, the artery and vein of the thoracic and abdominal walls, and the latesal cutaneous branch of the 4th intercostal nerve is distributed. Indications: Thoracic pain, cough, breast carbuncle, shortage of lactation. Puncture: 1. 5 cm with moxa cone or 5—10 minutes with warming moxibustion.

Tianliao (TE 15) 天髎 [tiān liáo] A point of Triple Energizer Meridian of Hand-*shaoyang* and Connecting Vessel of Yin. Location: At the upper corner of the scapula, 3 cm directly below Jianjing (GB 21). Regional anatomy: The trapezius muscle and levator muscle of scapula are below. There is the descending branch of the transverse cervical artery. The muscular branch of the superior artery of the scapula is in the deeper. The branches of the accessory nerve and the superior nerve of the scapula are distributed. Indications: Pain in the shoulder and arm, stiffness and pain in the neck, anxiety and fullness in the chest. Puncture: 1. 5—3 cm perpendicularly. Moxibustion: 3—7 moxa cones or 5—15 minutes with warming moxibustion.

Tinghe 听呵 [tīng hē] An alternate term for Tinghui (GB 2)

tinnitus and deafness 耳鸣耳聋 [ěr míng ěr lóng] The symptoms of abnormal hearing. The former refers to the patient's feeling of his or her ears while deafness refers to decreas or disappearing of hearing ability. The former is often the sign of the latter.

tiao cao zi 挑草子 [tiāo cǎo zǐ] I. e., pricking treatment.

Tinggong (SI 19) 听宫 [tīng gōng] A point of Small Intestine Meridian of Hand-*taiyang*. The confluence of hand-*shaoyang*, foot-*shaoyang*, and hand-*taiyang* meridians. Also termed Duosuowen. Location: Anterior to the tragus at the posterior edge of the condylar process of the mandible, in the depression when the mouth is open. Regional anatomy: There is the anteroauriuclar branch of the superial temporal artery and vein. The branch of the facial nerve and the aurciucular temporal nerve are distributed. Indications: Tinnitus, deafness, toothache, mania, aphonia, deaf-mutism, otitis media, epilepsy, inflammation of the external auditory meatus, aural vertgio, facial paralysis, inflammation of the mandibular joint. Puncture: 2. 5—4. 5 cm perpendic-

ularly with the mouth open. Moxibustion:
1—3 moxa cones or 5—10 minutes with
warming moxibustion.

Tiantu (CV 22) 天突 [tiān tū] A point of CV,
the confluentce of Connecting Vessel of
Yin and CV, also termed Yuhu, Tianqi. Location: In the centre of the deepression at
the superior edge of the sternal notch. Regional anatomy: At the left and right sides
of the deeper venous arc and the artery
branch of the inferior thyroid gland. The
anterior branch of the supraclavicular nerve
is distributed. Indications: Deafness, tinnitus, sore throat, obstruction of throat,
swelling in the cheek, goiter, swelling in the
head and neck, vomiting. Puncture: 1.5—
3 cm perpendicularly. Moxibustion: 3—5
moxa cones or 5—10 minutes with warming moxibustion. (Fig 135)

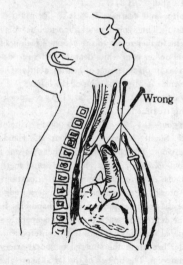

Fig 135

Tiancong 天聪 [tiān cōng] An extra point, located on the midline of head, in the hairline
of 1/2 of the distance from the tip of nose
to the hair line. Puncture: 1.5 cm horizontally. Moxibustion: 1—3 moxa cones or 3—
5 minutes with warming moxibustion.

Tianqu 天瞿 [tiān qú] An alternate term for
Tiantu (CV 22).

Tianqupang point 天瞿旁穴 [tiān qú páng
xué] Tianqi is another name of Tianding
(LI 11). Administer moxibustion on Tiantu
(CV 22) with a large moxa cone, the base
diameter of which is 1 cm.

tibia 胫 [jíng] The big bone of the leg.

Tingtou 亭头 [tíng tóu] An extra point, located 13.5 cm directly below one transverse
crease lateral to the centre of umbilicus. Indication: Prolapse of uterus. Puncture:
1.5—3 cm perpendicularly.

Tinghui (GB 27) 听会 [tīng huì] A point of
Gallbladder Meridian of Foot-*shaoyang*, also termed Tinghe, Houguan, Ermen. Location: In the depression anterior to the inte-
ragic incisure and posterior to the condylar
process of the mandible. Regional anatomy:
There is the anteroauricular branch of the
superficial temporal artery. The greater auricular nerve and the facial nerve are distributed. Indications: Tinnitus, deafness,
headache, toothache, deviated mouth and
eye, dislocation of the mandibular pain in
the face. Punctuer: 1—1.5 cm perpendicularly, with the mouth open. Moxibustion:
3—5 minutes with waming moxibustion.

Tongli (HT 5) 通里 [tōng lǐ] A point of Heart
Meridian of Hand-*shaoyin*, the connecting
point of the meridian. Location: At the palmar side of the forearm. At the radial edge
of the ulnar flexor muscle of wrist, 3 cm
above the transverse crease of wrist.
Regional anatomy: Between the ulnar flexor
muscle of wrist and the digital superficial
muscle of finger, the ulnar artery passes
through it. The medial cutaneous nerve of
forearm is distributed. The ulnar nerve is in
the deeper. Indications: Sudden aphonia,
stiff tongue, palpitation with fright,
headache, vertigo, profuse mense, metrorrhagia, pains in the medial aspects of the
shoulder, ellbow and arm. Puncture: 1.5—
2.5 perpendicularly. Moxibustion: 1—4
moxa cones or 3—5 minutes with warming

moxibustion.

Tonggu 通谷 [tōng gǔ] The meridian points. One pertains to Kidney Meridian at the abdomen, the other pertains to Bladder Meridian at foot. For the convenience of differentiation, the former one is termed Futongu (KI 20) and the latter, Zutongu (BL 66).

Tongjian 通间 [tōng jiān] An alternate term for Sanyangluo (TE 8).

Tongguan 通关 [tōng guān] An alternate term for Yindu (KI 19).

Tongmen 通门 [tōng mén] A wrong form of Tongjian, an alternate term for Sanyangluo (TE, SJ 8).

Tongtian (BL 7) 通天 [tōng tiān] A point of Bladder Meridian of Foot-*taiyang*, also termed Tianjiu, Location: 12 cm into the frontal hairline at the midline of head, and 4.5 cm lateral to or 4.5 cm posterior to Chengguang (BL 6). Regional anatomy: At galea aponeurotica. There is the superficial temporal artery and vein and the anastomotic network of the occipital artery and vein. The branch of the greater occipital nerve is distributed. Indications: Headache, heaviness of the head, vertigo, deviated mouth, stuffy nose with thin nasal discharge, expistaxis, nasal sore, rhinitis, nasal obstruction, difficulty in moving the neck, goiter. Punctured: 1—1.5 cm horizontally. Moxibustion: 1—3 moxa cones or 3—5 minutes with warming moxibustion.

Tongli 通理 [tōng lǐ] An extra point "Tongli is located 6 cm above the small toe." It is used for treating metrorrhagia and profuse mense. Puncture: 0.6 cm. Moxibustion: 2—7 moxa cones. (Collection of Acupuncture) According to Illustrations of Extra Points, it is located at the dorsal foot, 1.5 cm anterior to the posterior end of the interspace between the 4th and 5th metatarsal bones.

Tangziliao 瞳子髎 [tóng zǐ liáo] A point of Bladder Meridian of Foot-*shaoyang*, the confluence of hand-*taiyang*, and hand-*shaoyang* meridians, also termed Zhiqu, Taiyang, Qianguan, Yuwei. Location: 1.5 cm lateral to the outer canthus, in the depression at the lateral edge of the orbital bone. Regional anatomy: Passing through the orbicular muscle of eye, reaching at the termporal muscle. There is the temporal artery and vein. The zygomatic and facial nerve and the temporal branch of the facial nerves are distributed. Indications: Headache, ocular pain, congestive eyes, photophobia, lacrimation, blurred vision, cataract, nebula. Puncture: 0.9—1.5 cm horizontally. Moxibustion: 3—5 minutes with warming moxibustion.

Tongue 舌 [shé] An ear point located slightly above the area between upper Palate and Lower Palate.

toad-interposing moxibustion 隔蟾灸 [gé chán jiǔ] A kind of moxibustion. The skin of a toad is used as the interposing thing for moxibustion.

Toe 趾 [zhǐ] An ear point slightly lateral to the end of the upper foot of the antihelix.

Tongxuan 童玄 [tóng xuán] An alternate term for Lieque (LU 7).

Tonsil₁ 扁桃体₁ [biǎn táo tǐ] An ear point lateral to the tip of ear, vertical to Tonsil at Lobre Zone₈.

Tonsil₂ 扁桃体₂ [biǎn táo tǐ] An ear point lateral to the helix between Tonsil on the lobre and Tonsil.

tonifying the deficient essence with nourishment 精不足者补之于味 [jīng bù zú zhě bǔ zhī yú wèi] The patients with insufficient yin essence should be treated with animal or plant food or drugs rich in nutrients. (yin tonic, blood tonic, etc.)

toad 虾蟆 [há má] A kind of interposing thing used for indirect moxibustion. Used as toad-interposing moxibustion. Use a living toad, get rid of its internal organs and miscelaneous things, then put its skin on cover on scrofula, and put a moxa cone on it for moxibustion 7—14 moxa cones, and then put a moxa cone on it for moxibustion through the interior of the body. It is used for treating scrofula.

toad's muscle 蛤蟆肉[hā mā ròu]Referring to biceps muscle of arm.

toothache 牙痛[yá tòng]A common symptom in the mouth trouble, which aggravates whenever the teeth encounter cold, heat, sour, and sweet stimulation.

tooth meridian 齿脉[chǐ mài] A name of meridian during early period, similar to hang-*yangming* meridian.

tongue, the windwo of the heart 心开窍于舌 [xīn kāi qiào yú shé] Some of the physiopathologic states of the heart may be manifested as changes of the tongue.

Toothache point 牙痛点[yá tòng diǎn]An ear point at the medial side of Brain Stem, apposite to Throat-Tooth.

total palpation 总按 [zǒng àn] To feel the pulse with the index, middle and ring fingers simultaneously at *cun*, *guan* and *chi* sections.

Toufeng 头风[tóu fēng] An extra point located on the lateral side of the thigh. Stand erect with the hand touching the thigh inferior to the midpoint of the edge of the web between the thumb and index finger. Puncture: 3—4 cm perpendicularly. Moxibustion: 3—7 moxa cones or 5—15 minutes with warming moxibustion.

Touchong 头冲[tóu chōng]An extra point located on the radial side of the biceps muscle of arm of the upper arm. Extend the hand forward,deviate the head to touch the arm. The point is where the tip of the nose touches.

Toujiao 头角[tóu jiǎo] Referring to the node of the parietal bone.

touching manipulation 揣法[chuǎi fǎ]An accessary acupuncture manipulation,referring to touching the point. Before acupuncture, the doctor first uses his or her fingers to touch the patient's body to explore the point, then inserts the needle.

thumb-tag needle 撅针 [qīn zhēn] A kind of cutantous needle.

Toufeng 头缝 [tóu fēng] A wrong form of Touwei (SI 8).

Toulinqi(GB 15) 头临泣 [tóu lín qì] A point of Gallbladder Meridian of Foot-*shaoyang*, the confluence of foot-*taiyang* meridian, foot-*shaoyang* meridian and Connecting Vessel of Yang. Location: With the eye look forward, directly above the pupil, 1.5 cm in the hairline, i. e., at the midpoint of the line connecting Shenting (GV 24) and Touqei (ST 8). Regional anatomy: In the frontal muscle. There is the frontal artery and vein. The anastomotic branch at the medial and lateral aspects of the frontal nerve is distributed. Indications:Headache, vertigo, congestive and painful eyes, lacrimation, nebula, stuffy nose, deafness, infantile convulsion, febrile diseases. Puncture: 1—2 cm horizontally. Moxibustion: 1—3 moxa cones or 3—5 minutes with warming moxibustion.

Touqiaoyin(GB 11) 头窍阴 [tóu qiào yīn] A point of Gallbladder Meridian of foot-*shaoyang*, the confluence of foot-*taiyang* meridian and foot-*shaoyang* meridian, also termed Zhengu. Location: At the crossing point of the lower 1/3 and middle 1/3 of the arc line connecting Tianchong (GB 9) anterior-superior to the mastoid process of the temporal bone and Wangu (GB 12), posteroinferior to the mastoid process. Regional anatomy: There is the branch of the posterial ear artery and vein. The greater occipital nerve and the lesser occipital nerve are distributed. Indications:Headache,vertigo, tinnitrs, stiffness deafness, and pain in the neck, thoracic and hypochondriac pain, bitter mouth, auricular pain. Puncture: 1—2 cm horizontally. Moxibustion: 1—3 moxa cones or 3—5 minutes with warming moxibustion.

towel needle 巾针 [jīn zhēn] A needling instrument in ancient times. It is therefore called because it is small, and is used to fix the towel.

Touwei(ST 8) 头维[tóu wéi]A point of Stomach Meridian of Foot-*yangming*, the confluence of foot-*shaoyang* and foot-*yangming* meridians. Location: Superiolateral to the temporal depression of the anterior hairline, 1.5 cm in the hairline or 13 cm larteral to Shenting (GV 24), 1.5 cm in the hairline of the midline of the head. Regional anatomy : At the temproral musle. There is the temporal branch of the superficial temporal artery and vein. The branch of the auriculotemporal nerve and the temporal branch of the facial nerve are distributed. Indications: Auricular pain, headache, vertigo, lacrimation, blurred vision, tremor of eyes. Puncture: 1—2 cm horizontally.

transverse bone above the shoulder 肩上横骨 [jiān shàng héng gǔ]Referring to the spine of scapula.

treatment before being sick 治未病 [zhì wèi bìng] The prevention and early treatment of disease.

treatment of emptying viscera diseases by the joining points 合治内府[hé zhì nèi fǔ]One of the principles of point selection. It implies that the joining points of six emptying viscera on the three yang meridians of foot are for emptying viscera diseases. This is because the branch of the three yang meridians of foot enters into the six emptying viscera from here. The joining points of six emptying viscera for stomach trouble, select Zusanli (ST 36); For small intestine trouble select Shangjuxu (ST 37); For small intestine trouble select Xiajuxu (ST39); For triple energizer trouble select Weiyang (BL 39); For bladder trouble select Weizhong (BL40); For gallbladder trouble select Yanglingquan (GB 34).

trigger puncture 报刺 [bào cì] One of the twelve needling techniques used for treating wandering pains puncture it directly and retain the needle until another painful area is pressed. Then withdraw the needle and puncture the second painful area.

triple energizer meridian of hand-*shaoyang* 三焦手少阳之脉 [sān jiāo shǒu shào yáng zhī mài] The original name of Triple Energizer Meridian of Hand-*shaoyang*.

true cold and false heat 真寒假热 [zhēn hán jiǎ rè]It denotes that the disease itself is of cold nature but exihibits some apparently heat symptoms and signs.

true heat and false cold 真热假寒 [zhēng rè jiǎ hán] It denotes that the disease itself is of heat nature but exhibits some apparently cold symptoms and signs.

true excess and false deficiency 真实假虚 [zhēng shí jiǎ xū] It denotes that the disease itself is an excess syndrome but exhibits some apparently deficiency symptoms and signs.

true deficiency and false excess 真虚假实 [zhēng xū jiǎ shí] It denotes that the diseases is deficiency syndrome but exhibits some apparently excess symptoms and signs.

tingkong 廷孔 [tíng kǒng] Referring to the vaginal orifice.

transmitory palpation 初持[chū chí]The time of feeling the pulse is relatively short for about one minute.

triangular needle 三棱针 [sān léng zhēn] An acupuncture instrument from the sharp needle in ancient China. Made with stainless steel in modern times, its shaft appears as a cone and its body appears as a traingular knife. Clinically used to break the superficial vein to cause little bleeding for treating diseases. Usually used for febrile diseases, inflammation, sunstroke, coma. Be cautious when it is used for the patient weak in constitution, the patient with anemia, the patient with hypotension, and pregnant women. It is not advisable to use it for the patient tending to bleeding, the patient with vascular tumor and the patient with hemophilia. (Fig 136)

triple puncture 齐刺[qí cì]One of the twelve needling techniques for treating a relatively snall and deep area caused by cold blockage. (obstruction of pathogenic cold to the body) It is to puncture the centre of the

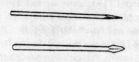

Fig 136

area one needle on both sides with two needles.

Triple Energizer Meridian of Hand-*shaoyang* (**TE**) 手少阳三焦经 [shǒu shào yáng sān jiāo jīng] One of the twelve meridians. The course: Starting from the end of the ring finger, ascending and emerging between the small finger and ring finger, running along the dorsal hand and emerging between the ulnar and radius of the extending side of the forearm, asending and passing through the tip of elbow, running along the lateral side of the upper arm, ascending to the shoulder, crossing and emerging from the posterior foot-*shaoyang* meridian, and emerging into the supraclavicular fossa, distributing over the diaphragm (Danzhong), connecting with the pericardium, passing through the diaphragm, and finally distributing over the uppper, middle and lower energizers. One branch ascends from the diaphragm, emerges from the supraclavicular fossa, ascends to the lateral neck, connects with the posterior ear, directly ascends and emerges from the upper corner of the ear, turns back and descends to the cheek, and finally reaches at the posterior eye. The other branch enters into the ear from the posterior ear, emerges from the anterior ear, passes through the anterior Shangguan (GB 35), crosses the cheek and reaches at the outer canthus. (connects with Gallbladder Meridian of Foot-*shaoyang*).

Jrapus point 耳屏点 [ěr bìng diǎn] An ear point located at the spot where the supratragic notch and the opening of the external antrum auris cross.

transverse head bone 头横骨 [tóu héng gǔ] Referring to the coccipital bone.

Trachea 气管 [qì guǎn] An ear point at the area where the opening of external antrum auris is at the level with Heart.

transverse crease 横纹 [héng wén] Referring to the wrinkle of shin, as the reason for locating the point. E. g. Chize (LU 5) is located above the transverse crease of elbow.

transverse puncture 横刺 [héng cì] See horizontal puncture.

transverse finger *cun* 横指寸 [héng zhǐ cùn] One of the proportional *cun* for selecting the point. The transverse diameter is taken as the standard of the measurement in selection of the point. Usually one thumb (referring to the transverse crease of the thumb) is taken as 3 cm, two tansverse fingers (the tranverse creases of the middle sections of the index and middle fingers) is taken as 4.5 cm, the four transverse fingers (the 2nd, 3rd, 4th and 5th) are taken as 9 cm. (I. e., four-finger widths measurement)

yuewen 约纹 [yuē wén] I. e., the transverse crease. Referring to the transverse crease at the articular portion.

transversely connecting collateral 横络之脉 [héng luò zhī mài] The branch meridian at the posterolateral side of the thigh of foot-*taiyang* meridian. It transversely passes through Huantiao (GB 30) and runs over Fuxi (BL 38) and Weiyang (BL 39), and meets at Weizhong (BL 40)

transmitting of the essence by six emptying viscera to the five storing viscera 腑俞精于脏 [fǔ shū jīng yú zàng] The stomach and small intestine of the six emptying viscera can transmit the essence from water and grain, after digestion and absorption, to the five storing viscera for storage.

transportation of nutritional fluids by the spleen for the stomach 脾为胃行其津液 [pí wéi wèi xíng qí jīn yè] After receiving the food the stomach must depend on the spleen to transport nutrient fluids to various parts of the body.

Treatment of Science of Chinese Acupuncture 中国针灸治疗学 [zhōng guó zhēn jiǔ zhì liáo xué] Compiled by Cheng Anru, containing general introductions, pills and powders were selected and recorded besides acupuncture treatment for auxiliary treatment, appended with the internal chapter and external chapter as the reference book for selecting the points according to different classifications. Later Sun Yanru supplemented therapeutic experiences to it as the "revised and enlarged edition", and published in 1931.

treating atrophy by only selecting the points on yangming meridians 治痿独取阳明 [zhì wěi dú qǔ yáng míng] The principle of selecting the point for treating atrophy in Internal Classic.

treatment directed at the disease 正治 [zhèng zhì] The method and drugs opposite to the nature of the disease are used for treatment. For instance, the cold symptoms are treated with drugs of hot nature, the heat ones with drugs of cold nature, the deficiency disease with tonification, and the excess ones with elimination.

Triple Energizer 三焦 [sān jiāo] An ear point among Medial Nose, Endocrine and Lung.

Treatise on External Medicine 串雅外篇 [chuàn yǎ wài piān] A book compiled by Zhao Xueming. Treatise on Medicine contains the Treatise on Internal Medicine of Treatise on External Medicine. (four volumes each) in which varieties of healing methods and remedies collected from folk healers were recorded. Treatise on External Medicine records empirical prescriptions, acupuncture-moxibustion, fumugating, washing and applying methods. Simple and convenient, it preserves quite a few experiences of folk medicine, phatmacology and acupuncture-moxibustion. It was completed in 1759.

triple energizer 三焦 [sān jiāo] One of the six emptying viscera, divided into the upper, middle and lower energizers. It acts as a water pathway, Triple Enerigizer Meridian of Hand-*shaoyang* pertains to the triple energizer while Pericardium Meridian of Hand-*jueyin* connects with it. Its back-*shu* point is Sanjiaoshu (BL 22), its anterior-referred point is Shimen (CV 5), and its lower-joining point is Weiyang (BL 39). Following viewpoints have recently been advanced. It refers to: 1. The body cavity (including the chest cavity, abdominal cavity and pelvic cavity); 2. The lymphatic system; 3. The omentum; 4. A name with nonexistent structure. At present, the concensus leans toward considering it the functional sections of the body cavity but not the actual organs. In general, the segment above the diaphragm, including the heart and lungs belongs to the upper energizer, that between the diaphragm and umbilicus, including the liver, stomach and spleen, belongs to the middle energizer, and that below the umbilicus including the kidneys, bladder and small and large intestines, belongs to the lower energizer.

Tuanggang 团冈 [tuán gǎng] An extra point. "When the abdominal heat is not blocked, difficult defecation and micturition occur, and lumbago involes the chest. Do moxibustion at Tuanggang 10 moxa cones. It is located at 6 cm below and 9 cm lateral to Xiaochangshu (BL 27). Moxibustion: 3—7 moxa cones or warming moxibustion."

Tunzhong 臀中 [tún zhōng] An extra point located at the hip. To take the line connecting the greater trochanter of femur and the node of sciatic as the base line and form a equilateral triangle. Its top point is the point. Indications: Sciatica, paralysis of lower limbs, urticaria. Puncture: 4.5—7.5 cm perpendicularly. Moxibustion: 3—7 moxa cones or 5—15 minutes with warming moxibustion.

Tuoji 佗脊 [tuó jí] Referring Huantuo's paravertebral points.

turbid *qi* 浊气 [zhuó qì] 1. The concentrated and turbid part of the refined materials of grain and water; 2. Air exhaled from the lungs and flatus from anus.

tuoju 脱疽［tuō jǔ］Gangrene of the fingers or toes with excruciating pain at first, and after rather a long time necrosis and sloughing off the skin, subcutaneous tissues, muscles and bones, resembling thronboamgiitis obliteration.

tuberculosis point 结核点［jié hé diǎn］An ear point in the centre of Lung Zone.

twelve manipulations 十二手法［shí èr shǒu fǎ］Including fingernail press (*zao qie*), finger holding (*zhi chi*), warming with mouth (*kou wen*), needle insertion (*jin zhen*), finger palpation (*zhi xun*), fingernail pinching (*zao nie*), needle withdrawal (*zhen tui*), finger kneading (*zhi chuo*), finger twirling (*zhi lian*), finger retention (*zhi liu*), needle shaking (*zhi yao*) and finger pulling (*zhi ba*).

twenty-eight pulses 二十八脉［èr shí bā mài］A collective term for 28 varieties of the commonly-seen pulses.

twelve meridians 十二经脉［shí èr jīng mài］The major part of the meridians. Each meridian internally pertains to a certain viscus (that pertaining to the emptying viscus connects with the emptying one and that pertains to the emptying one connects with the storing one externally), and is distributed over the four limbs, trunk, head and face. They are divided into the three yin and three yang meridians of hand and foot, namely, 1. Lung meridian of Hand-*taiyin*；2. Large Intestine Meridian of Hand-*yangming*；3. Stomach Meridian of Hand-*yangming*；4. Spleen Meridian of Foot-*taiyin*；5. Heart Meridian of Hand-*shaoyin*, 6. Small Intestine Meridian of Hand-*taiyang*；7. Bladder Meridian of Foot-*taiyang*；8. Kidney Meridian of Foot-*shaoyin*；9. Pericardium Meridian of Hand-*jueyin*；10. Triple Energizer Meridian of Hand-*shaoyang*；11. Gallbladder Meridian of Foot-*shaoyang*；12. Liver Meridian of Foot-*jueyin*. Their sources are connective.

twelve myotendinous meridians 十二经筋［shí èr jīng jīn］A collective term for the my-

ofascial system which is distributed along the courses of the twelve meridians. Their distribution is almost the same with that of the twelve meridians. They are divided into the three yang ones of hand and foot and three yin ones of hand and foot, start from the four limbs and end at the joints. The yang one is distributed over the body surface while the yin enters into the chest and abdomen, but does not enter into the viscera. They symptoms are mainly contraction, blockage and pain, flaccidity and spasm, etc.

twelve wells of hand 手十二井［shǒu shí èr jīng］The well-like points of the six meridians of hand.

twenty-first vertebra 第二十一椎［dì èr shí yī zhuī］Referring to the 4th sacral vertebra.

twenty-second vertebra 第二十二椎［dì èr shí èr zhuī］Referring to the 5th sacral vertebra.

Twelve branch meridians 十二经别［shí èr jīng bié］The major branches of the twelve meridians, circulating through the deeper part of the body, communicated with the head, chest and abdomen. They form six pairs, called the six correspondenses, the foot-*taiyin*, foot-*shaoyang* and foot-*jueyin* are the 1st, the foot-*shaoyang* and foot-*jueyin* are the 2nd, the food-*yangming* and foot-*taiyin* are the 3rd, the hand-*taiyang* and the hand-*shaoyin* are the 4th, the hand-*shaoyang* and the hand-*jueyin* are the 5th, the hand-*yangming* and the hand-*taiyin* are the 6th. They enlarge the scale of the course of the twelve meridians, forming the branching, joining and emerging relationship of the meridians. It stresses the explanation that the yin meridians join the yang ones and are upwardly communicated with the heart and head.

twelve trends 十二从［shí èr cóng］Referring to the sequence of the trend of the twelve meridians.

twelve cutaneous regions 十二皮部［shí èr pí bù］The surface of the whole body is divided into twelve regions according to the meridians. Refer cutaneous regions.

twelve needlings 十二刺 [shí èr cì] Also called *shier jieci*. They are anteroposteriorly coupled puncture, trigger puncture, lateral puncture, triple puncture, quintuple puncture, perpendicular puncture, *shu* puncture, short puncture, superficial puncture, yin puncture, side puncture and repeated shallow puncture.

two yang 二阳 [èr yáng] Referring to *yangming* meridians.

two yin 二阴 [èr yīn] 1. Referring to *shaoyin* meridians; 2. Referring to external genitalia (anterior yin) and anus (posterior yin).

twelve source points 十二原穴 [shí èr yuán xué] It is collectively called the twelve source points that the five viscera have the two source points pulse those of *gao* and *huang*, i. e., the source point of the lung—Taiyuan (LU 9), that of heart—Daling (PC 7), that of the spleen—Taibai (SP 3), that of liver—Boyang (Qihai) (CV 6).

Twelve Meridians	Source Points
Lung	Taiyuan (LU 9)
Large Intestine	Hegu (LI 4)
Stomach	Chongyang (ST 42)
Spleen	Taibai (SP 3)
Heart	Shenmen (HT 7)
Small Intestine	Wangu (GB 12)
Bladder	Jinggu (BL 64)
Kidney	Taixi (KI 3)
Pericardium	Daling (PC 7)
Triple Energizer	Yangchi (TE 4)
Gallbladder	Qiuxu (GB 40)
Liver	Taichong (LR 3)

twelve prohibitions 十二禁 [shí èr jìn] Some prohibitions before/after acupuncture. It is not advisable to puncture in the condition of disordered pulse and *qi* caused by different reasons. "Don't puncture before/after sexual activity. Don't puncture before/after drinking. Don't puncture before/after labore. Don't puncture before/after the stomach is full. Don't puncture before/after being thirst. Puncture after the patient who is astonished or in great terror has a rest so that his or her *qi* remains normal. Puncture after the patient who comes to see the doctor on foot has a rest by sitting a while. "

(Miraculous Pivot)

twelve wells of foot meridians 足十二井 [zú shí èr jǐng] Referring to the well-like points of six meridians of foot.

twelve wells 十二井 [shí èr jǐng] A general term for the well-like points of the twelve meridians. Each is located at the end of the four limbs, i. e., Shaoshang (LU 11) (lung), Zhongchong (PC9) (pericardium), Shaoshang (HT 9) (heart), Shangyang (LI 1) (large intestine), Guanchong (HT 9) (heart), Shangyang (LI 1), (large intestine), Guanchong (TE 1) (triple nergizer), Shaoze (SI 1) (small intestine), Yinbai

(SP 1)(spleen), Dadun(LR 1)(liver), Yongquan(KI 1)(kidneys), Lidui(ST 45) (stomach), Qiaoyin (gallbladder), zhiyin (BL 67)(bladder). Clinically they are used to treat high fever, mental convulsion, etc. Puncture: Superficially without needle retention or prick to cause little bleeding. (Fig 137)

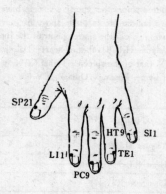 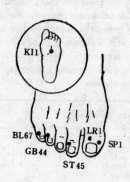

Fig 137

twenty-seven *qi* 二十七气 [èr shí qī qì] A general term for *qi* of the twenty-seven meridians and fifteen collateral meridians.

twirling technique 捻转法 [niǎn zhuǎn fǎ] Also called '*nian*' or '*zhuang*'. Pinch the handle of the needle with the thumb, index finger and middle finger and rotate it forward and backward.

two yin 二阴 [èr yīn] A collective term for the anterior yin (external genitalia) and the posterior yin (anus).

tympanic pulse 革脉 [gé mài] The pulse that is extremely taut but hollow, giving a feeling of the head of a drum. It is often seen in a post-hemorrhagic state or after spermatorrhea.

U

ultraviolet-ray point-radiated method 紫外线
穴位照射法 [zǐ wài xiàn xué wèi zhào shè
fǎ] To treat disease by using the ultraviolet
ray to radiate the point. For the adult, it be-
gins to 2 biological doses to gradually add
to 5—6 while for the aged and weak patients, it may be properly reduced, for the
infants the average biological dose of the
lamp is adopted. It can be used for treating
asthma, chronic bronchitis, influenza,
epistalsis, etc. But it is prohibited in the
cases of hemophilia, dysfunction of liver
and kidney, skin diseases that are hypersen-
snsitive to the utraviolet ray.

ulna-radius 臂骨 [bì gǔ] Referring to ulna and
adius.

umbilicus-sealed moxa 封脐艾 [fēng qí ài] A
kind of moxibustion technique. It can be
used for treating coldness and pain in the
umbilical abdomen, diarrhea of the senile
person, weak person, woman and child.

umbilicus-fumigated method 炼脐法 [liàn qí
fǎ] A kind of indirect moxibustion. It was
thought that moxibustion on the umbilicus
according to certain method can play a role
in promoting health preservation. The formula: musk 25 g.

umbilicus-warmed method 温脐法 [wēn qí
fǎ] A kind of indirect moxibustion. The
drugs of trogopferus dung, dahurian angelica root, dar-green salt 10 g each, musk 0. 5
g (ground into powder) are mixed with
'buckwheat powder and water and formed
as a circle that is put on the umbilicus.
Then the previous drug is put in it and finally do moxibustion on it.

umbilicus-fumigated moxibustion 熏脐法 [xūn
qí fǎ] To administer indirect moxibustion at
the umbilicus.

Universal Benevolent Prescriptions 普济方
[pǔ jì fāng] A medical book chiefly compiled by Zhu. Di. The original contains 168
volumes. It is extremely rich in medical ref-

erence data and is the highest formulary
book that have been preserved in China. Of
them 25 volumes deal with acupuncture,
Mingtang Moxibustion Classic, Bronze Figure Classic Acupuncture Classic,
Acupuncture Classic of Midnight-noon
Ebb-flow, Experiences of Acupuncture
were recorded. What's more the works
written by Dou Hanqin and others were
recorded. It was completed in 1406.

**unobstructing meridians and connecting with
qi** 通经接气 [tōng jīng jiē qì] 1. Referring
to respiratory times of puncturing various
meridians; 2. Some manipulations to promote flow of *qi* in meridians.

unusual internal organs 奇恒之府 [qí héng
zhī fǔ] A collective term for brain, spinal
cord, bone, blood vessels, gallbladder, and
uterus. It is because they differ from not
only the fine storing viscera but the six
emptying viscera as well as to the unusual
internal organs because the bile stored in it
is clear and not turbid. Differing from the
turbid contents of the stomach, the intestine and the bladder.

unit of bone 骨度 [gǔ dù] In ancient China the
lengths and widths of various portions of
the body were measured by mainly taking
the bone segments as the main landmarks
and by basing on this the location of the
meridian is ascertained. The lengths recorded in Miraculous Pivot has been adhered in
later point-location in acupuncture and was
applied as the proportional *cun* of various
portions of the body, i. e., within a certain
portion they are converted as the same
length no matter the body is tall or short,
fat or thin. For convenience of locating the
point, the length of a few portions were
corrected in latter generations. As for the
unit of bone commonly used at present are
seen from the following table. (Fig 138)

Upper abdomen 上腹 [shàng fù] An ear point

Division	Starting and finishing points	Number of cm	Notes
Head & Face	Anterior hair to posterior hairline	36	Used for locating the points between the aterior and posterior hairlines
	The length between the mastoid process of the two temporal bones	27	The transverse length between the two Wangu equals to that between two Touwei
	From the anterior hairline line to *yi* (laterosuperior to chin, lateroinferior to the angle of the mouth)	30	
Neck & Nape	From the posterior hairline to Dazhui (GV 14)	7.5	In locating the point, it is changed into 9 cm.
	From Adam's Apple to the superior notch of stern	12	
Chest, abdomen and Hypo-chondrium	From the superior notch of stern to Qigu (the point where two bones branch off)	27	Refer the location in the intercostal space in the way of selecting the point
	From Qigu to the interior umbilicus	24	Used for locating the point at the upper abdomen
	From the inferior Tiansh (ST 25) to Henggu (KI 11)	19.5	It is changed into 24 cm in selecting the point, used for the transverse measurement of the chest and abdomen
	Between the two nipples (transverse length)	28.5	It is changed into 24 cm in selecting the point, used for the transverse measurement of the chest and abdomen
	From axilla to the hypochondrium	36	
	From the 11th rib to the superior great trochanter	18	
Upper Limbs	From Dazhui (GV 14) to the tip of elbow	51	It is taken as 24 cm from Dazhui (GV 14) to the shoulder joint and 27 cm from the the shoulder to the tipe of elbow
	From elbow to wrist	37.5	It is changed into 36 cm in selecting the point
	From wrist to the metacarpophalangeal joint	12	
	From the metacarpophalangeal joint to the end of the middle finger.	13.5	
Lower Limbs	From the superior edge of pubis to the superomedial condyle of femur	54	Used for locating the point at foot meridian of yin
	From the superomedial condyle of femur to that of tibia	10.5	
	From the inferior edge of Neifu to the medial ankle	39	
	From the inferior ankle to the ground	19	
	From the great tranchter to Xiyan	57	Used for locating the point at foot meridian of yang
	From the knee to the lateral ankle		
	From the central cubital fossa to the superior edge of Achilles	48	

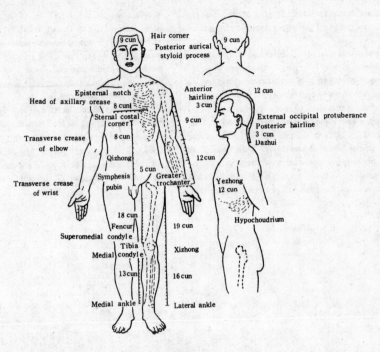

Fig 138

below the medial edge of the external antrum auris.

Upper back 上背 [shàng bèi] An ear point near the upper edge of the protruding auricular concha of the back of the ear.

Urethra 尿道 [niào dào] An ear point at the helix at the level with Bladder.

Urethra duct 输尿管 [shū niào guǎn] An ear point between Bladder and Kidney.

uroschesis 癃闭 [lóng bì] The symptom complex with the chief manifestations of difficulty of urination, distension and fullness of the lower hypochogastrium, even anuria.

urinary bladder 膀胱 [páng guāng]One of the six emptying viscera. Its action is to store urine. Discharge of urine depends on the function of the bladder *qi*. Bladder Meridian of Foot-*taiyang* pertains to the bladder and the foot-*shaoyin* meridian connects with the

bladder. Back *shu* point is Pangguangshu (BL 28), the anterior referred point is Zhongji (CV 3), and the connecting point is Weizhong (BL 40).

Urticarrhea point 寻麻疹点 [xún má zhěn diǎn] An ear point located between Finger and Wrist.

utrerus 女子胞 [nǚ zǐ bāo] It involves the functions of the entire genital system (including uterus, ovary and oviduct).

uterus 子宫 [zǐ gōng] 1. Name of the internal organ, also termed *zichu*, baogong; 2. Referring to Zigong (EX-CA 1). 3. Uterus, an ear point at the most hollow part of the deltoid fossa.

uterine collateral meridian 胞脉 [bāo mài] The meridian connecting the uterus. Chiefly referring to Vital Vessel.

upper bo 上膊 [shàng bó] The arm.

upper-lower eyelids 目纲 [mù gāng] Respectively termed the upper eyelid and the lower eyelid.

upper arm 臑 [nào] Referring to the upperarm, mainly referring to the biceps muscle.

upper eyelid 目上纲 [mù shàng gāng] Also termed *mu shang wang*, pertaining to myofascial meridian of foot-*taiyang*.

upper-lower points-combined method 上下配 穴法 [shàng xià pèi xué fǎ] One of the points-combined methods. Referring to the cooperative application of the points of the upper and lower limbs. E. g. , for stomach trouble, Neiguan (PC 6) of the upper limb is selected and Zusanli (ST 36) of the lower limb selected; For throat trouble, Hegu (LI 4) of the upper limb is selected and Neiting (ST 44) of the lower selected. The method of combining eight points of eight meridians recorded in ancient literatures belongs to this category.

upward flaming of cardiac fire 心火上炎 [xīn huǒ shàng yán] The febrile symptoms of the heart, reflected in the upper part of the body. The main symptoms are dark red tongue, ulcers of the mouth and tongue, flushed face, dysphoria, insomnia, etc.

V

various symptom complexes before/after menstrual pause 绝经前后诸证 [jué jīng qián hòu zhū zhèng] They are disordered menstrual cycle, dizziness, palpitation, anxiety, sweating, abnormal emotion, etc.

vascular bolockage 脉闭 [mài bì] A bockage syndrome charecterized mainly with the symptoms of the blood vessels. The chief manifestations are irregular fever, burning sensation of the skin, pain of the muscles of the joints and erythematous rash.

vertigo 眩晕 [xuán yūn] Dizziness and dimness of the eyesight. The clinical manifestations may be of the excess type or the deficiency type. The latter is more commonly seen.

vertebra 脊椎 [jí zhuī] A general term for the spinal bone.

Vertex 巅 [diān] An ear point approx. 0. 15 mm below Occiput.

vibrating manipulation 震颤法 [zhèn zhàn fǎ] An acupuncture manipulation. To make the needle vibrate slightly, up and down, by pinching the body of the needle so as to strengthen needling sensation.

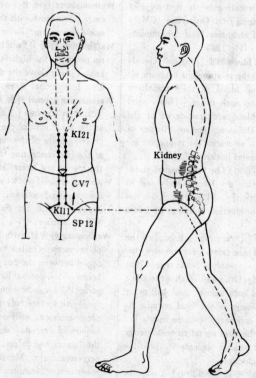

Fig 139

Vital Vessel 冲脉 [chōng mài] One of the eight extra vessels. The course: Originating from the inside of the lower abdomen (uterine) ascending from the artery in the groove along foot-*shaoyin* meridian lateral to the abdomen, reaching at the inner chest and spreading, ascending to join CV, distributing itself over the lips, mouth, head and face (five sense organs), descending together with foot-*haoyin* meridian through the medial aspect of the cubital fossa, entering deep into the lateral tibia and the posterial aspect of the medial ankle, penetrating through three yin meridians, emerging anteriorly between the dorsal foot and the great toe, ascending posteriorty to the spine, communicating with foot-*taiyang* meridian, starting from Guanyuan (CV 4) in the front of abdomen, and communicating with CV. (Fig 139)

vital essence and blood 精血 [jīng xuè] Usually referring to the relationship between vital essence and blood as they transform themselves into each other. Thus, vital essence and blood are considered of the same origin. Deficiency and insuffiiency of them manifests as one of the important indicators of general health.

vital essence 精 [jīng] The fundamental material to constitute the human body and to mantain its activities of life. It includes the essence of reproduction and that of water and grain.

vital portal 命门 [mìng mén] It implies the gate of life. There exists a contraoversy towards its actual meaning. Some regard it as the right kindy; Others think that there is a vital portal in both kideys; and still other think two kidneys is the vital portal. At present, the concencus tends to equate the functions of the vital portal to renal yang. Experimental studies indicate its possible relation to endocrine.

Wailing (ST 26) 外陵 [wài líng] A point of Stomach Meridian of Foot-*yangming*. Location: 6 cm lateral to Yinjiao (RN 7), 3 cm below the umbilicus. Regional anatomy: There are the branches of the 1st intercostal artery and vein and that of the artery and vein below the abdominal wall. The branch of the 10th intercostal nerve is distributed. Indications: Abdominal pain, hernia, dysmenorrhea, pains in the umbilicus due to cardialgia. Puncture: 4 cm perpendicularly. Moxibustion: 5—7 moxa cones or 10—20 minutes with warming moxibustion.

waiting for proper time 候时 [hòu shí] Referring to waiting for proper time before acupuncture.

Waiyang 外阳 [wài yáng] I. e., Fuyang (BL 59).

Waihuaishang 外踝上 [wài huái shàng] An extra point same with the tip of the lateral ankle in location. Refer Waihuaijian.

Waihuaijian 外踝尖 [wài huái jiān] 1. An extra point. At the highest point of the lateral ankle, 7 cm above the tip of the lateral ankle. Indications: Sapasm, foot *qi*.

Waihuaiqianjiaomai 外踝尖前交脉 [wài huái juān qián jiāo mài] An extra point located at the ankle joint of the dorsal foot, at the crossing point of the medial and lateral 1/4 of the line connecting the highest points of the medial and lateral ankle.

Waixiyan 外膝眼 [wài xī yán] An extra point, contrary to Neixiyan, collectively termed Xiyan (EX-LE 5). Same with Dubi (ST 35) in location.

Wailaogong 外劳宫 [wài láo gōng] An extra point, recently called Xiangqiang point. Locatied between the 2nd and 3rd metacarrpal bones on the dordsal hand, contrary to Laogong (PC 8). Indications: Indigestion, diarrhea with loose stool, acute/chronic infantile convulsion, stiff neck, inability of the fingers to extends, numbness and itch of the fingers and palms. Puncture: 1. 2 cm perpendicularly. Moxibustion: 1—3 moxa cones or 4—5 minutes with warming moxibustion. (Fig 140)

Waigou 外沟 [wài gōu] An alternate term for

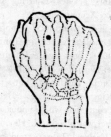

Fig 140

Futu (ST 32).

waiting for *qi* 候气 [hòu qì] 1. Referring to waiting for needling sensation at a proper depth during acupuncture, also called *dei qi*; 2. Referring to waiting for *qi* in four seasons; 3. Referring to diagnosing pulse *qi* (pulse indications).

Waishu 外枢 [wài shū] An alternate term for Weidao (GB 28).

Waijinjinyuye 外金津玉液 [wài jīn jīng yù yè] An extra point, located 3—4 cm directly above Lianquan (RN 23) between the thyroid cartilage and the hyoid bone, 1 cm bilateral. There is locally the branch of the external carotid artery and that of the carotid nerve. Indications: Aphasia due to apoplexy, salivation, ulcer on the surface of tongue, paralysis or spasm of the muscle of tongue, stomatitis. Puncture: 3—4 cm obliquely toward the root of tongue.

Waiguan (TE 5) 外关 [wài guān] A point of Energizer Meridian of Hand-*shaoyang*, the connecting point of the meridian, one of the eight confluence points, communicated with Connecting Vessel of Yang. Location: Between the radius and ulna, 6 cm above the transverse crease of the dorsal wrist, selected with the hand downward. Regional anatomy: Passing through the common extensor muscle of the index finger. There are the interossous dorsal artery and vein of forearm and, the basic stem of the palmar artery and vein are in the deeper. The cuta-

neous nerve at the dorsal side of the forearm is distributed. There is the interossous dorsal nerve of the radial nerve and the interosseous palmar nerve of the central nerve are in the deeper. Indications: Febrile disease, headache, pain in the cheek, tinnitus, deafness, congestive and painful eyes, hypochondriac pain in the elbow, arms, and fingers, tremor of hands. Puncture: 1. 5—3 cm perpendicularly. Moxibustion: 3—5 moxa cones or 5—10 minutes with warming moxibustion.

Waiqiu (GB 36) 外丘 [wài qiū] A point of Gallbladder Meridian of Foot-*shaoyang*, the gap-like point of the meridian. Location: 3 cm anterior to Yangjiao (GB 35) at the anterior edge of fibula, 21 cm above the tip of the lateral ankle. Regional anatomy: Passing through the long fibular muscle and long extensor muscle of toe, reaching at the short fibular muscle. There are the branches of artery and vein anterior to the tibia. The superficial fibular nerve is distributed. Indications: Headache, stiff neck, fullness in the chest and hypochondrium, flaccidity with cold limbs and blockage, epilepsy, vomiting up frothy saliva, foot *qi*, hepatitis, cholecystitis, sciatica. Puncture: 3—4. 5 cm perpendicularly. Moxibustion: 3—5 moxa cones or 5—10 minutes with warming moxibustion.

wandering moxibustion 回旋灸 [huí xuán jiǔ] One of wandering moxibustions to make the moxa stick hanging over the point and spiralling, so as to give the patient warm heat in a large scale. (Fig 141)

Wang Ji (1463—1539) 汪机 [wāng jī] A medical exert in Ming Dynasty (1368—1644), born at Qimenpushu, Anhui province. He wrote varieties of medical books of which Questions and Answers of Acupuncture describes the basis and concrete methods of acupuncture in the form of questions and answers, unique in his viewpoints.

Wang Ang (1615—?) 汪昂 [wāng áng] A medical expert in Qing Dynasty (1644—

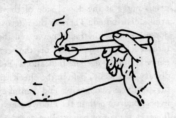

Fig 141

1911), born at Xiuning, Anhui Province. He praised highly Meridians, a chapter of Miraculou Pivot as the guiding principle of syndromes and treatments, purposefully selected Li Dongheng's Rhythmed Meridians (12 articles), polished and noted it, and then wrote one volume of Rhythymed Extra Vessels, which is concise, simple, direct, and practical for those learning basic theories of acupuncture. He also wrote a variety of medical books.

Wang Weiyi 王唯一 [wáng wéi yī] (Approx. 987—1067) An acupuncture expert in Northern Song Dynasty (960—1127). During 1023—1063 he was once a medical official. In 1026 he was officially appointed as the chief editor of Illustrated Acupunctue Classic on *Shu* Points on Newly-remoulded Bronze Figure and carved on the bone. Next year he conducted to remould two bronze figures, "which is a great creation in the development of acupuncture."

Wang Bin 王冰 [wáng bīn] A medical expert in Tang Dynasty (618—907). During 726—763 he was an official but studied medicine very hard. He spent over 12 years in compiling and took notes to Plain Questions (9 volumes). Since the 7th volume of the original has been lost, he had to supplemented it and edited it into 24 volumes, and completed it in 762 A.D., which is the present popular edition. In taking notes to the points in the book, he cited Illustrated Classic on the Points of Meridians and Qi Flow and Illustrated Classic of Meridians

and Points besides referring Systematic Classic on Acupuncture.

Wang Tao 王焘 [wáng tāo] (Approx. 670—755) A medical expert in Tang Dynasty (618—907), born in Mei County, Shanxi Province. He suffered from illness very frequently in his childhood, but was very interested in medical science. He more frequently contacted with famous doctors as his mother was always ill. He once worked in the National Library and read many books about the prescriptions. So he wrote the Medical Secrets of an Official (40 volumes), one volume of which is Mingtang Moxibustion Techniques.

Wangu (SI 4) 腕骨 [wǎn gǔ] A point of Small Intestine Meridian of Hand-*taiyang*. The source point of the meridian. Location: At the ulnar side of the wrist, in the depression between the posteriror end of the 5th base of the 5th metacarpal bone and the hamate bone. Regional anatomy: At the starting point of the extensor muscle of the small finger. There is the dorsal wrist artery of wrist (branch of the ulnar artery) and the dorsal venous network of hand. The dorsal branch of the ulnar nerve is distributed. Indications: Headache, stiff neck, tinnitus, nebula, spasm of the fingers and pain in the arms, jaundice, febrile disease with no sweat, malaria, hypochondriac pain, swelling of the neck, emaciation-thirst disease, lacrimation. Puncture: 1—1.5 cm perpendicularly. Moxibustion: 3—5 moxa cones or 5—10 minutes with warming moxibustion.

Wangu (GB 12) 完骨 [wán gǔ] 1. A point of Gallbladder Meridian of Foot-*shaoyang*. The confluence of foot-*taiyang* and foot-*shaoyang* meridians. Location: In the depression below the styloid process of temple, approx. at the level with Fengfu (GV, DU 20). Regional anatomy: Posterosuperior to the appending part of the sternocleudomastoidous muscle. There is the posteroauricular artery and vein. The main trunk of the lesser occipital nerve distributed. Indications: Headache, swelling cheek, toothache, sore throat, pain and stiffness of the neck, mania, toothache, insomnia, epilepsy. Puncture: 1—1.5 cm obliquely, Moxibustion: 1—3 moxa cones or 5—10 minutes with warming moxibustion. 2. The mastoid process of the temporal bone.

warming moxibustion apparatus 温灸器 [wēn jiǔ qì] A moxibustion instrument made of metal. To make a sylinder with the metal, and make dozens of small holes at its bottom, put a smaller sylinder with over ten small holes into it, and put moxa floss or drug powder into the small sylinder, and then ignite them and put the sylinder on the area where moxibustion is done, so as to make heat power exude into the skin. It has the action of regulating *qi* and blood, warming the middle energizer and eliminating pathogenic cold. It is particularly suitable for the women, children and those who fear acupuncture. (Fig 142)

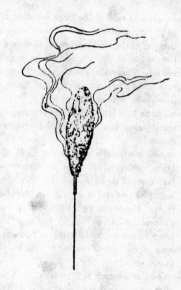

Fig 143

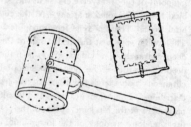

Fig 142

warming the ematicated with *qi* 形不足者温之于气 [xíng bù zú zhě wēn zhī yú qì] An emaciated patient as caused by insufficienty of yang *qi* should be treated with remedies of warm tonification and to tongnfy *qi*.

warming moxibustion 温灸 [wēn jiǔ] I. e., mild moxibustion.

warming needling 温针 [wēn zhēn] A kind of needling technique. After acupuncture, wind the tail of the needle with moxa floss and ignite it to warm the needle. (Fig 143)

water needling 水针 [shuǐ zhēn] I. e., point injection.

water moxibustion 水灸 [shuǐ jiǔ] The technique to treat disease by rubbing the body surface with garlic.

water-cupping technique 水罐法 [shuǐ guàn fǎ] A kind of cupping technique to get rid of air by making use of steaming air so as to form the negative pressure within the cup that can absorb the skin. The bamboo cup is usually used, first put it into clear water or drug liquid, then wipe out boiling water on the opening of the cup with a towel quickly, and make it cover the selected area, which can absorb the point.

walking cupping 走罐法 [zǒu guàn fǎ] I. e., pushing cupping technique.

weakness of both heart and spleen 心脾两虚 [xīn pí liǎng xū] The main symptoms are palpitation, amnesia, insomnia, frequent dreams, reduced appetite, loose stools, abdominal distension and fullness, fatigue and weakness, sallow complexion, emaciation, pale tongue with whitish coating, faint and weak pulse, etc.

weakness and cold of the large intestine 大肠虚寒 [dà cháng xū hán] The pathologic changes of the cold syndrome, as caused by the decline of the function of the large intestine. The main symptoms are diarrhea, cold limbs, vague pain of the abdomen relievable by heat and massage.

weak pulse 弱脉 [ruò mài] The soft, deep, and small pulse. It indicates the deficiency syndrome.

weakness and chills of bladder 膀胱虚寒 [páng guāng xū hán] The pathologic manifestations of the cold syndrome accompanying the impairment of the bladder functions. The major symptoms are frequency of urination, enuresis, light urine or dribbling of urine, cold feeling in hypogastrium, whitish moist coating of tongue, faint pulse, etc.

weakness of stomach 胃虚 [wèi xū] Pathologic changes due to gastric weakness, including deficiency of gastric *qi* and deficiency of gastric yin.

weakness due to exhaustion of refined *qi* 精气夺则虚 [jīng qì duó zé xū] When antipathogenic *qi* is exhausted, the deficiency syndrome will result.

Weidao (GB 28) 维道 [wéi dào] A point of Gallbladder Meridian of Foot-*shaoyang*, the confluence of foot-*shaoyang* meridian and Girdle Vessel, also termed Waishu. Location: Below the anterior iliac spine, 1.5 cm anterioinferior to Wushu (GB 27). Regional anatomy: There is the superficial deep iliac circumflex artery and vein. The iliohypogastric nerve is distributed. The needle passes through the external oblique muscle of abdomen and the internal oblique muscle of abdomen to reach at the transverse muscle of abdomen. Indications: Pain in the waist, pain in the bilateral lower abdomen, prolapse of uterus, hernia, leukorrhea, irregular menstruation, edema, pain in the bilateral lower abdomen, Puncture: 1.5—4.5 cm perpendicularly. Moxibustion: 3—5 moxa cones or 5—10 minutes with warm-ing moxibustion.

Weigong 维宫 [wéi gōng] An extra point. located at the lower abdomen, medioinferior to the anterosuperior illiac spine at the level with Guanyuan (CV, RN 4) or 3 cm medial and oblique to Weidao (GB 28). Indications: Prolapse of uterus, herniac pain, dysfunction of the intestines. Puncture: obliquely along the ligament of the groin, 4.5—6 cm. Moxibustion: 5—10 minutes with warming moxibustion.

Weiqionggu 尾穷骨 [wěi qióng gǔ] 1. Referring to coccyx; 2. an extra point. Located 3 cm above the tip of coccyx and 3 cm bilateral to the tip, 3 in total. Indications: Lumbago, pain in the coccyx, constipation, enuresis, hemorroids. Moxibustion: 3—5 moxa cones or 5—10 minutes with warming needling.

Weizhong (BL 40) 委中 [wěi zhōng] A point of Bladder Meridian of Foot-*taiyang*, the sea-like (earth) point of the bladder, also termed Xuexi, Zhongxi. Location: At the midpoint of the transverse crease of the cubital fossa. Regional anatomy: At the cubital fossa. There is vena femoropoplitea. The cubital vein is at the medial side of the deeper stratum. The cubital artery is in the deepest stratum. The posterior temporal cutaneous nerve and the tibial nerve are distributed. Indications: Lumbago, difficult movement of the hip joint, spasm of the politeal tendon, atrophy of the lower limbs, apoplexy and coma, hemiplegia, abdominal pain, vomiting, malaria, epistaxis, enuresis, dysuria, spontaneous sweating, night sweat, erysepilas, deep-rooted sore. Puncture: 1.5—3 cm perpendicularly or prick to cause little bleeding at the superficial vein.

Weizhu 尾组 [wěi zǔ] An alternate term for Changqiang (GV 1).

well-like points 井穴 [jǐng xué] One of the five *shu* points, located at the end of the four limbs. It can be used in the case of pathogenic *qi* staying at the srorring viscera with the symptoms such as fever, coma, anxiety, and depression of the chest. Frequently used in first aid and examination of the meridians. It is also the root of the twelve meridians.

Weibao 维胞 [wéi bāo] An extra point. Located at the hypogastric area, inferomedial to the anterosuperior spinal process of ilium, 3 cm below Weidao or 6 cm medial and inferior to Weidao (GB 28). Indications: Prolapse of uterus, intestinal hernial pain, pelvitis, dysfunction of the intestinal function. Puncture: 1. 5—3 cm perpendicularly. Moxibustion: 3—5 moxa cones or 5—10 minutes with warming moxibustion.

Weicui 尾翠 [wěi cuì] An extra point. Located 9 cm directly above the tip of the coccyx. Indications: Infantile malnutrition and emaciation, indigestion, abdominal pain and diarrhea, prolapse of anus. Puncture: 1. 5—3 cm horizontally. Moxibustion: 3—7 moxa cones or 5—15 minutes with warming needling.

Weicang (BL 50) 胃仓 [wèi cāng] A point of Bladder Meridian of Foot-*taiyang*. Location: 9 cm lateral to the interspace between the 12th spinal processes of the thoracic vertebra and the 1st lumbar vertebra. Regional anatomy: At the broadest muscle of back and the iliocostal muscle. There is the posterior branch of the infracostal artery and vein. The lateral branch of the posterior branch of the 11th thoracic nerve is distributed. Indications: Stomachache, abdominal distension, indigestion, pains in the back spine, edema, constipation, malaria. Puncture: 1. 5—2. 5 cm obliquely. Moxibustion: 5—7 moxa cones or 10—20 minutes with warm needling.

Weizhongyang 委中央 [wěi zhōng yāng] I. e., Weizhong (BL 40).

Weiyang (BL 39) 委阳 [wěi yáng] A point of Baldder Meridian of Foot-*taiyang*, the lower joining point of the triple energizer. Location: At the crossing spot between the end of the lateral aspect of the transverse crease of the cubital fossa and the medial edge of the biceps muscle of thigh, or 3 cm lateral to Weizhong (BL 40). Regional anatomy: At the medial side of biceps muscle of thigh. There is the suprolateral artery and vein of knee. The branches of the posterior femoral cutaneous nerve and that of common femoral peroneal nerve are distributed. Indications: Stiffness and pain in the lumbar spine, distension and fullness in the lower abdomen, dysuria, contracture, spasm and pain of the legs and feet. Puncture: 3—4. 5 cm perpendicularly. Moxibustion: 3—5 moxa cones or 5—10 minutes with warming moxibustion.

Wenliu (LI 7) 温溜 [wēn liū] A point of Large Intestine Meridian of Hand-*yangming*, the gap-like point of the meridian, also termed Nizhu, Shetou. Location: At the radial side of the dorsal forearm, on the line connecting Yangxi (LI 5) and Quchi (LI 11), 15 cm above Yangxi (LI 5). Regional anatomy: Between the radial extensor muscle of wrist and the long adductor muscle of thumb. There is the muscular branch of the radial artery and the cephalic vein. The dorsal cutaneous nerve of forehead and the deeper branch of the radial nerve are distributed. Indications: Headache, swollen face, epistaxis, sore throat, swelling and pain in the mouth and tongue, pains in the shoulder and back, borborygmus, abdominal pain, mania, wagging of the tongue. Puncture: 1. 5—3 cm perpendicularly. Moxibustion: 3—5 moxa cones or 5—10 minutes with warming moxibustion.

Weicuigu 尾翠骨 [wěi cuì gǔ] Referring to ccocyx.

Weiyi 尾翳 [wěi yì] An alternate term for Jiuwei (GV 15).

Weilu 尾闾 [wěi lǘ] 1. I. e., coccyx; 2. Referring to Changqiang (GV 1).

weizhen 煨针 [wèi zhēn] I. e., fire puncture.

Weixiashu 胃下俞 [wèi xià shū] I. e., Weiguanxiashu (EX-B 3).

Weihui 维会 [wéi huì] Referring to Baihui (GV 20) or Shenque (CV 8).

Wenliu 温流 [wēng liǔ] I. e., 温溜, Wenliu (LI 7).

Wenliu 温留 [wēn liǔ] I. e., 温溜, Wenliu (LI 7).

Weishu (BL 21) 胃俞 [wèi shū] A point of Bladder Meridian of Foot-*taiyang*, the back *shu* point of the stomach. Locations: 4. 5 cm lateral to the interspace between the spinal processes of the 12th thoracic vertebra and the 1st lumbar verbar vertebra. Regional anatomy: At the longest muscle and the iliocostal muscle. The medial branch of the dorsal branch of the posterior branch of the 12th thoracic nerve is in the deeper. Indications: Spermatorrhea, impotence, enuresis, frequent urination, irregular menstruation, leukorrhea, soreness and pain in the waist and kness, blurred vision, tinnitus, deafness, dysuria, edema, diarrhea, cough, short breath. Puncture: 1. 5—2. 5 cm obliquely. Moxibustion: 5—7 moxa cones or 10—20 minutes with warming moxibustion.

Weiwan 胃脘 [wèi wǎn] 1. An alternate term for Shangwan (CV 13) or an alternate term for Zhongwan (CV 12); 2. Epigastrium.

Weiwei 胃维 [wèi wéi] An alternate term for Dicang (ST 4).

Weiguan 胃管 [wèi guǎn] Referring to Zhongwan (CV 12).

Weiguanxiashu 胃管下俞 [wèi guǎn xià shū] An extra point, located 4. 5 cm lateral to the interspace between the spinal processes of the 8th and 9th thoracic vertebra. Indications: Emacition-thirst disease, dry throat, abdominal pain and vomiting, intercostal neuralgia. Puncture: 1—1. 5 cm obliquely. Moxibustion: 5—7 moxa cones or 10—20 minutes with warming moxibustion.

'white tiger shakes its head' 白虎摇头 [bái hǔ yáo tóu] One of the four manipulations contrary to 'dark green tiger sways its tail'. According to Rhythmed Golden Needle it is to insert the needle to a proper depth, and shake the needle left and right in combination of lifting, repeatedly 18 times, so as to make *qi* flourishing. (Fig 144)

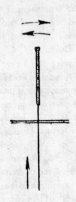

Fig 144

white mustard seed 白芥子 [bái jiè zǐ] One of the drugs used for dressing on the skin. Dried wippened seed of Sinpis alba. It can make the skin hot and blistering. To grind white mustard seed into powder and mix it with water, and dress it on the skin. In clinic it is usually used to treat cold blockage of the joint by dressing it on the affected area.

whooping cough 顿咳 [dùn ké] An infectious disease frequently seen in children, caused by seasonal pathogens with obstruction of the air passages by putrid phlegm, and characterized clinically by phlegm, and characterized clinically by chronic paroxyxmal spasmodic cough.

wheat-seed moxibustion 麦粒炙 [mài lì jiǔ] I. e., moxibustion with smaller moxa cone. To administer moxibustion with smaller moxe cone like the seed of wheat.

withdrawing of needle 发针 [fā zhēn] I. e., withdrawing the needle.

wind the premier pathogen 风为百病之长 [fēng wéi bái bìng zhī zhǎng] Wind is the number one pathogenic *qi* and of primary importance in causing diseases.

wind skin rash 风疹 [fēng zhěn] A common disease of children with skin rash caused by seasonal pathogenic wind-heat, clinically manifested by generalized skin rash which spreads all over the body within 24 hours after onset, the skin ash fades in 2—3 days without desquamation and scarring, and is accompanied by a mild cough and fevre.

withdrawing manipulation 退法[tuì fǎ]Referring to withdrawal of the needle from the deep stratum to the subcutaneous region and pulling the needle.

wrist-ankle needling 腕踝针 [wǎn huái zhēn] A therapeutic method to puncture the six specific points above the wrist joint or ankle joint to treat diseasess. It was seen in the report in 1976. The points are from the transverse finger widths to the upper wrist and upper ankle. Repeatedly for diseases at the various parts of the body. While puncturing insert the needle 4 cm along the subcutaneous region upwardly. It needs not occurrence of induction and the needle is retained over half an hour. It can be used for treating functional disorders and neuralgia. (Fig 145)

Wrist 腕[wǎn]An ear point located in the 4th equicalent zone superior to clavicle.

Wuyi (ST 15) 屋翳 [wū yì] A point of Stomach Meridian of Foot-*yangming*. Location: In the 2nd costal space, 12 cm lateral to Zigong (CV 19) at the midline of the chest. Regional anatomy: In the greater and lesser pectoral muscles. There is the acromion artery and vein of chest and the branches of the lateral artery and vein of chest. The branch of the greater pectoral muscle of the anterior pectoral nerves is distributed. Indications: Cough and asthmatic breath, coughing up blood, breast carbuncle, purulent bloody sputum, distension and pain in the chest and hypochondrium, pain in the skin, puffiness of the body. Puncture: 1—1. 5 cm obliquely. Moxibustion: 3—5 moxa cones of 5—10 minutes with warming moxibustion.

Wuli 五里 [wǔ lǐ] A name of the meridian points. One pertaining to Large Intestine Meridian at the upper arm; The other pertaining to Liver Meridian at the medial side of thigh. For convenience of differentiating them, the former is called Shouwuli (LI 13) while the latter, Zuwuli (LR 10); 2. Another name of Laogong (PC 8).

Wuming 无名 [wú míng] An extra point, i. e. , Erzhuixia.

Wushu (GB 27)五枢[wǔ shū]A point of Gallbladder Meridian of Foot-*shaoyang*, the confluence of foot-*shaoyang* meridian and Girdle Vessel. Location: 1 dm below, and anteroinferior to Girdle Vessel, anterior to the anterosuperior process of ilium at the level with Guanyuan (RN 4). Regional anatomy: Passing through the internal and external trapezius muscles of abdomen, reaching the transverse muscle of abdomen. There are the superifical and deep circumflex artery and vein. The iliohypogastric nerve is distributed. Indications: Prolapse of uterus, leukorrhea, irregular menstruation, hernia, pain in the lower abdomen and waist. Puncture: 3—4. 5 cm perpendicularly. Moxibustion: 3—5 moxa cones or 5—10 minutes with warming moxibustion.

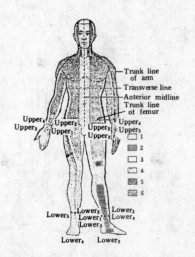

Trunk line of arm
Transverse line
Anterior midline
Trunk line of femur

Upper₄ Upper₅
Upper₃ Upper₂
Upper₁
Upper₁ Upper₂
Upper₃ Upper₄ Upper₅

☐ 1
▦ 2
☐ 3
▭ 4
▨ 5
▩ 6

Lower₅ Lower₁ Lower₂
Lower₁ Lower₄
Lower₃
Lower₄ Lower₃

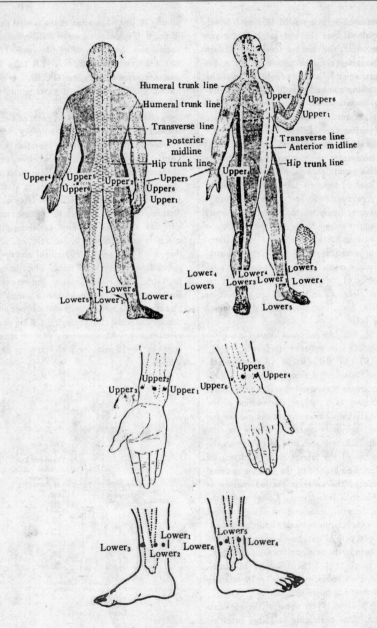

Fig 145

Wuchu (BL 5) 五处 [wǔ chù] A point of Bladder Meridian of Foot-*taiyang*. Location: On the midline of head, 4.5 cm lateral to Shangxing (GV, DU 23), 3 cm in the hairline. Regional anatomy: At the frontal muscle. There are the frontal artery and vein. The lateral branch of the frontal nerve is distributed. Indications: Headache, vertigo, blurred vision, epilepsy, infantile convulsion. Puncture: 1.5—3 cm horizontally. Moxibustion: 3—9 moxa cones or 3—5 minutes with warming moxibustion.

Wubu 五虎 [wǔ hǔ] An extra point. In modern times, it was located according to Supplementary Illustration, i. e. , at the highest point of the small hesd of the 2nd and the metacarpal bones of the dorsal hand. Moxibustion: 3—5 moxa cones.

Wuqueshu 五怯俞 [wǔ qué shū] An alternate term for Yixi (BL 45)

Wuhui 五会 [wǔ huì] 1. An alternate term for Renying (ST 9); 2. An alternate term for Baihui (GV 20).

X

xi (gap-like) points 郄穴 [xī xué] The name of the classified meridian points. It means the interspace where *qi* and blood in the meridians gather. The twelve meridians and Motility Vessel of Yin, Motility Vessel of Yang, Connecting Vessel of Yin and Connecting Vessel of Yang have such a point each at the four limbs, totally 16. In clinic they are usually used for treating actue cases, e. g., for vomiting Kongzui (LU 6) is cooperated, for cardialgia Ximen (PC 4) is cooperated, for stomachache Liangqui (ST 34) is cooperated. (See the picture and chart following) (Fig 146)

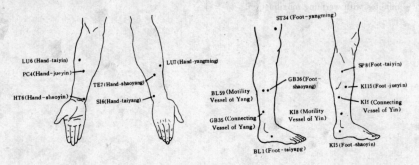

Fig 146

Xiaqihai 下气海 [xià qì hǎi] Contrary to Shangqihai. Referring to Qihai (CV 6).

Xiafengchi 下风池 [xià fēng chí] I. e., Xinshe.

Xiasifeng 下四缝 [xià sì fèng] See Zhigen.

Xiadicang 下地仓 [xià dì cāng] An alternate term of Xiachengjiang.

Xiayao 下腰 [xià yāo] An extra point, located between the spinal process of the 2nd sacrum and that of the 3rd. Indications: Chronic enterites, chronic dysentery, distocia. Moxibustion: 3—5 moxa cones or 5—10 minutes with warming moxibustion.

Xiahuang 下肓 [xià huāng] An alternate term for Qihai (CV, RN 6).

Xiaji 下极 [xià jí] 1. Originally implying the lowest place; 2. An alternate term for Henggu (KI 11); 3. Referring to Huiyin (CV, RN 1).

Xiajizhishu 下极之俞 [xià jí zhī shū] 1. Referring to Changqiang (GB, RU 1) or Huiyin (CV, RN 1), or Xiajishu point; 2. Referring to Xiajishu.

Xiajishu 下俞 [xià jí shū] An extra point. Located on the posterior midline below the spinal process of the 3rd lumbar vertebra. Indications: Abdominal pain, lumbago, diarrhea, cystitis, enteritis. Puncture: 1.5—3 cm perpendicularly. Moxibustion: 3—5 moxa cones. Moxibustion: 5—10 minutes with warming moxibustion.

Xialin 下林 [xià lín] I. e., Xiajuxu (ST 39).

Xiakunlun 下昆仑 [xià kūn lún] 1. An extra point. Located at the anterior edge of Achilles tendon, 3 cm below at the level with the top of the lateral ankle. Indications: Cold blockage syndrome, lumbago, Hemiplegia, paraplegia, heaviness and pain in the foot. Puncture: 1.5 cm perpendicularly. Moxibustion: 5—7 moxa cones of 10—15 minutes with warming moxibustion; 2. An alternate term for Kunlun (BL

60).

Xiadu 下都 [xià dū] An extra point. One of baixie (EX—UE 9). "Baxie points are locate between the five fingers, 4 at either hand ⋯ the fourth one is Xiadu (two points) located between the ring finger and the small finger, called Zhongzhu, which is located 1. 5 cm below Yemen (TE, SJ 2)." Indications: Congestive and swelling arm. Punctured 0. 3 cm and 5 moxa cones can be used by warming moxibustion on it. "

Xialing 下陵 [xià líng] I. e. , Zusanli (ST 36).

Xiawan (CV 10) 下脘 [xià wán] A point of Conception Vessel, the conluence of foot-*taiyin* meridian and Conception Vessel. Location: On the abdominal midline, │6 cm above the umbilicus. Regional anatomy: At the white abdominal line, there is the inferior artery and vein of the abdominal wall. The anterior cutaneous branch of the 8th costal nerve is distributed. Indications: Epigastric pain, abdominal distension, borborygmus, vomiting, diarrhea, indigestion, puffiness due to asthenia, indigestion, hiccup, abdominal mass. Puncture: 3—5 cm perpendicularly. (Be cautious for the pregnant woman) Moxibustion: 3—7 moxa cones or 5—15 minutes with warming moxibustion.

Xialian (LI 8) 下廉 [xià lián] 1. A point of Large Intestine Meridian of Hand-*Yangming*. Location: 1. 2 dm below Quchi (LI 11) on the line connecting Yangxi (LI 5) and Quchi (LI 11), on the radial side of the dorsal forearm. Regional anatomy: In the radial long extensor muscle of wrist and supinator muscle. There is the muscular branch of the radial artery and the cephalic vein. The dorsal cutaneous nerve of forearm and the deep branch of the radial nerve are distributed. Indications: Headache, vertigo, ocular pain, pains in the elbows and arms, indigestion, pain in the breast. Puncture: 1. 5—3 cm perpendicularly: Moxibustion: 3—5 moxa cones of 5—10 minutes with warming

moxibustion; 2. Referring to Xiajuxu (ST 39).

Xiaguan 下管 [xià guǎn] I. e. , Xiawan (CV 10) from Classic of Pulse.

Xiaheng 下横 [xià héng] An alternate term for Henggu (KI 11).

Xialiao (BL 34) 下髎 [xià liáo] A point of Bladder Meridian of Foot-*taiyang*, in the 4th posterior foramen on the lateral side of the median sacral crest or on the inferior edge of the spinal segment of the 4th sacral vertebra, select it 1. 5 cm to the sacral midline. Regional anatomy: At the starting point of the great muscle of hip. There are the branches of the inferior gluteal artery and vein. The posterior branch of the 4th sacral nerve is distributed. Indications: Lumbosacral pain, difficult urination, constipation, hematochezia, pain in the lower abdomen, borborygmus and diarrea, dysuria, constipation, Leukorrhea. Puncture: 3— 3. 5 cm perpendicularly. Moxibustion: 5— 7 moxa cones or 5—15 minutes with warming moxibustion.

xianliu **paste** 香硫饼 [xiāng liú bǐng] A kind of material used for moxibustion. Indications: Pathogenic cold and damp. The formula can be seen from Thong Fu Tang Gong Xian Liang Fang (volume II).

Xiangu (ST 43) 陷谷 [xiàn gǔ] A point of Stomach Meridian of Foot-*yangming*, the stream-like (wood) point of the meridian, also called Xiangu. Location: In the depression anterior to the connective part of the 2nd and 3rd metatarsal bones or 6 cm above Neiting (ST 44) at the end of the suture crease of toe. Regional anatomy: At the interosseous muscle of the 2nd metatarsal bone. There is the dorsal venous network of foot. The medial cutaneous nerve of the dorsal foot is distributed. Indications: Puffiness of the face and eyes, edema, borborygmus, abdominal pain, swelling and pain in the dorsal foot. Puncture: 1. 5—3 cm perpendicularly. Moxibustion: 3—7 moxa cones or 5—15 minutes with warming moxibustion.

Xiangu 陷骨 [xiàn gǔ] I. e., Xiangu (ST 43).

Xiaoluo (TE 12) 消泺 [xiāo luò] A point of Triple Energizer Meridian of Hand-*shaoyang*. Location: At the dorsal side of the upper arm. At the midpoint of the line connecting Qinglengyuan (TE 11) and Naohui (TE 13). When the forearm is anteriorly rotated, it is located at the inferior edge of the protruding lateral head of the brachial triceps muscle or 9 cm above Qinglengyuan (TE 13). Regional anatomy: At the triceps muscle. There is the accessary artery and vein at the middle side. The dorsal cutaneous nerve of arm and the muscular branch of the radial nerve are distributed. Indications: Headache, stiffness neck, toothache, pain in the arm, epilepsy. Puncture: 1.5—3.5 cm perpendicularly. Moxibustion: 3—7 moxa cones or 5—15 minutes with warming moxibustion.

Xiaoli 消疬 [xiāo lì] An extra point located at the back.

Xia Ying 夏英 [xià yīng] An acupuncture expert in Ming Dynasty (1368—1644), born at Hang Zhou City. In 1497 he noted Miraculous Pivot with a chapter of Meridians of The Expounding of Fourteen Merichans and completed the book, supplement to Meridians of Miraculous Pivot.

Xiabai (LU 4) 侠白 [xiá bái] A point of Lung Meridian of Hand-*taiyin*. Location: At the anterolateral side of the upper arm, 15 cm above the transverse crease of the elbow, at the radial edge of the biceps muscle of arm, or 3 cm directly below Tianfu (LU 3). Regional anatomy: At the lateral side of biceps muscle of arm. There are the muscular branches of the cephalic vein, and the muscular cutaneous nerve are distributed. Indications: Cough, short breath, dry vomiting, anxiety, cardialgia, pain in the medial aspect of the upper arm. Puncture: 1.5—3 cm perpendicularly. Moxibustion: 3—5 moxa cones or 5—10 minutes with warming mox-

ibustion.

Xiachengjiang 侠承浆 [xiá chéng jiāng] An extra point, also called Xiadicang, Keliao. Located 3 cm lateral to Chengjiang (CV 24), at the mental foramen of the mandible. There is the orbicular muscle of mouth. The quadrate muscle of the lower lip, the branches of the facial and mental artery and vein, and the branches of the facial nerve and mental nerve. Indications: Jaundice, pestilence, facial paralysis, toothache, deep-rooted sore at the mouth and lips. Puncture: 1—1.5 cm perpendicularly. (Fig 147)

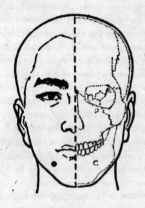

Fig 147

Xiaxi (GB 43) 侠溪 [xiá xī] A point of Gallbladder Meridian of Foot-*shaoyang*, the spring-like (water) point of the meridian. Location: At the doral foot, at the end of the articular crease of the 4th and 5th toes. Or select it at the midpoint above the toe web. Regional anaomy: There is the dorsal digital atery and vein. The doral digital nerve of foot is distributed. Indications: Headache, vertigo, tinnitus, deafness, pain in the outer canthi, swelling and pains in the chest and hypochondrium, swolen cheek, pain in the knee and thigh, swelling and pain in the dorsal boot, malaria. Puncture: 1—1.5 cm perpendicularly. Moxibustion: 1—3 moxa cones or 3—5 minutes with warming moxibustion.

Xiaoerjixiong point 小儿鸡胸穴 [xiǎo ér jī xiōng xué] An extra point. Location: Between the 2nd, 3rd and 4th intercostal space, 3—4 cm to the thoracic midline, 6 in total. Indication: Pigeon chest. Moxibustion: 3 moxa cones, or 5—10 minutes with warming moxibustion.

Xiaoerguixiong point 小儿龟胸穴 [Xiǎo ér guī xiōng xué] I.e., Xiaerjixiong point.

Xiaoershixian 小儿食痫 [xiǎo ér shí xián] An extra point. Location: On the abdominal midline, 2.5 dm above the umbilicus. Indications: Epilepsy. Moxibustion: 3—5 moxa cones. Moxibustion: 5—10 minutes with warming moxibustion.

Xiaoerganli 小儿疳痢 [xiǎo ér gān lì] See Weicui.

Xiaoerganshou 小儿疳瘦 [xiǎo ér gān shòu] See Weicui.

Xiaoershuijin 小儿睡惊 [xiǎo ér shuì jīn] An extra point. Location: 1 cm directly above the end of the radial side of the cubital transverse crease. Select it with the elbow slightly flxed. Indications: Infantile fright during sleep, pains in the elbow and arm. Moxibustion: 1—3 moxa cones or 3—5 minutes with warming moxibustion.

Xiaotianxin 小天心 [xiǎo tiān xīn] An extra point. Location: At the root of the palm and the part connecting greater *yuji* and smaller *yuji*, 1.5 cm to Daling (PC 7). Indications: Convulsion, high fever and mental confusion, anuria, angina pectoris, rheumatic heart disease. Puncture: 1—1.5 cm perpendicularly of press with the fingernail.

Xiaoji 小吉 [xiǎo jí] An alternate term for Shaoze (SI 1).

Xiaozhu 小竹 [xiǎo zhú] An alternate term for meichong (BL 3).

Xiaohai (SI 8) 小海 [xiǎo hǎi] A point of small Intestine Meridian of Hand-*taiyang*, the sea-like (earth) point of the meridian it pertains to. Location: In the depression between the olecranon and mediosuperior condyle of humerus at the groove of ulnar nerve. Select it with the elbow flexed. Regional anatomy: There are the ulnar superior and inferior accessary artery and vein and ulnar recurrent artery and vein. The branch of the medial cutaneous nerve of forearm and the ulnar nerve are distributed. Indications: Headache, vertigo, stuffy nose, epistaxis, pains in the waist and back, weakness of the leg, hemorrhoidal pain, mania. Puncture: 3—5 cm perpendicularly. Moxibustion: 3—5 moxa cones or 5—10 minutes with warming moxibustion.

Xiaochangshu (BL 27) 小肠俞 [xiǎo cháng shū] A point of Bladder Meridian of Foot-*taiyang*, the back-*shu* point of the small intestine. Location: At the level with the posterior foramen of the first sacrum, 4.5 cm lateral to the sacral midline, in the depression of the medial edge of the posterosuperior ilium and sacrum. Regional anatomy: At the starting portion of the sacrospinal muscle and the great muscle of the hip. There are the posterior branches of the lateral artery and vein of sacrum. The lateral branch of the posterior branch of the 1st sacral nerve is distributed. Indications: Spermatorrhea, enuresis, hematuria, leukorrhea, distension and pain in the lower abdomen, diarrhea, dysentery, malaria, hernia, pains in the waist and leg. Puncture: 3—5 cm perpendicularly or 5—15 minutes with warming moxibustion.

Xiaozhizaowen 小指爪纹 [xiǎo zhǐ zǎo wén] An extra point, located on the dorsal side of the small finger, at the midpoint of the root of the fingernail.

Xiaozhijian 小指尖 [xiǎo zhǐ jiān] An extra point, located at the tip of the small finger. Puncture: 3—6 mm. Moxibustion: 3—7 moxa cones. Indication: Pertussis.

Xiaogukong 小骨空 [xiǎo gú kōng] An extra point, located on the dorsal side of the small finger, at the midpoint of the transverse side crease of the proximal interphalangeal articulation of hand. Select it with the finger flexed. Indications: Ocular trouble, deafness, sore throat, pain in the fingers. Moxibustion: 3—5 moxa cones. (Fig 148)

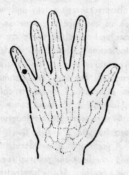

Fig 148

Xiaji 下纪 [xià jì] "Xiaji refers to Guanyuan (CV 4)." (Plain Questions).

Xiashangxing 侠上星 [xià shàng xīng] An extra point.

Xianhguan (**ST 7**) 下关 [xià guān] A point of Stomach Meridian of Foot-*yangming*, the confluence of foot-*yangming* and foot-*shaoyang* meridians. Location: In the depresion foramen by the zygomatic arc and the mandibular notch. Regional anatoy: There is the facial transverse artery and vein. The maxillary artery and vein are in the deeper. The zygomatic branch of the facial nerve and the branch of the audio-temporal nerve are distributed. Indications: Toothache, lockjaw, deafness, tinnitus, pain in the ears, otitis media, deviated mouth and eyes, vertigo. Puncture: 1. 5—3 cm perpendicularly. Moxibustion: 5—10 minutes with warming moxibustion.

Xiguan (**LR 7**) 膝关 [xī guān] A point of Liver Meridian of Foot-*jueyin*. Location: Posteroinferior to the medial ankle of the tibia, 3 cm posterior to Yinlingquan (SP 9). Regional anatomy: There is the posterior tibial artery in the deeper. The branch of the medial cutaneous nerve of the gastrocnemius

muscle is distributed. The tibial nerve is in the deeper. Indications: Distension and pain the knees, atrophic debility, rheumatic arthralgia. Puncture: 3—4. 5 cm perpendicularly. Moxibustion: 3—5 moxa cones or 5—10 minutes with warming moxibustion.

Xiasanli 下三里 [xià sān lǐ] I. e., Zusanli (ST 36).

Xiajuxu (**ST 39**) 下巨虚 [xià jù xū] A meridian point, called Juxuxialian in Internal Classic, the lower joining point of the small intestine. Location: 2. 7 dm cirectly below Dubi (ST 35) on the lateral side of the patellar liganent, i. e., 1. 8 dm below Zusanli (ST 36) on the lateral side of tibia. Reginal anatomy: Between the anterior muscle of tibia and the long exterior muscle of toe. There is the anterial tibial artery and vein. The branch of the superficial femoral nerve and deep femoral nerve are distributed. Indications: Pain in the lower abdomen, lumbovertebral pain referring to the testicles, breast carbuncle, atophy of the lower limbs, diarrhea, suppurative and bloody stools. Puncture: 3—5 cm perpendicularly. Moxibustion: 5—7 moxa cones or 5—15 minutes with warming moxibustion.

Xieliao 胁髎 [xié liáo] An alternate term for Zhangmen (LR 13).

Xietang 胁堂 [xié táng] An extra point, located 6 cm below the anxillary fossa, 3 cm obliquely anterosuperior to Yuanye (GB 22). Select it when the arm is raised. Indications: Fullness of the chest and hypochondrium, asthmatic breath, abdominal distension, yellow eyes, intercostal neuralgia. Puncture: 1—1. 5 cm obliquely. Moxibustion: 3—5 moxa cones or 5—10 minutes with warm needling.

***Xifangzi Mingtang* Moxibustion Classic** 西方子明堂灸经 [xī fāng zǐ míng táng jiǔ jīng] The book written by the unknown person. Consisting of 8 volumes. Chiefly deeling with the indications of moxibustion techniques on the *shu* points of the whole body, and appeared with the figuers. The

1st volume contains the figure of the face, the figure of the chest, and the figure of the abdomen. The 2nd and the 3rd volumes contains the figure of the prone head. The 5th and the 6th volumes contain the figures of the prone head and foot. The 7th, the figure of the lateral head and that of the hypochondrium and that of hands. The 8th, the figure of foot. Whether moxibustion is administered or not on the points at the above-mentioned portion was described, it was first published in 1368, collected into the Complete Book of the Four. There was the collected edition at the end of Qing Dynasty (1644—1911).

Xijie 膝解［xī jiě］Referring to the knee joint.

Ximen (PC 4) 郄门［xī mén］A point of Pericardium Meridian of Hand-*jueyin*, the gap-like point of the meridian. Location: At the palmar side of the forearm, 15 cm above the transverse crease of the wrist, between the long palmar muscle and the radial flexor muscle of wrist, select it by making the hand supine. Regional anatomy: There is the central artery and vein of forearm. The palmar interosseous artery and vein of the forearm are distributed. The central nerve is in the deeper. The palmar interosseous nerve of forearm is in the deepest. Indications: Cardialgia. palpitation, thoracalgia, anxiety, hemoptysis, epistaxis, deep-rooted sore, mania. Puncture: 2—3 cm perpendicularly. Moxibustion: 3—5 moxa cones or 5—10 minutes with warming moxibustion.

Ximu 膝目［xī mù］An alternate term for Xiyan.

Xinshi 新识［xīn shí］I. e., Xinshe.

Xinzhu 心主［xīn zhǔ］Referring to Pericardium Meridian of Hand-*jueyin* or its source point.

Xinglong 兴隆［xīn lóng］An extra point, 3 cm obliquely superior to the corner of the umbilicus, approx. 3 cm lateral to Shuifen (CV 9). Puncture: 1. 5—3 cm perpendicularly. Moxibustion: 3—5 moxa cones or 5—10 minutes with warming moxibustion.

Xinzhong 囟中［xìn zhōng］An extra point. Almost the same with Xinhui (GV 22) in location.

Xinhui (GV 22) 囟会［xìn huì］A GV point, also termed Dingmen. Location: 6 cm anterior to Baihui (GV 20). Regional anatomy: In galea aponeurotica at the confluential part of the corner suture and the sagital suture of the cranital bone. There are the superficial temporal artery and vein and the anastomotic network of the temporal artery and vein. The branch of the temporal nerve is distributed. Indications: Headache, vertigo, rhintis, pain in the nose, nasal poply, epistaxis, epilepsy, infantile convulsion. Puncture: 0. 9—1. 5 cm obliquely. Moxibustion: 3—6 moxa cones or 5—10 minutes with warming moxibustion.

Xinshu (BL 15) 心俞［xīn shū］A point of Bladder Meridian of Foot-*taiyang*, the back-*shu* point of the heart. Location: 3—4 cm lateral to Shendao (GV 11) between the styloid processes of the 5th and 6th thoracic vertebrae. Regional anatomy: Passing through the trapezius muscle and rhomboid muscle to reach the longest muscle. There are the medial branches of the dorsal branch of the 5th intercostal artery and vein. The medial cutaneous branch of the posterior branch of the 5th thoracic nerve is distributed. The lateral cutaneous branch of the posterior branch of the 5th thoracic nerve is in the deeper. Indications: Mania, epilepsy, palpitation with fright, insomnia, chest pain, nocturnal emission, schizophrenia, intercostal neuralgia. Puncture: 1. 5—2 cm obliquely (It is not advisable to puncture deep) Moxibustion: 3—5 moxa cones or 5—15 minutes with warming moxibustion.

xin in yang 阳中隐阴［yáng zhōng yǐn yīn］An acupuncture manipulation contrary to the manipulation of earlier reinforcing and later reducing. There is to puncture the needle first at the superfiial region, with swift insertion and slow thrusting at times of number 'nine' till the patient feels slightly hot, then to insert the needle into the deep region with swift thrusting and slow insertion at times of number 'six' to acquire *qi*. Used for the symptom of earlier cold and later heat. (Fig 149)

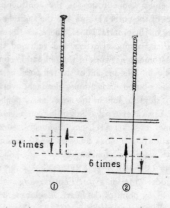

① Swift insertion and slow thrusting
② Swift thrusting and slow insertion

Fig 149

Xinxin Point 惺惺穴 [xīng xīng xué] 1. An alternate term for Duoming Point; 2. Referring to Fengfu (GV 16).

Xingjian (LR 2) 行间 [xíng jiān] A point of Liver Meridian of Foot-*jueyin*, the spring-like (fire) point of the meridian. Location: At the end of the suture crease between the 1st and 2nd toes. Regional anatomy: There is the artery and vein of the 1st dorsal toe. Just at the nerve of the dorsal toe divided by the superficial peroneal nerve and deep peroneal nerve. Indications: Profuse mense, amenorrhea, dysmenorrhea, vertigo, congestion, swelling and leukorrhea, pain in the public region, enuresis, hernia, fullness and pain in the chest and hypochondrium, hiccup, cough, diarrhea, toothache, congestive and painful eyes, apoplexy, epilepsy, insomnia, deviated mouth, swollen knees, pain in the medial aspect of the lower limb, swelling and pain in the dorsal foot. Punc-

ture: 1.5—3 cm obliquely. Moxibustion: 3—5 moxa cones or 5—10 minutes with warming moxibustion.

Xinjian 新建 [xīn jiàn] An extra point, located at the hip, between the greater protuberance of the femur and the anterosupraspinal process of the ilium in the extensor muscle of fascia lata. Indications: Inflammation of the lateral cutaneous nerve of femur, arthralgia of thigh, neuralgia of thigh. Puncture: 3—4.5 cm perpendicularly. Moxibustion: 3—5 moxa cones or 5—10 minutes with warming moxibustion.

Xiongxue 胸薛 [xiōng xué] An alternate term for Xuexi.

Xiongtonggu 胸通谷 [xiōng tōng gǔ] An extra point, 6 cm below the nipple. Indications: Cardialgia, thoracalgia, hypochondriac pain, mastitis.

Xiongtang 胸堂 [xiōng táng] Referring to Danzhong (CV 17), also an extra point located between the two nipples, at the bilateral side of the stern. Indications: Cough, asthmatic breath, hemoptysis, palpitation with fright, insufficient lactation, pain in the breast, bronchitis, spasm of esophagus, stomatitis. Moxibustion: 3—5 moxa cones or 5—10 minutes with warming moxibustion.

Xixia 膝下 [xī xià] An extra point, located at the knee, at the patella ligament, at the lower edge of the tip of the patella. Indications: Pain in the tibia. Moxibustion: 1—3 moxa cones or 3—5 minutes with warming moxibustion.

Xiyangguan (GB 33) 膝阳关 [xī yáng guān] A point of Gallbladder Meridian of Foot-*shaoyang*, also termed Yangling, Hanfu. Originally termed Yangguan, recently called Xiyangguan. Location: At the lateral side of knee, 9 cm directly above Yanglingquan (GB 34), in the depression at the edge of the laterosuperior condyle of the femur. Regional anatomy: Posterior to the iliotibial tract, anterior to the biceps muscle of thigh. There is the superolateral artery and vein of knee. The terminal branch of thelateral cutaneous nerve of thigh is distributed. Indications: Congestion, swelling and pain in the knees, spasm of the popliteal muscle, numbness of the legs. Puncture: 3—4. 5 cm perpendicularly. Moxibustion: 5—15 minutes with moxa stick.

Xiyan 膝眼 [xī yǎn] An extra point. Located at the extensor side of the knee joint, in the depression bilateral to the patella ligament. The medial one is called Neixiyan, the lateral one, Waixiyan, i. e. , Dubi, 4 in total. Indications: Pain in the knee, heaviness and pains in the legs and feet, beriberi, numbness of the lower limbs. Puncture: 1. 5—3 cm obliquely toward the knee, or from Neixiayan to Waixiayan. (Fig 150)

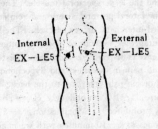

Fig 150

Xizhong 郄中 [xī zhōng] Referring to Weizhong (BL 40).

Table for Sixteen *xi* (Gap-like) Points

	Six Meridians of Hand	Six Meridians of Foot	Motility Vessel, Connecting Vessel
Yin Meridian	Hand-*taiyin*: Kongzui (LU 6) Hand-*shaoyin*: Yinxi (HT 6) Hang-*jueyin*: Ximen (PC 4)	Foot-*taiyin*: Diji (SP 8) Foot-*shaoyin*: Shuiquan (KI 5) Foot-*jueyin*: Zhongdu (LR 6)	Motility Vessel of Yin: Jiaoxin (KI 8) Connecting Vessel of Yin: Zhubin (KI 9)
Yang Meridian	Hang-*yangming*: Wenliu (LI 7) Hang-*taiyang*: Yanglao (ST 16) Hand-*shaoyang*: Huizong (TE, SJ 7)	Foot—*yangming*: Liangqiu (ST 34) Foot-*taiyang*: . Jinmen (BL 63) Foot-*shaoyang*: Waiqiu (GB 36)	Motility Vessel of Yang: Fuyang (BL 59) Connecting Vessel of Yang: Yangjiao (GB 35)

Xuemen 血门 [xué mén] An extra point located, 9 cm lateral to Zhongwan (CV, RN 12). Indications: Clots in the woman's abdomen, stomachache, indigestion. Puncture: 3—4. 5 cm perpendicularly. Moxibustion: 3—5 moxa cones or 5—15 minutes with warming moxibustion.

Xuehui 血会 [xué huì] One of the eight confluent points. "Blood confluence, Geshu (BL 17). It corresponds with the diaphragm, the upper point of which is Xinshu (BL 15) (the heart controls blood). It is therefore called blood confluence. Clinically used for hemoptysis, spitting blood, insufficiency of blood.

Xuexi 血郄 [xué xī] 1. Referring to Weizhong (BL 40); 2. Another name of Baicongwo (EX-LE 3).

Xuefu 血府 [xué fǔ] I. e. , Jijupikuai point.

Xiongzhiyinshu 胸之阴俞 [xiōng zhī yīn shū] An alternate term for Changqiang (GV 1).

Xiongxiang (SP 19) 胸乡 [xiōng xiāng] A point of Spleen Meridian of Foot-*taiyin*. Location: 18 cm lateral to Yutang (CV 18), at the midline of the chest. In the 3rd intercostal space. Regional anatomy: At the lateral aspects of the greater pectoral muscle and the lesser pectoral muscle. There are the lateral pectoral artery and vein and the 3rd intercostal artery and vein. The lateral cutaneous branch of the 3rd intercostal nerve is distributed. Indications: Distension and pain in the chest and hypochondrium, thoracic pain referring to the back. Puncture: 1—1.5 cm obliquely (Deep puncture is prohibited). Moxibustion: 3—5 moxa cones or 5—10 minutes with warming moxibustion.

Xipang 膝旁[xī páng]An extra point, located at the two ends of the medial and lateral creases of the transverse crease of the cubital fossa, 4 in total. Indications: Lumbago, soreness of the feet to stand persistently. Puncture: 1.5—3 cm perpendicularly. Moxibustion: 3—5 moxa cones or 5—10 minutes with warming moxibustion.

Xishang 膝上 [xī shàng] An extra point located at the upper part of the knee joint, each on either depression bilateral to the straight muscle of thigh at the superior edge of patella, 4 in total. Indications: Inflammation of the knee joint. Puncture: 1.5 cm perpendicularly. Moxibustion: 3—7 moxa cones or 5—15 minutes with warming moxibustion.

xiu 畜 [xù] Referring to posterior nazis.

Xiwai 膝外 [xī wài] An extra point, located at the end of the lateral aspect of the transverse crease of the cubital fossa, at the anterior edge of the biceps muscle. Indications: Pain in the knee joint, ulcer of the lower limns. Puncture: 1.5—3 cm perpendicularly. Moxibustion: 3—7 moxa cones or 5—15 minutes with warming moxibustion.

Xixue 溪穴 [xī xué] 1. An alternate term for Guilai (ST 29); 2. I. e., Xixue, an alternate term for Chengqi (ST 1).

Xuehai (SP 10) 血海 [xué hǎi] A point of Spleen Meridian of Foot-*taiyin*, also termed Baocongwo. Location: At the protruding point of the muscle at the medial side of thigh, 6 cm above the mediosuperior

condyle of femur. Select it when the knee is flexed. When the knee is flexed to form a right angle, the doctor presses the knee with the palm at the opposite side, extend the 2nd—5th fingers toward the upper knee, and obliquely put his thumb to form a 45° angle, the end of the thumb is the point. Regional anatomy: There are the muscular branches of the femoral artery and vein at the lower part of the medial femoral muscle. The muscular branches of the anterofemoral cutaneous nerve and femoral nerve are distributed. Indications: Irregular menstruation, dysmenorrhea, amenorrhea, metrorrhagia, pain in the medial thigh, abdominal distension and adverse flow of *qi*, dribbling of urine, erysepilas, anemia, excema, urticaria, skin itch. Puncture: 3—6 cm perpendicularly. Moxibustion: 3—5 moxa cones or 5—10 minutes with warming moxibustion.

Xuechou 血愁 [xué chóu] See Zhuzhang.

Xunyuan 循元 [xún yuán] An alternate term for Tianshu (ST 25).

Xunji 循际 [xún jì] An alternatet term for Tianshu (ST 25).

Xunji 循脊 [xún jǐ] An alternate term for Tianshu (ST 25).

Xuanlu (GB 5) 悬颅[xuán lú]A point of Gallbladder Meridian of Foot-*yangming*. Location: At the temporal corner, at the midpoint of the arc line connecting Touwei (at the hairline corner of the forehead) and Qubin (in the temporal hair anterior to the root of ear), i. e., between Hanyan (GB 4) and Xuanli (GB 6). Regional anatomy: There is the superficial temporal artery and vein. The temporal branch of the parietal branch of the aural temporal nerve is distributed. The temporal muscle is in the deeper. Indications: Migraine, pain in the outer canthus, toothache, swollen face. Puncture: 1—1.5 cm horizontally. Moxibustion: 1—3 moxa cones or 3—5 minutes with warming moxibustion.

xuanyang 悬阳 [xuán yáng] Referring to the

nasal region.

Xuanshu (GV 5) 悬枢 [xuán shū] A GV point. Location: Between the spinal processes of the 1st and 2nd lumbar vertebrae at the midline of waist. Regional anatomy: Passing through the myofascia of the waist and back and the superaspinal ligament, reaching at the interspinal ligament. There is the posterior branch of the lumabr artery. The medial branch of the posterior branch of the lumbar nerve is distributed. The lower end of the spinal cord is in the deeper. Indications: Stiffness and pain in the lumbar spine, abdominal distension, abdominal pain, indigestion, diarrhea, dysentery. Puncture: 1.5—3 cm obliquely. Moxibustion: 3—5 moxa cones or 5—10 minutes with warming moxibustion.

Xuanming 悬命 [xuán mìng] An extra point, also termed Guilu. Located at the midpoint of the frenulum of the superior lip. Indications: Mentol confusion and delirium, infantile convulsion. Puncture: 0.3—0.6 cm perpendicularly. (Fig 151)

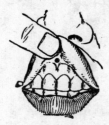

Fig 151

Xuanzhu 悬柱 [xuán zhù] I.e., Xuanshu (GV 5).

Xuanji 旋玑 [xuán jī] I.e., 璇玑, Xuanji (CV 21).

Xuanji 旋机 [xuán jī] I.e., 璇玑 (Xuanji, CV 21).

Xuexi 薛息 [xuē xī] I.e., Rugen (ST 18), also termed Xiongxue.

Xuli 虚里 [xū lǐ] The big collateral meridian of stomach, at the pulsation spot of the tip

of the heart.

Xuanli (GB 6) 悬厘 [xuán lí] A point of Gallbladder Meridian of *shaoyang*, the confluence of *shaoyang* and *yangming* meridians of hand and foot. Location: At the temporal corner, at the crossing point of the lower 1/4 and upper 3/4 of the line connecting Touwei (at the corner of the hairline at the lateral forehead) and to Qubin (in the temporal hair anterior to the root of the ear), between Xuanlu (GB 5) and Qubin (GB 7). Regionaal anatomy: At the temporal muscle. There is the parietal branch of the temporal superficial artery and vein. The temporal branch of the temproral nerve is distributed. Indications: Migraine, pain in the outer canthus, swollen face, tinnitus, pains in the upper teeth. Puncture: 1—1.5 cm horizontaly. Moxibustion: 1—3 moxa cones or 3—5 minutes with warming moxibustion.

Xuanzhong (GB 39) 悬钟 [xuán zhōng] A point of Gallbladder Meridian of Foot-*shaoyang*, the confluence of the bone marrow of the eight confluential points, also termed Juegu. Location: 9 cm directly below the tip of the lateral ankle, at the anterior edge of the fibula. Regional anatomy: Between the short muscle of fibula and the long extensor muscle of toe. There is the branch of the anterior tibial artery and vein. The superficial fibular nerve is distributed. Indications: Hemplegia, stiffness and pain in the neck, distension and fullness in the chest and abdomen, pain in the hypochondrium, pains in the knees and legs, foot *qi*, swelling below the axilla. Puncture: 3—4 cm perpendicularly. Moxibustion: 3—5 moxa cones or 15 minutes with warming moxibustion.

Xuanquan 悬泉 [xuán quán] An alternate term for Zhongfeng (LR 4).

Xuanjiang 悬浆 [xuán jiāng] An alternate term for Chengjiang (CV, RN 24)

Xuanji (CV 21) 璇玑 [xuán jī] A CV point. Location: At the thoracic midline, at the centre of the manubranium of sternun, or 3 cm below Tiantu (CV 22). Regional anatomy: There is the anterior perforating branch of the inferior breast artery and vein. The anterior branch of the supraclaviscular bone and the anterior branch of the 1st intercostal nerve are distributed. Indications: Cough and asthmatic breath, fullness and pain in the chest, something accumulating in the stomach, sore throat. Puncture: 1—1. 5 cm horizontally. Moxibustion: 3—5 moxa cones or 5—10 minutes with warming moxibustion.

Y

Yafengtong 牙风痛 [yá fēng tòng] I. e., Fengcitong.

Yamen (GV 15) 哑门 [yǎ mén] A GV point, the confluence of GV and Connecting Vessel of Yang, also termed Sheheng, Sheyan. Location: At the posterior midline of the nape, 1.5 cm above the posterior hairline. Regional anatomy: There is the nuchal ligament, the interspinal ligament, and the branches of the occipital artery and vein. The 3rd occipital nerve is distributed. The upper end of the spinal cord is in the deeper. Indications: Aphonia, aphasia, mania, epilepsy, heaviness of the head, headache, stiff neck and spine, apoplexy, hysteria, epistaxis, vomiting. Puncture: 1.5—3 cm perpendicularly or downwardly obliquely (It must not puncture superoanteriorly deeply). Moxibustion is prohibited.

Yangling 阳陵 [yáng líng] 1. An abbreviation Yanglingquan (GB 34); 2. Another name of Xiyangguan (GB 33).

Yanglingquan (GB 34) 阳陵泉 [yáng líng quán] A point of Gallbladder Meridian of Foot-*shaoyang*, the sea-like (earth) point of the meridian, the confluence of eight confluential points. Regional anatomy: Between the long peroneal muscle and the long extensor muscle of toe. There is the inferior lateral artery and vein of kee. The lateral cutaneous nerve of flibula and the superficial and deep peroneal nerve are distributed. Location: In the depression anterior-inferior to the small head of fibula. Indications: Swelling, fullness and pain of the chest and hypochondrium, swollen face, mainia, pain in the knee and thigh, atrobhy of the lower limbs. Puncture: 3—4.5 cm perpendicularly. Moxibustion: 3—5 moxa cones or 5—10 minutes with warming moxibustion.

Yangfu (GB 38) 阳辅 [yáng fǔ] A point of

Gallbladder Meridian of Foot-*shaoyang*, the rive-like (dfire) point of the meridian, also termed Fenrou, Jugn. Location: At the anterior edge of fibula, 12 cm above the lateral ankle. Regional anatomy: Between the long extensore muscle of toe and the short peroneal muscle. There are the branches of the anterior tibial artery and vein. There the superficial peroneal nerve is distributed. Indications: Migraine, pain in the outer canthi, pain in the supraclavicular fossa, pain in inferior axilla, scrofula, pains in the chest, hypochondrium and the lateral aspect of the lower libms, malaria, hemiplegia. Puncture: 3—4.5 cm perpendicularly. Moxibustion: 3—5 moxa cones or 5—10 minutes with warming moxibustion.

Yangwei 阳维 [yáng wéi] 1. Connecting Vessel of Yang; 2. Yangwei, the extra point located at the root of the auricle, at the wirylike tendon appearing posteriorly to the root of ear when the ear is pulled forward by the hand. Indication: Tinnitus, deafness, Puncture: 0.3—0.6 cm perpendicularly. Moxibustion: 1—3 moxa cones or 3—5 minutes with warming moxibustion.

Yangwei point 阳维穴 [yáng wéi xué] 1. The confluential point of Connecting Vessel of Yang according to the records of Systematic Classic of Acupuncture; 2. Referring to Waiguan (TE 5).

Yangxi (LI 5) 阳溪 [yáng xī] A point of Large Intestine Meridian of Hand-*yangming*, the river-like (fire) point of the meridian, also termed Zhongkui. Location: At the end of the radial side of the transverse crease of the dorsal wrist, in the depression between the long extensor muscle of thumb and the short extensor muscle of thumb when the thumbs are up. With the hands crossed the end of the thumb is the point. Regional anatomy: Between the extensor muscle of thumb of the short extensor muscle of thumb. There is the cephalic vein, the radial artery and the dorsal carpal branch. The superficial branch of the radial nerve is distributed. Indications: Headache, deafness, tinnitus, sore throat, pain in dental carrier, congestive eyes, nebula, febrile diseases and anxiety, pain in the arm and wrist, mania, epilepsy, insanity. Puncture: 1. 5—1. 8 cm perpendicularly. Moxibustion: 3—5 moxa cones or 5—10 minutes with warming moxibustion.

Yangku 阳窟 [yáng kū] The wrong form of Changku. Another name of Fujie (SP 14).

Yangze 阳泽 [yáng zé] I. e., Guichen. Another name of Quchi (LI 11).

yang collateral meridian 阳络 [yáng luò] Contrary to yin collateral meriadians, referring to the collateral meridians in the superficial part of the body.

Yangshi 羊矢 [yáng shǐ] 1. The name of the location. It originally means sheep's stool. It is therefore called because the lymphatic node that can be touched at the superiomedial aspect of thigh and below the groove resembles sheep's stool; 2. An extra point located in the transverse.

Yangqiao 阳跷 [yáng qiào] 1. Referring to Motility Vessel of Yang; 2. Referring to Shenmai (BL 65).

Yangqiao point 阳跷穴 [yáng qiào xué] The confluential point to Motility Vessel of Yang.

Yang Shangshan 杨上善 [yáng shàng shàn] A medical expert during Sui and Tang dynasties (618—907 A. D.). His birth place is unknown. He once compiled and noted Yellow Emperor's Internal Classic, *Taisu*, and *Huangdi Neijing Mingtang Leicheng*.

yangbai 杨白 [yáng bái] A wrong form of Yangbai (GB 14).

Yang Jizhou 扬继州 [yáng jì zhōu] An acupuncture expert in Ming Dynasty (1368—1644), born in Qu County, Zhejiang Province. His grandfather was once the royal doctor and there were many medi-

cal books in his family. He once learned medicine very conscientiously and later he worked at the Imperial Health Institute. In 1601, basing on the book handed down from his family and combining with his own experiences and medical records and selecting and recording acupuncture literatures of various schools, he completed the book Compendium of Acupuncture. In the book a lot of acupuncture techniques and extra points were recorded and described, the materials were selected widely, the contents are rich, which has made a great contribution to the development of acupuncture science.

Yangming **meridian** 阳明脉 [yáng míng mài] The name of the meridian during the early period. Referring to foot.

Yangzhilingquan 阳之陵泉 [yáng zhī líng quán] I. e., Yanglingquan (GB 34).

Yangjiao (GB 35) 阳交 [yáng jiāo] A point of Gallbladder Meridian of Foot-*shaoyang*, the gap-like point of Connecting Vessel of Yang, also termed Bieyang, Zuliao. Location: Approx. 3 cm above the tip of the lateral ankle. Regional anatomy: At the long fibular muscle. There are the branches of the fibular artery and vein. The lateral cutaneous nerve of calf is distributed. Indications: Distension, fullness and pain in the chest and hypochondrium, swolen face, mania, pain in the knees and thigh, atrophy of lower limbs. Puncture: 3—4. 5 cm perpendicularly. Moxibustion: 3—5 moxa cones or 5—10 minutes with warming moxibustion.

Yangguan 阳关 [yáng guān] A GV point. One located at the waist; The other pertains to Gallbladder Meridian and is located at the knee. In modern times it is usually called Yaoyangguan (GV 3) and Xiyangguan (GB 33).

Yangchi (TE 4) 阳池 [yáng chí] A point of Triple Energizer Meridian of Hand-*shaoyang*, also termed Bieyang, the source point of the meridian, also called Bieyang. Location: In the depression at the edge of the ulnar side of the common extensor muscle of fingers on the transverse crease of the dorsal wrist. Regional anatomy: At the long fibular muscle. There are the branches of the fibular artery and vein. The lateral cutanous nerve of calf is distributed. Indications: Pain in the wrist, pains in the shoulder and arm, deafness, malaria, emaciation-thirst disease, dry mouth, sore throat. Puncture: 1—1.5 cm perpendicularly. Moxibustion: 3—5 moxa cones or 5—10 minutes with warming moxibustion.

Yanggu (SI 5) 阳谷 [yáng gǔ] A point of Small Intestine Meridian of Hand-*taiyang*, the river-like (metal) point of the meridian. Location: In the depression anterior to the smaller end of ulna at the ulnar end of the transverse crease of the dorsal wrist. Regional anatomy: Swollen neck, pain in the lateral aspect of the arm, pain in the wrist, febrile disease without sweat vertigo, congestive and painful eyes, mania, hypochondriac pain, scabies and wart, hemorrhoids, deafness, tinnitus, toothache. Puncture: 1—2 cm perpendicularly. Moxibustion: 3—5 moxa cones or 5—10 minutes with warming moxibustion.

Yanggang (BL 48) 阳纲 [yáng gāng] A point of Bladder Meridian of Foot-*taiyang*. Location: 9 cm lateral to Zhongshu (GV 7) below the spinal process of the 10th thoracic vertebra. Regional anatomy: passing through the broadest muscle of back, reaching at the iliocostal muscle. There is the posterior branch of the 10th intercostal artery and vein. The lateral branches of the posterior branches of the 9th thoracic nerves are distributed. Indications: Jaundice, borborygmus, diarrhea, abdominal pain, emaciation-thirst disease. Puncture: 1.5—2 cm obliquely. (deep puncture is not proper) Moxibustion: 3—5 moxa cones or 5—15 minutes with warming moxibustion.

Yangbai (GB 14) 阳白 [yáng bái] A point of Gallbladder Meridian of Foot-*shaoyang*, the confluence of foot-*shaoyang* meridian and

Connecting Vessel of Yang. Location: With the eyes look straight forward, directly above the pupil 3 cm above the eyebrow. Regional anatomy: At the temporal muscle. There are the lateral branches of the temporal artery and vein. The lateral branch of the temporal nerve is distributed. Indications: Headache, vertigo, ocular pain in the outer canthi, tremor of eyelids, contraction of the visional field. Puncture: 1—1.5 cm horizontally. Moxibustion: 1—3 moxa cones or 3—5 minutes with warming moxibustion.

Yanggang 阳刚 [yáng gāng] 1. I. e., 阳纲; 2. The extra point located 3 cm lateral to Mingmen (GV, DU 14). Indications: emaciation-thirst disease, jaundice, melena due to intestinal hemorrhoids, affection, lumbago, enuresis, nocturnal emission. Puncture: 1.5—3 cm perpendicularly. Moxibustion: 3—7 moxa cones or 5—15 minutes with warming moxibustion.

yang in yin 阴中隐阳 [yīn zhōng yǐn yáng] An acupuncture manipulation, symetrical to yin in yang. The manipulation of first reducing and then reinforcing. That is to first practicing acupuncture in the deep by swiftly thrusting the needle but slowly inserting it at the times of number of 'six'. After the patient feels slightly cool, withdraw the needle to the superficial area to practice acupuncture by swiftly inserting the needle but slowly thrusting it at the times of the number of 'nine', so as to acquire *qi*. It can be used for treating the symptom of earlier fever and later chilliness. (Fig 152)

yanhou 咽喉 [yān hóu] A collective term for the pharynx and larynx.

Yankou 燕口 [yàn kǒu] An extra point, located at the dorsal-palmar boundary between the two corners of mouth. Indications: Mania, deviated mouth and eyes, infantile spasm, constipation, anuresis, triangular neuralgia. Puncture: 1—1.5 cm horizontally.

Yanglao (SI 6) 养老 [yǎng lǎo] A point of

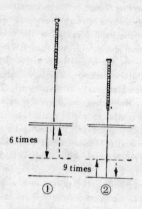

① Swift thrusting and slow lifting
② Swift lifting and slow thrusting
Fig 152

Small Intestine Meridian of Hand-*taiyang*, the gap-like point of the meridian. Location: In the inteosseous space at the radial side of styloid process of ulna, at the dorsum of the small head of ulna. While locating it, take the palm toward the chest. Regional anatomy: Between the ulnar extensor muscle of wrist and the proper extensor muscle of small finger. There are the terminal branches of the interosseous dorsal artery and vein of forearm and the dorsal vein network of wrist. The dorsal cutaneous nerve of forearm and the commissure branch of the dorsal branch of the ulnar nerve are distributed. Indications: Blurred vision, pains in the shoulder, back, elbow and arm, acute lumbago. Puncture: 1—1.5 cm perpendicularly or obliquely. Moxibustion: 3—5 moxa cones or 5—10 minutes with warming moxibustion.

yanmen 咽门 [yān mén] The opening of the pharynx.

yanzi 研子 [yán zǐ] An abbreviation of *liang shou yan zi gu*.

Yao zhu 腰注 [yāo zhù] An alternate term for Yaoshu (GV 2).

Yaoshu (GV 2) 腰俞 [yāo shū] A GV point, also termed Jijie, Suikong, Yaohu, Yaozhu, Suishu. Location: At the sacral midline, in the hiatus of the sacral canal. Regional anatomy: Passing through the sacrococcygeal ligament, reaching at the hiatus of the sacral canal. There are the branches of the sacral artery and vein. The branch of the coccygeal nerves is distributed. Indications: Stiffness and pain in the lumbar spine, diarrhea, constipation, hemarrhoids, prolapse of anus, hemafecia, epilepsy, irregular menstruation, atroply of the lower limbs. Puncture: 1.5—3 cm obliquely puncture. Moxibustion: 3—7 moxa cones or 5—15 minutes with warming moxibustion.

Yaoyan 腰眼 [yāo yǎn] An extra point, also termed Guiyan, Yaomuliao. Located 9—12 cm lateral to the spinal processes of the 4th and 5th lumbar vertebrae, in the depression of the waist. Indications: Consumptive disease, lumbago, pain in the lower abdomen, renoptosis, testitis, lumbar sprain, strain of the lumbar soft tissue. Puncture: 3—4.5 cm perpendicularly. Moxibustion: 5—7 moxa cones or 10—20 minutes with warming moxibustion. (Fig 153)

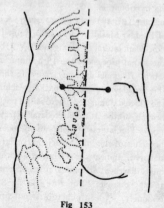

Fig 153

Yaohu 腰户 [yāo hù] An alternate term for Yaoshu (GV 2)

Yaokong 腰孔 [yāo kǒng] An alternate term for Shiqizhui (EX-B8).

Yaomu 腰目 [yāo mù] An extra point located 4.5 cm below Shenshu (BL 23), bilateral to the spine. Used for treating emaciation-thirst disease and frequent urination. Moxibustion: 3—7 moxa cones or 5—15 minutes with warming moxibustion.

Yaoyangguan (GV 3) 腰阳关 [yāo yáng guān] A point of GV, originally termed Yangguan. The character 'yao' was added later. Location: At the midline of the lumbar region, between the spinal processes of the 4th and 5th lumbar vertebrae, approx., at the level with the iliac spinal crest. Regional anatomy: Passing through the lumbar myofascia, reaching at the superior spinal ligament and the interspinal ligament. There is the posterior branch of the lumbar artery. The medial branch of the posterior branch of the lumbar nerve is distributed. Indications: lumbosacral pain, atrophy of the lower limbs, irregular menstruation, lueukorrhea, spermatorrhea, hemafecia, impotense. Puncture: 1.5—3 cm obliquely. Moxibustion: 3—7 moxa cones or 5—15 minutes with warming moxibustion.

Yaoqi 腰奇 [yāo qí] An extra point located 6 cm directly above the tip of the coccyx. Indication: Epilepsy. Puncture: 6—9 cm horizontally.

Yeguang 夜光 [yè guāng] An alternate term for Zanzhu (BL 2).

Yejian 掖间 [yè jiān] An alternate term for the extra point, Yemen (TE 2).

Yellow Emperor's *Mingtang* **Moxibustion Classic** 黄帝明堂灸经 [huáng dì míng táng jiǔ jīng] A medical book. The original occurred before Tang Dynasty (618—907 A.D.), written by an unknown person. It was compiled into Peaceful Holy Benevolent Prescriptions by Wang Huaiyin.

Yellow Emperor 黄帝 [huáng dì] The legendary ancestor of the Chinese nation. Internal Classic was written in the form of questions and answers between the Yellow Emperor and Qi Bo, etc. According to Han Book, the books of various schools that had been inscribed with the Yellow Emperor have 21 kinds, most of which deal with formulary. Yellow Emperor's Internal Classic is one of them. During the Warring States Periods (770—221 B. C.) and the beginning of the Han Dynasty (206 B. C. —220 A. D.) the Yellow Emperor and Laozi's works were mentioned simultaneously, called 'Huanglao'.

Yellow Empeoror's Internal Classic 黄帝内经 [huáng dì nèi jīng] A medical book briefly termed Internal Classic, including Miraculous Pivot and Plain Questions, formed approx. from the Warring States Periods (770—221 B. C.) to Qin and Han dynasties (221B. C. —220A. D.), in the name of Yellow Emperor. It is a theoretical medical work that has been preserved in China. The descriptions concerning acupuncture-moxibustion in the book have laid a solid foundation for the development of acupuncture moxibustion science in latter generations.

Yemen 掖门 [yè mén] I. e., Yemen (TE, SJ 2), an extra point, located at the midline of axilla, 3 cm below the axillary fossa. Select it when the arm is lifted. Indications: Headache, congestive eyes, ocular pain, tinnitus, deafness, sore throat, malaria, pain in arms. Puncture: 1—1.5 cm. Moxibustion can be done.

Yemen (TE 2) 液门 [yè mén] A point of Triple Energizer Meridian of Hand-*shaoyang*, the spring-like (water) point of the meridian. Location: At the dorsal hand, between the 4th and 5th fingers, in the depression anterior to the metacarpophalangeal joint, at the dorsopalmar boundary. Regional anatomy: There is the digital dorsal artery coming from the ulnar artery. The dorsal branch of the ulnar nerve is distributed. Indications: Headache, vertigo, congestive eyes, ocular pain, deafness, tinnitus, sore thoat, pains in the shoulder, back and elbow, inability of the fingers to move, pain in the spine, febrile disease. Puncture: 1—1.5 cm perpendicularly. Moxibustion: 1—3 moxa cones or 3—5 minutes with warming moxibustion.

Yemen 腋门 [yè mén] 1. Yemen (TE 2); 2. An alternate term for Daju (ST 27).

Yeqi 腋气 [yè qì] An extra point. It is located at the acea where the black spot appears when it is painted with starch powder. Moxibustion: 3—5 moxa cones. Indications: Bramhydrosis.

Yexia 腋下 [yè xià] An extra point, located at the lateral chest, on the axillary midline, 4.5 cm below the axillary fossa. Indications: Bromhydrosis, intercostal neuralgia. Puncture: 1—1.5 cm obliquely. Moxibustion: 3—5 moxa cones or 5—10 minutes with warming moxibustion.

yi 颐 [yí] The area lateropposterior to the *chin*, and lateroinferior to the angle of the mouth, over the lateralosuperior part of the mandible.

yi 嗌 [yì] Referring to the upper esophagus.

Yi Huan 医缓 [yī huǎn] A medical expert in Qin Kingdom during the Spring Autumn and Warring States Periods. According to *Zuo Juan*, Jin Hou was ill and went to Qin Kingdom for medial care. Yi Huan went to treat him and said, "Your disease can not be treated because it is located above *huang* and below *gao*, which can not be treated neither by moxibustion nor by acupuncture or drug." That is the early record on treating disease with acupuncture and moxibustion in the historical book concerned.

Yifeng (TE 17) 翳风 [yì fēng] A point of Triple Energizer Meridian of Hand-*shaoyang*, the confluence of hand-*shaoyang* and foot-*shaoyang* meridians. Location: At the posterior process of the temple and mandible. Regional anatomy: There is the posterior au/rical artery and vein and the lateral cervical vain. The greater nerve of ear is distributed. The deeper stratum is where the stem of the facial nerve penetrates from the styloid mastoid foramen. Indications: Tinnitus, deafness, deviated mouth and eyes, closejaww, swollen cheek,

scrofula. Puncture: 1.5—3 cm perpendicularly. Moxibustion: 1—3 moxa cones or 5—10 minutes with warming moxibustion.

yige 噎嗝 [yí gé] Feeling obstruction of swallowing in the throat is called '*yi*', while diffculty of blockage of the swallowed food in the chest, '*ge*'. They are considered collectively and may be seen in carcinoma of the stomach, carcinoma of esophagus, esophagostenosis, esophagus spasm, etc.

Yiming 翳明 [yì míng] An extra point, located posterior to the ear, in the fibre anterior to the sternocleidomastoidous muscle, i.e., approx. 3 cm posterior to Yifeng (TE, SJ 17). There is the posterior aural artery and vein. The sympathetic nerve 16 in the deeper. The vagus nerve and the supracervical nerve mode of the sympathetic trunk are distributed. Indications: Myopia, hyperopia, night blindness, headache, tinnitus, vertigo, insomnia, cateract, glaucoma, atrophy of the visual nerve, mumps, mental trouble. Puncture: 3—4.5 cm perpendicularly. (Fig 154)

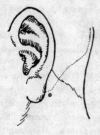

Fig 154

yin blockage 阴闭 [yīn bì] 1. Referring to pain blockage and heavy blockage as caused by pathogenic cold and dampness; 2. The blockage of the five storing viscera because the five storing viscera belong to yin.

ying (**nutrition**) and *wei* (**defense**) 营卫 [yíng wèi] A collective term for nutritional *qi* and defensive *qi*. Both of them pertain to *qi* derived from refined cereals. The former has the nutritional action on the internal organs while the latter has the action of defending the body surface.

Yingtu 应突 [yīng tū] An extra point, located 3 cm below the 6th intercostal space, 18 cm lateral to the middle of stern. Punctured: 1—1.5 cm horizontally. Moxibustion: 3—5 moxa cones or 5—10 minutes with warming moxibustion.

Yingchi 营池 [yíng chí] An extra point located in the depression anterioposterior to the inferior edge of the medial ankle. Each foot has two, four in total. Indications: Profuse menstruation, leukorrhea. Puncture: 0.6—0.9 cm perpendicularly. Moxibustion: 3—7 moxa cones or 5—15 minutes with warming moxibustion.

Yinnangxiahengwen 阴囊下横纹 [yīn náng xià héng wén] An extra point located at the midpoint of the 1st transverse crease below the scrotum. Moxibustion: 3—5 moxa cones or 5—10 minutes with warming moxibustion.

Yingzhongwaishu 膺中外俞 [yīng zhōng wài shū] Referring to Yunmen (LU 2) and Zhongfu (LU 1).

Yingzhongshu 膺中俞 [yīng zhōng shū] An alternate term for Zhongfu (LU 1).

Yingshu 膺俞 [yīng shū] 1. Referring to various points of the 3rd lateral line of the chest; 2. Generally referring to various meridian points of the chest; 3. Referring to Zhongfu (LU 1).

Yinmen (BL 37) 殷门 [yīn mén] A point of Bladder Meridian of Foot-*taiyang*. Location: 18 cm directly below Chengfu (BL 36) at the midpoint of the transverse crease of the hip. Regional anatomy: Between the biceps muscle and the semitendinous muscle. There is the 3rd perforating branch of the deep femoral artery and vein at its lateral aspect. The posterior femoral nerve is distributed. The sciatic nerve is in the deeper. Indications: Stiffness and pain in the lumbar spine, pain in thigh. Puncture: 3—4.5 cm perpendicularly. Moxibustion: 5—15 minutes with warming moxibustion.

Yinlingquan (SP 9) 阴陵泉 [yīn líng quán] A point of Spleen Meridian of Foot-*taiyin*, the sea-like (water) point of the meridian. Location: In the depression at the inferior edge of the ankle at the medial aspect of the tibia. Regional anatomy: At the posterior edge of tibia, passing between the anterior semimenmbranous muscle and the gastrocnemious musle, reaching at the starting point of the soleus muscle. There is the great saphenous vein and the supreme genicular artery. There is the posterial tibial artery and vein in the deeper. The medial cutaneous nerve of leg is distributed. The tibial nerve is in the deeper. Indications: Abdominal distension, abdominal pain, edema, jaundice, vomiting, loose stool, difficulty or incontinence of urine, urethra infection, nocturnal emission, foot *qi*, pain in the knee, atrophic blockage of the lower abdomen. acute/chronic enteritis, bacterial dysentery, rentention of urine, infection of the urethral duct, hypertension, disorder of the soft tissues surrounding the knee joint. Puncture: 3—6 cm perpendicularly. Moxibustion: 3—5 moxa cones or 5—10 minutes with waming moxibustion.

Yinwei point 阴维穴 [yīn wéi xué] 1. The confluential point of Connecting Vessel of Yin. According to Systematic Classic of Acupuncture, acupuncture treatment of acute bacterial dysentery with Yinlingquan (SP 9) can make the index of the white cells remarkably increase; 2. Referring to Neiguan (PC 6); 3. An alternate term for Dahe (KI 12).

Yinnangfeng 阴囊缝 [yīn náng fèng] An extra point, also termed Nangxiafeng, located on the midline at the inferior scotum.

Yinjiao 断交 [yīn jiāo] I.e., Yinjiao (GV 28).

yinjin 婴筋 [yīn jīn] Referring to the big tendon, i.e., the anterior part of the sternocleidomastoidous muscle.

Yindu (KI 19) 阴都 [yīn dū] 1. A point of Kidney Meridian of Foot-*shaoyin*, the confluence of Vital Vessel. Foot-*shaoyin* meridian, also termed Shigong, Tongguan. . Location: 1. 5 cm lateral to Zhongwan (CV 12), 12 cm above the umbilicus. Regional anatomy: At the medial edge of musculus rectus femoris. There are the branches of the superior epigastric artery and vein. The 8th intercostal nerve is distributed. Indications: Abdominal distension, abdominal pain, belching, vomiting, borborygmus, difficulty in defecation, sterility. Puncture: 3—4. 5 cm perpendicularly. Moxibustion: 5—7 moxa cones or 10—15 minutes with warming moxibustion; 2. The extra point, i. e., Jingzhong.

Yinling 阴陵 [yīn líng] A brief term for Yinlingquan (SP 9).

Yingjiao (GV 28) 龈交 [yíng jiāo] A GV point. Location: In the upper lip, at the connective junction between the frenunum of the superior lip and gum. Regional anatomy: There is the artery and vein of the upper lip. The branch of the superior alveolar nerve is distributed. Indications: Swollen and painful gums, deviated mouth and lockjaw, foul mouth, epistaxis, rhinitis, flushed face and swollen cheek, stiffness in the corner of the mouth, facial sore and tinea, sores at the bilateral cheek, mania, stiff neck. Puncture: 0. 6—0. 9 cm obliquely. Moxibustion is prohibited.

ying 瘿 [yīng] An enlargement of the thyroid gland.

Yingchuang (ST 16) 膺窗 [yíng chuāng] A point of Stomach Meridian of Foot-*yangming*. Location: At the 2nd lateral line of the chest, in the 3rd intercostal space, 1. 2 dm lateral to Yutang (CV, RN 18) at the thoracic midline. Regional anatomy: At the greater thoracic muscle and the lesser thoracic muscle. There is the lateral artery and vein of the chest. The branch of the anterior sternal nerve is distributed. Indication: Cough, asthmatic breath, distension and pain of the chest and hypochondrium, breast carbuncle. Puncture: 1—1. 5 cm

obliquely. Moxibustion: 3—5 moxa cones or 5—10 minutes with warming moxibustion.

Yingxiang (LI 20) 迎香 [yíng xiāng] A point of large Intestine Meridian of Hand-*yangming*, the confluence of *yangming* meridians of hand and foot, also termed Chongyang. Location: In the nasolabial groove, at the level with the lateral edge of ala nasi. Regional anatomy: At the quadrate muscle of the upper lip. There is the facsial artery and vein and the branches of the infraorbital artery and vein. The anastomotic branch of the facial nerve and the infraorbital nerve are distributed. Indications: Stuffy nose, epistaxis, nasal polyp, deviated mouth and eyes, facial itch, puffy face.

Yingu (KI 10) 阴谷 [yīn gǔ] A point of Kidney Meridian of Foot-*shaoying*, the sea-like (water) point of the meridian. Location: At the medial aspect of the transverse crease of the cubital fossa when the knee is flexed between the semitendinous muscle and semimembranous muscle. Regional anatomy: There is the superomedial artery and vein of knee. The medial cutaneous nerve of thigh is distributed. Indications: Impotence, hernia, pain, irregular menstruation, metrorrhagia, dysuria, pain in the pubic region, mania, pain in the medial aspect of the knee and thigh. Puncture: 3—4. 5 cm perpendicularly. Moxibustion: 3—5 moxa cones or 5—10 minutes with warming moxibustion.

Yinbao (LR 9) 阴包 [yīn bāo] A point to Liver Meridian of Foot-*jueyin*. Location: On the medial aspect of the thigh, at the posterior edge of the cubital fossa 12 cm directly above Ququan (LR 8) at the end of the transverse crease of the sartorius muscle. Select it when the knee is flexed. Regional anatomy: Passing through the midpoint of the long adductor muscle, reaching at the short adductor muscle. There is the femoral artery and vein on the lateral side of the deeper region. There is the superficial branch of the medial circumflex femoral artery. The anterial cutaneous nerve of thigh, and the anterier branch of the obductor muscle are distributed. Indications: Irregular menstruation, dysuria, lumbosacral pain referring to the lower abdomen. Puncture: 3—6 cm perpendicularly. Moxibustion: 3—5 moxa cones or 5—10 minutes with warming moxibustion.

Yinshi (ST 33) 阴市 [yīn shì] A point of Stomach Meridian of Foot-*yangming*, also termed Yinding. Location: 9 cm above the base of patella on the line connecting the antero-superior illiac process at the anterolateral thigh. Regional anatomy: Between musculus rectus femoris and the lateral femoral muscle. There is the descending branch of the lateral femoral circumflex artery. The femoral rectal cutaneous nerve, the la-teral femoral cutancous nerve and the muscular branch of the femoral nerve are distributed. Indications: Distension, abdominal pain, numbness, pain and dfficult movement, pains in the knees, foot *qi*, paralysis of the lower limbs, lumbago, cold hernia, abdominal distension and pain. Puncture: 1. 5—3 cm perpendicularly. Moxibustion: 3—5 moxa cones or 5—10 minutes with warming moxibustion.

yin-yang 阴阳 [yīn yáng] 1. One of the basic theories in traditional Chinese medicine. Originally from the ancient philospohical thought, which divides everything and phenomenon as the two aspects, yin and yang, and possesses the primitive dialectic viewpoint. They are the basic rule of the natural world, and are the guiding priniciple of everything, and the source of which the biological objects grow, develop and change. In acupuncture science. *Shu* points, diagnostic techniques and treatments all can not depart from them; 2. Yinyang, an extra point, at the crease of the medial aspect of the metatarrsal joint of the thumb. Indications: Syncope, diarrhea. Puncture: 0. 6—0. 9 cm perpendicularly. Moxibustion: 3—5 moxa cones or 5—10 minutes with warming mox-

ibustion; 3. Another name of Yingchi, the extra point.

yin-yang point-combined method 阴阳配穴法 [yīn yáng pèi xué fǎ] One of the pointcombind methods. Referring to the combination and application of the points of yin and yang meridians. E. g. , Neiguan (PC 6) combines with Zusanli (ST 36) to treat stomach trouble; Sanyinjiao(SP 6)combines with Zusanli (ST 36) to treat indigestion, Lieque (LU 7) combines with Hegu (LI 4)to treat common cold, etc. It is called *biao li pei xue fa* (external-internal point-combined method) if the two meridians the combined points pertain to are related externally and internally. Location: 3 cm below the mubilicus on the midline of the abdomen. Regional anatomy: In the white abdominal line. There are the branches of the superficial artery and vein of the abdominal wall and those of the inferior artery and vein of the abdominal wall. The anterial cutaneous branch of the 10th intercostal nerve is distributed. The small intestine is in the deeper. Indications: Abdominal pain, diarrhea, irregular menstruation, metrorrhagia, leukorrhea, dysemenorrhea, itch of the pubic region, sterility, hernia, edema, bacterial dysentery, intestinal paralysis, functional bleeding of uterus. Puncture: 3— 4. 5 cm perpendicularly. (Be cautious for the pregnant woman) Moxibustion: 3—7 moxa cones or 10—15 minutes with warming moxibustion.

Yinguan 阴关 [yīn guān] An alternate term for Dahe (KI 12) and Changfu (BL 36).

Yinxi 饮郄 [yǐn xī] An extra point. Located in the 6th intercostal space 18 cm to the sternal midline. Indications: Abdominal pain, borborygum, pains in the chest and hypochondrium. Puncture: 1—1. 5 cm obliquely, or 5—10 minutes with warming moxibustion.

Yintang 印堂 [yìn táng] An extra point located at the midpoint of the line connecting the two end of the eyebrows. There is musculus corrugator supercilli. There are the branches of the artery and vein at the interior aspect of the forehead on the bilateral side. The superior pulpebral branch of 4th supratrochlear nerve is distributed. Indications: Headache, vertigo, vomiting, insomnia, rhinitis, epistaxis, ocular pain, blurred vision, pain in the supraorbital area, facial deep-rooted sore, acute/chronic infantile convulsion, postpartum anemic fainting, eclapsia, common cold, rhinitis, hypertension, triangular neuralgia. Puncture: 1.5—3 cm horizontally. Moxibustion: 5—10 minutes with warming moxibustion. (Fig 155)

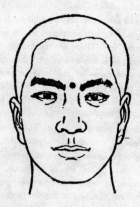

Fig 155

Yinzhilingquan 阴之陵泉 [yīn zhī líng quán] I. e., Yinlingquan (SP 9).

Yinji point 阴基穴 [yīn jī xué] An extra point, also termed Shitou. Located at the superior to the urethra. Indications: Epilepsy, withdarwal of the genitalia. Moxibustion: 5—10 minutes with warming moxibustion.

yin puncture 阴刺 [yīn cì] One of the twelve needling techniques for treating cold *jue* syndrome of the lower limb due to exhaustion of yang *qi*. It is to puncture bilaterally Taixi (KI 3) of Kidney Meridian of Foot-*shaoyin* behind the medial malleolus of the foot. The left and right points are cooperated and used widely in clinic.

Yinxi (HT 6) 阴郄 [yīn xī] 1. A point of Heart Meridian of Hand-*shaoyin*, the gap-like point of the meridian. Location: At the palmar side of the forearm, 1.5 cm above the transverse crease of the wrist, at the radial aspect of the ulnar flexor muscle of wrist. Regional anafomy: Passing through between ulnar flexor muscle of wrist and the superficial flexor muscle of fingers, reaching at the deep flexor muscle of finger and the quadrate pronator muscle. The ulnar artery passes through it. The medial cutaneous muscle of forearm is distributed. The ulnar nerve is in the deeper. Indication: Cardialgia, fright, palpitation, steaming of bones, spitting blood, epistaxis, aphasia. Puncture: 1.5—2.5 cm perpendicularly. Moxibustion: 1—3 moxa cones or 3—5 minutes with warming moxibustion.

yin collateral meridians 阴络 [yīn luò] Contrary to yang collateral meridians, referring to the collateral meridians in the deep part of the body. The yin collateral meridians in the deeper part of the body are similar to the meridians while the yang ones in the superficial are of different in color due to flourishing and decline of *qi* and blood.

Yinlian (LR 11) 阴廉 [yīn lián] A point of Liver Meridian of Foot-*jueyin*. Location: On the medial side of thigh, 6 cm directly below Qichong (ST 30), 6 cm lateral to the midpoint of the superior edge of symphysis pubis. Regional anatomy: There are the branches of the medial circumflex artery and vein at the long and short abductor muscles. The genral femoral nerve and the medial cutaneous nerve of thigh are distributed. The anterior branch of the obductor muscle is in the deeper. Indications: Irregular mensturaton, leukorrhea, pain in the bilateral lower abdomen, pain in the medial aspect of the thigh, spasm of the lower limbs. Puncture: 2—6 cm perpendicularly. Moxibustion: 3—5 moxa cones or 5—

10 minutes with warming moxibusion.

Yinding 阴鼎［yīn dǐng］An alternate term for Tinshi（ST 33）.

yin organ 阴器［yīn qì］Referring to external genitalia, also termed the anterior yin.

Yinqiao point 阴跷穴［yīn qiào xué］1. The confluential point of Motility Vessel of Yin. They are Zhaohai（KI 16）and Jiaoxin（KI 8）where Motility Vessel of Yin converges into foot-*shaoyin* meridian, and Jingming（BL 1）of foot-*taiyang* meridian above which it meets motility vessel of Yang; 2. Referring to Zhaohai（KI 16）, one of the eight confluential point.

Yishe（BL 49）意舍［yì shè］A point of Bladder Meridian of Foot-*taiyang*. Location: 9 cm lateral to Jizhong（GV, DV 6）between the spinal processes of the 11th and 12th thoracic vertebrae. Regional anatomy: Passing through the broadest muscle of back, reaching at the iliolumbar muscle. There are the posterior branches of the 11th intercostal artery and vein. The lateral branch of the posterior branch of the 10th and 11th thoracic vertebrae is distributed. Indications: Abdominal distension, borborygmus, vomiting, anorexia. Puncture: 1.5—2.5 cm obliquely. (It is not advisable to puncture deep) Moxibustion: 5—7 moxa cones or 10—20 minutes with warming moxibustion.

Yishanmen 一扇门［yī shàn mén］A massage point located at the radial aspect of the 3rd metacarpal bone. It can relieve fever and has the diaphoretic action. Indications: Infantile anhidrosis, persistent fever, acute convulsion, deviated mouth and eyes.

Yishu 胰俞［yí shū］An alternate term for Weiguangxiashu.

Yiwofeng 一窝风［yī wō fēng］A massage point located at the midpoint of the transverse crease of the dorsal wrist. Indications: Abdominal pain, acute/chronic convulaion, dearrhea, pathogenic wind and heat by diaphoresis.

Yixi（BL 45）噫嘻［yì xī］A point of Bladder Meridian of Foot-*taiyang*. Location: 9 cm lateral to Lingtai（GV 10）between the spinal processes of the 6th and 7th thoracic vertebrae. Regional anatomy: Passing through the lateral edge of the trapezius muscle, reaching at the iliocostal muscle. There are the posterior branches of the 6th intercostal nerve artery and vein. The medial cutaneous branch of the posterior branches of the 5th and 6th thoracic vertebrae is distributed. The lateral branches of the posterior branches of the 5th and 6th thoracic nerves are in the deeper. Indications: Cough, asthmatic breath, pains in the shoulder and back, hypochandriac pain referring to the bilateral side, malaria, branchial astma, lower abdomen, vertigo, epistaxis, malaria, febrile disease with no sweat. Puncture: 1.5—2.5 cm obliquely. (It is not advisable to puncture deep) Moxibustion: 3—5 moxa cones or 5—15 minutes with warming moxibustion.

Yongquan（KI 1）涌泉［yǒng quán］A point of Kidney Meridian of Foot-*shaoyin*, the well-like point of the meridian, also termed Dichong. Location: At the sole. In the depression when the metatarsopohalangeal joint is flexed. Regional anatomy: Passing through the short flexor muscle of toe, the long flexor muscle of toe, and the lumbrical muscle, reaching at the interosseous muscle. There is the medial artry of the sole and the plantar arch. The common nerve of the 2nd plantar toe is distributed. Indications: Vertical pain, dizziness, blurred vision, aphonia, dysuria, difficulty in defecation, infantile convulsion, feverish sensation in the soles, mania, cholera with cramp, syncope. Puncture: 1.5—3 cm perpendicularly. Moxibustion: 1—3 moxa cones or 5—10 minutes with warming moxibustion.

Youmen（KI 21）幽门［yōu mén］A point of Kidney Meridian of Foot-*shaoyin*, the confluence of Vital Vessel and foot-*shaoyin* meridian, also termed Shangmen. Location: 1.5 cm lateral to Juquen（CV 14）, 18 cm

above the umbilicus. Regional anatomy: At
the medial edge of the straight muscle of
thigh. There is the branch of the superficial
epigastic artery and vein. The 7th intercostal nerve is distributed. Indications: Distension and fullness on in the chest and abdomen, anxiety, vomiting, belching, indigestion, abdominal pain and diarrhea, dysentery. Puncture: 1. 5—3 cm perpendicularly.
(It is not advisable to puncture deeply)
Moxibustion: 5—7 moxa cones or 5—15
minutes with warming moxibustion.

Youguan 右关 [yòu guān] I. e., Shiguan (KI
18).

Youyuye 右玉液 [yòu yù yè] See Jinjin (EX-
HN 12), Yuye (EX-HN 13).

yu 鱼 [yú] The proinene of the palm proximal
to the thumb or that of the sole proximal to
the big toe. It is so called because its shape
is like the fish belly. The thenar eminence
of the hand.

yu collateral meridain 鱼络 [yú luò] Referring
to the collateral meridian at the dorsal
thenar eminence. The thenar eminence pertains to Lung Meridian of Hand-*taiyin*,
passes through the opening of the stomach
and externally-internally related to Stomach Meridian of Hand-*yangming*. So,
stomach trouble can be diagnosed and examined from the variation of the color of
the collateral meridian at the thenar eminence.

Yuanzhu 元柱 [yuán zhù] I. e., Yuanzhu, another name of Zanzhu (Bl 2)

Yuanzhu 员柱 [yuán zhù] An alternate term
for Zanzhu (BL 2).

Yuan Jue 圆觉 [yuán jué] A monk in the end
of Qing Dynasty (1644—1911). He was
very experienced in acupuncture and *qigong*
(Chinese deep breathing exercises) and
handed his techniques down to Huang Ship-
ing.

Yuanzhai 员在 [yuán zhài] An alternate term
for Zanzhu (BL 2)

Yuaner 元儿 [yuán ér] An alternate term for
Danzhong (CV 17).

Yuanye （GB 22） 渊液 [yuān yè] A point of
Gallbladder Meridian of Foot-*shaoyang*.
Location: At the axillary line, in the interspace of the 5th intercostal space. Select it
when the arm raised. Regional anatomy: At
the serratus anterior muscle. There is the
thoracoepigastric artery and vein. The lateral cutaneous branch of the 4th intercostal nerve and the branch of the long thoracic nerve are distributed. Indications:
Fullness in the chest, pain in the hypochondrium, swelling beneath the axilla, pain in
the shoulder and arm. Puncture: 1. 5—2. 5
cm obliquely or horizontally. Deep puncture
is prohibited. Moxibustion: 3—5 minutes
with warming moxibustion.

Yuchang 鱼肠 [yú cháng] I. e., Yufu, an alternate term for Chengshan (BL 57).

Yuhuan 玉环 [yù huán] Name of the location.
It refers to the area between the heart, kidneys, liver and spleen, opposite to the umbilicus according to Taoist viewpoints.

Yuhu 玉户 [yù hù] An alternate term for
Tiantu (CV 11).

Yuhuanshu 玉环俞 [yù huán shū] An alternate
term for Baihuanshu (BL 30).

Yuji 鱼际 [yú jì] 1. Yuji (LU 10), A point
of Lung Meridian of Hand-*taiyin*, the
spring (fire) point of the meridian. Location: At the thenar eminance, in the midpoint of the 1st palmer metacarpal bone, at
the dorso-palmar boundary. Regional
anatomy: In the short-addouctor muscle of
thumb and the opposing muscle of thumb.
There is the venous branch that flows from
the thumb to the cephalic vein. The superficial radial branch of the radial nerve is distributed. Indications: Cough, hemoptysis,
aphonia, sore throat, general fever, breast
carbuncle, spasm of the ellows, feverish
sensation in the palm. Puncture: 1. 5—3 cm
perpendicularly. Moxibustion: 3—5 moxa
cones or 5—10 minutes with warm
needling; 2. An anatomical location. It is
called '*yu*' or '*shouyu*' that the protuberance formed by the globoid muscle of

thumb. The dorso-palmar boundary is called '*yu*'.

Yumentou 玉门头 [yù mén tóu] An extra point, also Nuyinfeng, located on the head of the clitoris of the woman's external genitalia. Indications: Women's yin sore, mania. Puncture: 1 cm deep. Moxibustion: 3—7 minutes with moxa stick.

Yuyao 鱼腰 [yú yāo] An extra point, located in the centre of the eyeblow. When looking straight forward, it is directly above the pupil. There is the lateral branch of the frontal artery and vein and the lateral branch of the frontal nerve. Indications: Migraine and vertical headache, swelling and congestion of eyes, nebula, myopia, as well as keratitis and conjunctivitis, paralysis of ocular muscle, supraorbital neuralgia. Puncture: 1—1.5 cm horizontally.

Yuying 玉英 [yù yīng] An alternate term for Yutang (CV 18).

Yuzhong 彧中 [yù zhōng] An extra point. Located at the face. One is located at the anterior edge of the process of the helix. The other is located at the level with the inferior edge of the lobre.

Yuzhong 彧中 [yù zhōng] I. e. Yuzhong (KI 26).

Yuzhong (KI 26) 彧中 [yù zhōng] A point of Kindney Meridian of Foot-*shaoyin*. Location: 6 cm lateral to Huagai (CV, RN 20) at the midline of chest, in the 1st intercostal interspace. Regional anatomy: At the greater pectoral muscle. There is the 1st intercostal artery and vein. The anterior cutaneous branch of the 1st intercostal nerve and the anterior branch of the supraclavicular nerve are distributed. The 1st intercostal nerve is in the deeper. Indications: Cough, asthmatic breath, profuse sputum, fullness and distension in the chest and hypochondrium, vomiting, breast carbuncle, asthmatic breath, salivation. Puncture: 1—1.5 cm obliquely. (It is not advisable to puncture deep) Moxibustion: 3—5 moxa cones or 5—10 minutes with warming moxibustion.

ibustion.

Yuzhen (BL 9) 玉枕 [yù zhěn] A point of Bladder Meridian of Foot-*taiyang*. Location: 3.5 cm lateral to Naohu (GV, DU 17), on the superior edge of the external occipital protuberance, downwardly opposite to Tianzhu (BL 10). Regional anatomy: At the occipital muscle. There are the occipital artery and vein. The branch of the greater occipital nerve is distributed. Indications: Headache, aversion to wind and cold, vomiting, ocular pain, reduced vision, stuffy nose. Puncture: 1 cm horizontally. Moxibustion: 1—3 moxa cones or 3—5 minutes with warming moxibustion.

Yunmen (LU 2) 云门 [yún mén] A point of Lung Meridian of Hand-*taiyin*. Location: Laterosuperior to the anterior chest, at the inferior edge of the clavicle, 2 dm lateral to the thoracic midline, or 3 cm above Zhongfu (LU 1). Select it in the supine position. Regional anatomy: Between the broadest muscle of chest and the deltoid muscle. There are the cephalic vein, the thoracoacrominal artery and vein. The axillary artery is below. The middle and posterior branches of the supraclavicular nerve, the branch of the anterothoracic nerve and the lateral bundle of brachial plexus are distributed. Indications: Sudden blindness, deafness, tinnitus, pains in the shoulder and back, pains in the hypochondrium, vomiting, constipation, febrile diseases. Puncture: 3 cm perpendicularly. Moxibustion: 3—5 moxa cones or 5—10 minutes with warming moxibustion.

Yuquan 玉泉 [yù quán] 1. An alternate term for Zhongji (RN 3); 2. An extra point, located 2 dm below the umbilicus, on the root of the penis. Indications: Swelling of scrotum, testitis. Puncture: 1 cm perpendicularly. Moxibustion: 3—7 moxa cones or 5—15 minutes with warming moxibustion; 3. An extra point located 3.5 cm lateral to the midline of head, on the superior edge of the external occipital protuberance, 3 cm below Yuzhen (BL 9). Moxibustion: 1—3 moxa cones or 3—5 minutes with warming moxibustion.

Yutian 玉田 [yù tián] An extra point, located in the depression below the styloid process of the 4th thoracic vertebra. Indications: Dystocia, pain in the lumbosacral region. Puncture: 1.5—3 cm horizontally. Moxibustion: 3—5 moxa cones or 5—10 minutes with warming moxibustion.

Yutang (CV 18) 玉堂 [yù táng] A CV point also termed Yuying, located on the midline of chest, at the level with the 3rd intercostal space. Regional anatomy: In the proper sternal bone. There are the anterior perforating branches of the artery and vein in the mammary gland. The anterior cutaneous branch of the 3rd intercostal nerve is distributed. Indications: Thoracalgia, cough, asthmatic breadth, short breath, sore throat, vomiting, cold sputum, swelling and pain of the breast. Puncture: 1 cm horizontally.

Yuye (EX-HN 13) 玉液 [yù yè] See Jinjin, Yuye.

Yuwei 鱼尾 [yú wěi] 1. An extra point, located at the end of the transverse crease of the outer canthus. Indications: Headache, migraine, ocular trouble, facial paralysis, Puncture: 1—1.5 cm horizontally; 2. Referring to Tongziliao (GB 1).

Z

Zafeng 匝风 [zā fēng] An alternate term for Naohu (GV 17).

zanghui 藏会 [zàng huì] I. e. , Fuhui.

Zang-fu(staring-emptying)**organs** 脏腑[zàng fǔ]A collective term for internal organs, including the five storing viscera, six emptying viscera and unusual organs. *Zang* refers to being capable of storing refined principle; *'fu'* refers to being capable of receiving and transporting food.

Zangshu 藏俞 [zàng shū] An extra point, located at the posterior midline, at the end of the spinal process of the 5th thoracic vertebra. According to Prescriptions Worth of a Thousand Gold, its indications are aversion to wind, aphasia, muscular blocakge, and unconsciousness.

Zeqian 泽前 [zé qián] An extra point, located 3 cm below Chize (LU 5), directly opposite to the middle finger. Indications: Enlargement of the thyroid, paralysis of the upper limb, spasm of forearm. Puncture: 1.5— 3 cm perpendicularly. Moxibustion: 3—5 moxa cones or 5—10 minutes with warming moxibustion.

Zhangmen(**LR 13**)章门 [zhāng mén]A point of Liver Meridian of Foot-*jueyin*, the anterior referred point of the spleen, the *zang* confluence of the eight confluential points, the confluence of foot-*jueyin* meridian and foot-*shaoyang* meridian, also termed Changping, Xieliao. Location: At the lateral abdomen, at the lower end of the 11th rib. At the end of the tip of the rib when the elbow is flexed and the axilla is closed. Regional anatomy: At the terminal branch of the 10th intercostal space. There is the 10th intercostal nerve slightly below it. Indications: Vomiting, diarrhea, cough, jaundice, pains in the waist, back, and hypochondrium, abdominal pain, abdominal distension, edema, indigestion, masses, ma-

nia, unobstruction of defecation and micturition, hepatitis, enteritis, enlargement of liver, intercostal neuralgia. Puncture: 1. 3— 2. 5 cm perpendicularly (It is not advisable to puncture deep). Moxibustion: 3—5 moxa cones or 5—10 minutes with warming moxibustion.

Zhaohai（**KI 6**）照海 [zhào hǎi] A point of Kidney Meridian of Foot-*shaoyin*, the starting point of Motility Vessel of Yin. One of the eight confluential points, communicated with Motility Vessel of Yang. Location: 3 cm directly below the tip of the medial ankle, i. e. , 1. 2 cm below the inferior tibial artery and vein at the postero-inferior part. The medial cutaneous nerve of leg is distributed. The basic stem of the tibial nerve is in the deeper. Indications: Dry thoroat, epilepsy, insomnia, lethargy, congestion, swelling and pain of the eyes, irregular menstruation, leukorrhea, dysmenorrhea, prolaps of uterus, itch of the pubic region, hernia, frequent urination, insomnia, foot *qi*. Puncture: 1. 5—3 cm perpendicularly. Moxibustion: 3—5 moxa cones or 5—10 minutes with warming moxibustion.

Zhang Sanxi 张三锡[zhāng sān xī]A medical expert in Ming Dynasty （1368—1664）, born at Nanjing, Jiangshu Province. He learned medicine from Wang Kentang. In 1609 he wrote Six Key Points of Medicine. The 1st volume is Textral Study on Meridians, in which he brought out that in research on the formulary, pulse and acupuncture one should clear up the locations of the meridians and search for their origins. He had textually studied and expounded meridian theories.

Zhang Sanlei(1872—1934)张三雷[zhāng sān léi]A contemporary medical expert, born at Jiading (pertaining to Shanghai City at present). He did clinical and teaching work of traditional Chinese medicine with great efforts,and wrote a lot of books. On the basis of *Yixue Zhigui* written by Zhao Shutang in Qing Dynasty (1644—1911), he compiled New Textual Study on Meridians and *Shu* Points in 1027, etc. , and contributed to the expounding the meridian theory and textual study on *shu* points.

Zhang Jiebin (1562—1639) 张介宾 [zhāng jiè bīn] A medical expert in Ming Dynasty (1368—1644),born at Huiji(Shaoxin,Zheijiang Province at present). He learned medicine from Jin Mengshi and had studied Internal Classic for 30 years, and wrote Classified Classic, Illustratied Supplement of Classified Classic, Supplement of Classified Classic,of which the descriptions about acupuncture and meridians are rich. During his later age, he wrote Complete Book of Zhang Jingyue, to which special attention has been paid by the later medical expert in succeeding dynasties.

Zhang Zhongjing 张仲景 [zhāng zhòng jǐng] An outstanding medical expert at the end of Eastern Han Dynasty (25—220 A. D.), born at Nanyang county. (Henan Province at present) He "deligently searched for the ancients",doctrines and adopted many popular formulas widely, wrote Treatise on Cold Injury and Miscellaneous Diseases, which was systematized by the later scholars into two books,Synopsis of the Goldern Chamber and Treatise on Cold Injury. The application of differentiating the syndromes with the names of the six meridians is the expounding development of the meridian theory. The two books mainly deal with drug treatments, accompanied by acupuncture-moxibustion, including apropriateness, warming needling, burning needling, fumigation, ironing, etc.

Zhangzhong 掌中 [zhǎng zhōng] Referring to Laogong (PC 8).

Zanzhu(BL 2)攒竹[zàn zhú]A point of Bladder Meridian of Foot-*taiyang*, also termed Shiguang, Yeguang, Mingguang, Yuanzai.

Location: In the depression at the medial end of the eye brow, opposite to Jingming (BL 1). Regional anatomy: In the temporal muscle of the superciliary corrugator muscle. There are the temporal artery and vein. The medial branch of the teporal nerve is distributed. Indication: Headache, pain in the supra-orbital bone, vertigo, blurred vision, congestion, swelling and pain of the eyes, lacrimation, myopeia, tremor of eyelids, facial paralysis. Puncture: 1—1. 5 cm horizontally, or to prick to cause little bleeding. Moxibustion is prohibited.

Zhao Xi (1877—1938) 赵熙 [zhào xī] A comtemporary acupuncture expert born at Dai County, Shanxi province. He loved study from childhood, knew history very well and was good at medicine and pharmacology. He adopted the strengthens of various schools and treated diseases very effectively and paid special attention to medial morality, and did not search for benefits with medicine. He was once the lecturer of Shanxi Chinese Medicine Improving Research Association, and wrote Real Handing Down of Acupuncture by combining his individual experiences on the basis of Internal Classic, Difficult Classic, Systematic Classic of Acupuncture, and Cold Injury.

Zhengu 枕骨 [zhěn gǔ] 1. An alternate term for Touqiaoyin (GB 11); 2, Referring to the orccipital bone, located posterior to the cranial head.

Zheijin(GB 23)辄筋[zhé jīn]A point of Gallbladder Meridian of Foot-*shaoyang*. Location: 3 cm anterior to Yuanye (GB 22) at the crossing point of the axillary line and the 4th intercostal space. Select it when the arm is lifted. Regional anatomy: At the seratus anterior muscle. There are the lateral artery and vein of chest and the 4th intercostal vein. The lateral cutaneous branch of the 4th intercostal nerve is distributed. Indications: Pains in the chest and hypochondrium, asthmatic breath, vomiting, acid regurgitation, swelling of axilla, pains in the shoulder and arm. Puncture: 1—1.5 cm obliquely(deep puncture is prohibited). Moxibustion: 1—3 moxa cones or 3—5 minutes with warming moxibustion.

Zhengying (GB 17) 正营 [zhèng yíng] A point of Gallbladder Meridian of Foot-*shaoyang*, the confluence of foot-*shaoyang* meridian and Connecting Vessel of Yang. Location: With the eyes look forward, 3—15 cm directly above the pupil, 3—15 cm in the hairline, i. e. , 3 cm above Muchuang (GB 16). Indications: Headache, vertigo, dizziness, stiffness of the corner of the mouth, toothache, Puncture: 1—2 cm horizontally. Moxibustion: 3—5 moxa cones or 5—10 minutes with warming moxibustion.

zhichu(EX-CA 1) 子处[zhǐ chǔ]I. e. , uterus.

Zhihu 子户 [zhǐ hù] 1. An alternate term for Qixue (KI 13); 2. An extra point.

Zhigou(TE 6) 支沟[zhī gōu]A point of Triple energizer Meridian of Hand-*shaoyang*, the river-like (fire) point of the meridian it pertains to. Also termed Feihu. Location: 1 dm above the transverse crease of wrist, between the ulna and radius. Regional anatomy: Between the long extensor muscle of thumb and common extensor muscles. There are the interosseous dorsal artery and vein of forearm and the stems of palmar artery and vein. The cutaneous dorsal nerve of forearm is distributed. The interosseous dorsal nerve of the forearm of radius and the interosseous extensor nerve of the central nerve are in the deeper. Indications: Febrile diseases, headache, cardialgia, swollen thorat, tinnitus deafness, closejaw, sudden aphonia, vomiting, constipation, hypochondriac pain, angina pectoris, pleurasy, intercostal neuralgia. Puncture: 3—5 cm perpendicularly. Moxibustion: 3—5 moxa cones or 5—10 minutes with warming moxibustion.

Zhizheng (SI 7) 支正 [zhǐ zhèng] A point of Small Intestine Meridian of hand-*taiyang*, the connecting point of the meridian it pertains to. Location: On the line connecting

Yanggu (SI 5) and Xiaohai (LU 4), 15 cm above Yanggu(SI 5). Regional anatomy: At the ulner extensor muscle of wrist. There are the terminal branches of the interosseous dorsal artery and vein of forearm. The cutaneous medial branch of forearm is distributed. Indications: Chillss and fever, headache, vertigo, stiff neck, swollen cheek, spasmodic elbow, pains in the fingers, inability of the hands to raise, mania, neuroasthenia, auditory vertigo. Punctre: 1.5—3 cm perpendicularly or obliquely. Moxibustion: 3—5 moxa cones or 5—10 minutes with warming moxibustion.

Zhigen 指根[zhǐ gēn]An extra point, located at the midpoint of the transverse creases of the 2nd, 3rd, 4th and 5th metacpophalangeal joints, eight in total. Indication: Deep-rooted sore at the hand, pains in the five fingers, abdominal pain and vomiting, fever. Prick to cause little bleeding by a triangular needle.

Zhiyang (GV 9) 至阳 [zhì yáng] A GV point. Location: Between the spinal process of the 7th and 8th thoracic vertebrae on the midline of the back. Regional anatomy: Passing through the fascia of the waist and back, the supraspinal ligament and interspinal ligament. There is the posterior branch of the 7th intercostal artery. The medial branch of the posterior branch of the 7th thoracic nerve is distributed. The spinal cord is in the deeper. Indication: Distension and pain in the chest and hyochondrium, abdominal pain, jaundice, cough, asthmatic breath, pains in the waist and back, stiff spine, general fever. Puncture: 1.5—3 cm obliquely. Moxibustion: 3—5 moxa cones of 5—10 minutes with warming moxibustion.

Zhiyin (BL 67) 至阴 [zhì yīn] A point of Bladder Meridian of Foot-*taiyang*, the well-like (metal)point of the meridian. Location: Approx. 0.3 cm lateral to the corner of the toenail on the lateral side of the small toe. Regional anatkomy: There is the arterial network formed by arteriae digitales planteres and the proper plantar digital artery. The proper plantar digital nerve and the lateral cutaneous nerve of the dorsal foot are distributed. Indications: Headache, stuffy nose, epistaxis, ocular pain, feverish sensation in the sole, retension of the placenta, dystocia. Punctured: 0. 3—0. 6 cm obliquely to prick to cause little bleeding with a triangular needle. Moxibustion: 3— 5 moxa cones or 5—10 minutes with warming moxibustion.

Zhigong 至宫 [zhì gōng] The wrong form of Zhiying (BL 67).

Zhiying 至营 [zhì yíng] An alternate term for Muchuang (GB 16).

Zhichang 直肠 [zhí cháng] 1. The last segment of the large intestine; 2. An alternate term for Chenjin (BL 56).

Zhigu 直骨 [zhí gǔ] An extra point, located on the transverse crease directly below the nipple. Moxibustion: 3—5 moxa cones or 5—10 minutes with warming needling.

Zhichuan Point 治喘穴 [zhì chuán xué] An alternate term for Chuaixi Point.

Zhibian (BL 54) 秩边 [chì biān] A point of Bladder Meridian of Foot-*taiyang*. Location: 9 cm lateral to Yaoshu (GV 2) below the pseudo-spinal process of the 4th sacral vertebra. Regional anatomy: At the greatest gluteal muscle. At the inferior edge of piriformis. There is the inferior gluteal artery and vein. The inferior gluteal nerve, the posterior cutaneous nerve of thigh and the sciatic nerve are distributed. Indications: Lumbosacral pain, atrophy of the lower limbs, abnormal defecation and micturition, pains in the pubic region, hemorrhoids. Puncture: 3—6 cm perpendicularly. Moxibustion: 3—7 moxa cones or 5—15 minutes with warming moxibustion.

Zhishi (BL 52) 志室 [zhì shì] A point of Bladder Meridian of Foot-*taiyang*. Location: 9 cm lateral to Mingmen (GV, DU 4) between the 2nd and 3rd lumbar vertebrae. Regional anatomy: Passing through the broadest muscle of back, reaching at the il-

iocostal muscle. There are the posterior branches of the 2nd lumbar artery and vein. The lateral branch of the posterior branch of the 12th thoracic nerve and that of the 1st lumbar nerve are distributed. Indications: Spermatorrhea, impotence, pain and swelling in the pubic region, dribbling of urine, edema, stiffness and pain in the lumbar spine. Puncture: 1. 5—2. 5 cm obliquely. (Deep puncture is not proper.) Moxibustion: 5—7 moxa cones or 10—20 minutes with moxibustion.

Zhitang 志堂 [zhì táng] A wrong form of Zhishi (BL 52).

Zhongju 中矩 [zhōng jù] An extra point, also termed Chuiju. Located on the medial side of the mandible below the mouth cavity, at the midline of the transferring part of the base of the mouth and mucoid membrane of the gum.

Zhong zhijie 中指节 [zhōng zhǐ jié] Located on the dorsal side of the middle finger, in the depression slightly anterior to the midpoint of the transverse crease of the interphalangeal articulation of hand.

zhong 踵 [zhǒng] Referring to the root of Achilles.

Zhourong (SP 20) 周荣 [zhōu róng] A poin of Spleen Meridian of Foot-*taiyin*. Location: At the 2nd intercostal space, 18 cn lateral to Zigong (CV 19) at the midpoint of chest. Regional anatomy: Between the greatest and lesser muscles of chest. There are the lateral pectoral artery and vein and the 2nd intercostal artery and vein. The muscular branch of the anterior thoracic nerve and the lateral cutaneous branch of the 2nd intercostal nerve are distributed. Indications: Distension and pain in the chest and hypochondrium, poor appetite, cough and asthmatic breath, spitting suppurative blood. Puncture: 1—1. 5 cm obliquely (deep puncture is prohibited). Moxibustion: 3— 5 moxa cones or 5—10 minutes with warm needling.

Zhouying 周营 [zhōu yíng] I. e. , Zhourong

(SP 20)

Zhoujian 肘尖 [zhǒu jiān] 1. Referring to the tip of the protruding tip of the acromion, also used as an extra point. Indications: Scrofula, furuncle and carbuncle, deep-rooted sore; 2. Another name of Zhouliao.

Zhongdu (LR 6) 中都 [zhōng dū] 1. A point of Liver Meridian of Foot-*jueyin*, the gaplike point of the meridian, also termed Zhongxi. Location: 2 dm directly above the tip of the medial ankle, in the centre of the medial side of tibia. Regional anatomy: There is the posterior artery of tibia. The medial cutaneous branch of leg of the proper nerve and muscular branch of the tibial nerve are distributed. Indications: Hypochondriac pain, abdominal distension, diarrhea, hernia, pain in the lower abdomen, metrorrhagia, dystocia. Puncture: 1.5—2 cm horizontally. Moxibustion: 1—3 moxa cones or 3—5 minutes with warming moxibustion; 2. Another name of Shenmen (HT); 3. One of Baixie (EX-UE 9).

Zhonge 中恶 [zhōng è] An extra point. Indications: Abdominal pain, pains in the chest and hypochondrium, intercost neuralgia. Moxibustion: 3—5 moxa cones or 5—10 minutes with warming moxibustion.

Zhonglushu 中膂俞 [zhōng lǚ shū] I. e., Zhonglushu (BL 29).

Zhongwan (CV 12) 中脘 [zhōng wán] A point of CV, the anterior-referred point of the stomach, also the confluential point of hand-*taiyang* meridian, hand-*shaoyang* meridian, foot-*yangming* meridian and CV. The confluence of the emptying viscus of the eight confluential points in Difficult Classic, also termed Taichong, Weiwan, Shangji. Location: 1.2 dm above the umbilicus on the midline of the abdomen. Regional anatomy: In the white abdominal line. There is the hypognstric artery and vein. The anterior cutaneous branch of the 7th Epigastric pain, abdominal distension, vomiting, hiccup, acid regurgitation, indiges-

tion, infantile malnutrition, jaundice, borborygmus, diarrhea, constipation, firmness and pain below the hypochondrium, spitting blood due to the consumptive disease, asthma, headache, insominia, mania, epilepsy, convulsion. Puncture: 3—4 cm perpendicularly. (Cautiously used in the case of the pregnant woman) Moxibustion: 3—7 moxa cones or 10—20 minutes with warming moxibustion.

Zhongshang 中商 [zhōng shāng] One of Sanshang.

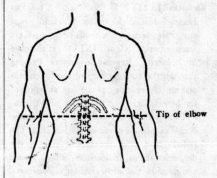

Tip of elbow

Fig 156

Zhouzhui 肘椎 [zhǒu zhuī] An extra point, located at the waist, let the patient take prone position, extend the arms. It is 3 cm lateral to the crossing point of the line connecting the tip of the elbow and the midline of the spin. Indications: Cholera, vomiting and diarrhea, convulsion, distension and pain in the epigastrium, vomiting and diarrhea. Puncture: 1.5—3 cm obliquely. Moxibustion: 3—5 moxa cones or 5—15 minutes with warming moxibustion. (Fig 156)

Zhoushu 肘俞 [zhǒu shū] An extra point, located posterior to the elbow joint, in the depression between the protuberance of acromion and the small head of radius. Indications: Disorders of the elbow joint and its surrounding tissurs. Puncture: 1 cm perpendicularly. Moxibustion: 3—5 moxa cones or 5—10 minutes with warming moxibustion. (Fig 157)

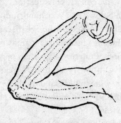

Fig 157

Zhouliao (LI 12) 肘髎 [zhǒu liáo] A point of Large Intestine Meridian of Hand-*yang-ming*, also termed Zhoujian. Location: 3 cm laterosuperior to Quchi(KI 11), at the edge of humerus. Reginal anatomy: Passing through the starting part of the brachioradial muscle, reaching at the lateral aspect of the brachial triceps muscle. There is the radial collateral artery and vein. There is the dorsal cutaneous nerve of the forearm. The radial nerve is in the medial side of the deeper stratum. Indications: Pain, spasm and numbross of ellow, lethargy. Puncture: 1.5—3 cm perpendicularly. Moxibustion: 3—5 moxa cones or 5—10 minutes with warming moxibustion.

Zhongji (CV 3) 中极 [zhōng jí] A point of CV, the anterior referred point of the bladder, the confluence of three yin meridians of foot and CV. Also termed Yuquan, Qiyuan. Location: 1.2 dm below the mbilicus on the midline of the abdomen. Regional anatomy: In the white abdominal line. There are the branches of the superficial gastric artery and vein and those of the hypogastric artery and vein. The branch of the iliohypogastric nerve is distributed. Indications: Nocturnal emission, premature ejaculation, impotence, enuresis, dysuria, irregular menstruation, dysmenorrhea, metrorrhagia, leukorrhea, prolapse of uterus, retention of placenta, edema. Puncture: 3—5 cm perpendicularly. (It must be cautious for pregnant women) Moxibustion: 3—7 moxa cones or 10—20 minutes with warming moxibustion.

Zhongzhu (TE 3) 中诸 [zhōng zhù] A point of Triple Energizer Meridian of Hand-*shaoyang*, the stream-like (wood) point of the meridian, also termed Xiadu. Location: In the depression posterior to the metacarpo-phalangeal joint between the 4th and 5th metacarpal bones on the dorsal hand. Regional anatomy: In the white abdominal line. There is the hypergastric artery and vein. The anterior cutaneous branch of the 7th intercostal nerve is distributed. Indications: Headache, tinnitus, congestive eyes, deafness, ocular pain, sore throat, febrile diseases, pains in the elbow and arm, inability of the fingers to extend, pain in the spine. Puncture: 1—2 cm perpendicularly. Moxibustion: 3—5 moxa cones or 5—10 minutes with warming moxibustion.

Zhongdu (GB 32) 中渎 [zhōng dú] A point of Gallbladder Meridian of Foot-*shaoyin*. Located: 1.5 dm at the horizontal line of the transverse crease of the cubital fossa, between the middle of the lateral side of the thigh, or 6 cm directly below Fengshi (GB 31). Regional anatomy: In the illotibial bundle and lateral muscle of thigh. There are the muscular branches of the lateral femoral circumflex artery and vein. The lateral femoral cutaneous nerve and the femoral branch of the femoral nerve are distributed. Indications: Hemiplegia, atrophy and numbness of the lower limbs. Puncture: 3—6 cm perpendicularly. Moxibustion: 3—5 moxa cones or 5—10 minutes with warming moxibustion.

Zhongdu 中犊 [zhōng dú] I. e., Zhongdu (GB 32).

Zhongguan 中管 [zhōng guǎn] I. e., Zhong-wan (CV 12).

Zhongkui 中魁 [zhōng kuí] 1. An alternate term for Yangxi (LI 15); 2. The extra point, located on the dorsal side of the middle finger, at the midpoint of the tansverse crease of the proximal phalangeal articulation of finger. Select it with the finger flexed. Indications: Vomiting, obstructive sensation of swallowing and difficult swallowing, epistaxis, toothache, vitiligo. Moxibustion: 3-7 moxa cones. (Fig 158)

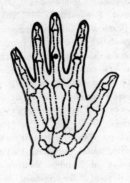

Fig 158

Zhongxi 中郄 [zhōng xī] 1. I. e., Zhongdu (LR 6) 2. I. e., Xizhong, another name of Weizhong (BL 40).

Zhongfu (LU 1) 中府 [zhōng fǔ] A point of Lung Meridian of Hand-*taiyin*, the anteriorreferred point of the lung, the conflunence of hand-*taiyin* and meridians. Location: 1. 8 dm lateral to the midline of the chest, at the level with the 1st intercostal space, laterosuperior to the chest, or 3 cm below Yumen (TE 2). Location: In the supine position. Regional anatomy: There is the axillary artery and vein and the thoracoacromial artery and vein. The central branch of the supraclavicular nerve, the branch of the anterothoracic nerve and the lateral branch of the 1st intercostal nerve are distributed. The needle passes through the broader and lesser thoracic muscles, reaches the 1st intercostal internal and external muscles. Indications: Cough, asthmatic breath, thoracalgia, full and suffocationg chest, sore throat, pain in the shoulder, abdominal distension, puffiness, pain in the shoulder and back. Puncture: 1. 5— 3 cm obliquely toward the lateral side of

the chest wall. Moxibustion: 3—5 moxa cones or 5—10 minutes with warming moxibustion.

Zhongzhu (KI 15) 中注 [zhōng zhù] A point of Kidney Meridian of Foot-*shaoyin*, the confluence of Vital Vessel and foot-*shaoyin* meridian. Location: 1. 5 cm lateral to Yinjiao (CV 7), 3 cm below the umbilicus. Location: Irregular menstruation, contipation, pains in the waist and abdomen, diarrhea, dysentery. Puncture: 3—5 perpendicularly. Moxibusti on : 3—5 moxa cones or 5—10 minutes with warming moxibustion.

Zhongzhu 中柱 [zhōng zhù] I. e., Zhanshu (GV 7).

Zhongquan 中泉 [zhōng quán] An extra point. Located on the transverse crease of the wrist of the dorsal hand, at the midpoint of the line connecting Yangchi (TE Sj 4) and Yangxi (LI 5). Indications: Cardialgia, fullness of *qi* in the chest that makes the patient fail to sleep, distension and fullness of the lungs, nebula, feverish sensation in the palms, adverse flow of gastric *qi*, spitting blood, *qi* pain in the abdomen. Puncture: 1—2 cm perpendicularly. Moxibustion: 3—7 moxa cones or 5—15 minutes with warming moxibustion.

Zhongting (CV 16) 中庭 [zhōng tíng] A point of CV, located on the thoracic midline, at the joining part of the stern and xiphoid process, 4 cm below Danzhong (CV 17). Regional anatomy: The anterior perforating branch of the internal mammary artery and vein. The anterior cutancous branch of the 6th intercostal nerve is distributed. Indications: Full chest hiccup, vomiting, cardialgia. Puncture: 1—2 cm horizontally. Moxibustion: 3—5 moxa cones or 5—10 minutes with warming moxibustion.

Zhonglushu 中膂俞 [zhōng lǚ shū] A point Bladder Meridian of Foot-*taiyang*, also termed Jineishu. Location: 3—4 cm lateral to the midline of sacral region, in the posterior foramen of the 3rd sacrum. Regional anatomy: Passing through the greater gluteal muscle, reaching the starting point of the sacrospinal muscle. There are the posterior branches of the lateral artery and vein of sacrum and the branches of the inferogluteal artery and vein. The lateral branches of the posterior branches of the lateral branches of the 3rd and 4th sacral nerves are distributed. Indications: Dysentery, hernia, stiffness and pain in the lumbar spine, hernia, emciation-thirst disease. Puncture: 3—4 cm perpendicularly. Moxibustion: 3—7 moxa cones or 5—15 minutes with warming moxibustion.

zhonglu 中膂 [zhōng lǚ] I. e., Zhong lushu (BL 29).

Zhongluneishu 中膂内俞 [zhōng lǚ nèi shú] I. e., zhong lushu (BL 29)

zhongliao (BL 33) 中髎 [zhōng liáo] A point of Bladder Meridian of Foot-*taiyang*, also termed Zhongkong. Location: In the posterior formamen of the 3rd sacrum, on the lateral side of the medial sacral crest, or at the lower end of the pseudospinal process of the 3rd sacrum, 2.4 dm to the sacral midline. Regional anatomy: There are the posterior branches of the lateral artery and vein of sacrum. The posterior branch of the 3rd sacral nerve is distributed. Indications: Irregular menstruation, leukorrhea, lumbago, dysuria, constipation. Puncture: 3—4 cm perpendicularly. Moxibustion: 3—7 moxa cones or 5—15 minutes with warming moxibustion.

Zhongshu (GV 7) 中枢 [zhōng shū] A point of GV. Location: Between the spinal processes of the 10th and 11th thoracic vertebrae on the midline of the back. Regional anatomy: Passing through the fascia of the waist and back, the supraspinal ligament and the intestinal ligament. The posterior branch of the 10th thoracic nerve is distributed. The spinal cord is in the deeper. Indications: Jaundice, vomiting, fullness of abdomen, stomachache, anorexia, pains in the waist and back. Puncture: 1.5—3 cm obliquely. Moxibustion: 3—5 moxa cones or

5—10 minutes with warming moxibustion.

Zhongfengbuyu point 中风不语穴 [zhōng fēng bù yǔ xué] An extra point located on the spinal process of the 2nd and 5th thoracic vertebrae. Indications: Apoplplexy, aphasia. Moxibustion: 3—5 moxa cones or 5—10 minutes with warming moxibustion.

Zhongping 中平 [zhōng píng] An extra point located on the centre of metacarpophangeal transverse crease of the middle finger. Indication: Stomaitis. Puncture: 0.6—0.9 cm perpendicularly. Moxibustion: 1—3 moxa cones or 3—5 minutes with warming moxibustion.

Zhongchong (PC 9) 中冲 [zhōng chōng] A meridian point, pertaining to Pericardium Meridian of Hand-*jueyin*, the well-like (wood) point of the meridian. Location: Approx. 3 cm lateral to the corner of the fingernail on the radial side of the middle finger, or in the centre of the tip of the middle finger. Regional anatomy: There is the network of the artery and vein formed by the digital-palmar proper artery and vein, the digital palmar proper nerve of the central nerve is distributed. Indications: Coma due to apoplexy, stiff tongue, sunstroke, fainting, infantile convulaion, febrile diseases swelling and pain below the tongue. Puncture: 0.3—0.6 cm perpendicularly, or prick to cause little bleeding. Moxibustion: 1—3 moxa cones or 3—5 minutes with warming moxibustion.

Zhongshou 中守 [zhōng shǒu] An alternate term for Shuifeng (CV 9).

Zhu lian 朱琏 [zhū lián] (1910—1978) A contemprary acupuncture spicialist, born in Suyang, Jianshu Province. At her earlier age, she took part in Chinese Revolution, carried on medical work and administrative health leading work. During the initial stage of the Anti-Japanese War, she learned acupuncture from Ren Zhotian at Yunan, Later she populariezed and applied it in the troops and held the training course to cultivate a lot of acupuncture practitioners. At the initial stag of the Liberation of China. She created the Experimental Research Institute of Acupuncture Therapy (the former institute of China's Academy Acupuncture). In 1954, she was the Vice President of China Academy of Traditional Chinese Medicine and President of Institute of Acupuncture Research. In 1960 she transferred to Nanjing City and created Nanjing Municipal Institute of Acupuncture Research and Nanjing Municipal Acupuncture College, and she herself taught the students. She also wrote New Acupuncture Science.

Zhuangu 转谷 [zhuǎn gǔ] An extra point. Located at the lateral chest directly below the plica of the anterior axilla, in the 3rd intercostal space. Indications: Fullness of the chest and hypochondrium, anorexia, vomiting, intercostal neuralgia. Puncture: 1—1.5 cm obliquely. Moxibustion: 3—5 moxa cones or 5—10 minutes with warm needling.

zhuan 纂 [zuǎn] Referring to the anal region.

Zhugu 拄骨 [zhù gǔ] See *zhu gu*. (柱骨)

Zhushi 疰市 [zhù shì] I.e., 注市.

Zhubin 筑滨 [zhú bīn] I.e., Zhubin (KI 9).

zhuo 䫏 [zhuō] Referring to the zygomatic region below the eye.

Zhuzhang 竹杖 [zhú zhàng] An extra point located on the posterior midline, above the spine, opposite to the umbilicus. Indications: Lumbago, hematuria, spitting blood, epistaxis, hemorrhoids, prolapse of anus, prolapse of uterine, difficulty in urination, chornic enteritis, difficulty in urination, chornic enteritis, intestinal tuberculosis, disorder of the spinal cord. Moxibustion: 3—5 moxa cones or 5—10 minutes with warming moxibustion. (Fig 159)

Zhi Cong 知聪 [zhī cōng] The pioneer who spread Chinese acupuncture over Japan, a monk. In 562 A. D., he brought 160 volumes of medicial books such as Mingtan Illustration, Systematic Classic of Acupuncture, etc., went eastword. The Japanese

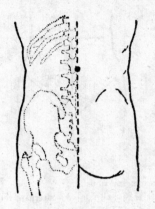

Fig 159

called him "The Wu person Zicong", he was the important person who had made contribution to the exchange between Chinese and Japanese culture during early period.

Zigong 子宫 [zǐ gōng] 1. The uterus; 2. Referring to Zigong point.

Zigong point 子宫穴 [zǐ gōng xué] An extra point. Location: 9 cm lateral to Zhongji (CV 3), 1.2 dm below the umbilicus. Indications: Prolapse of uterus, irregular menstruation, dysmenorrhea, sterility, anexitis, pelvic inflammation, systitis, pyelonephritis, testitis, appendicitis. Puncture: 3—5 cm perpendicularly. Moxibustion: 3—7 moxa cones or 5—15 minutes with warming mo-xibustion. (Fig 160)

Zigong (CV 19) 紫宫 [zǐ gōng] A CV point. Location: At the thoracic midline, at the level with the 2nd intercostal space. Regional anatomy: There is the anteriorly perforating branch of the medial mammary artery and vein. The anterior cutaneous branch of the 2nd intercostal nerve is distributed. Indications: Cough, asthmatic breath, fullness in the chest, sore throat, thoracalgia, spitting blood, anoxexia. Puncture: 1—1.5 cm horizontally. Moxibustion: 3—5 moxa cones or 5—10 minutes with

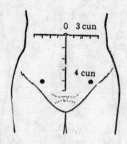

Fig 160

warming moxibustion.

Zimai 资脉 [zī mài] An alternate term for Chimai (TE 18).

Zhuang 壮 [zhuàng] 1. A unit of enumerable times of moxibustion with moxa cone. It is called one *zhuang* that moxibustion is done with one moxa cone; 2. Referring to the moxa cone. E. g., bigger *zhuang* moxibustion refers to administering moxibustion with a bigger moxa cone while small *zhuang* moxibustion refers to administering moxibustion with a small moxa cone.

Zhuiding 椎顶 [zhuī dǐng] An alternate term for Changgu.

Zhubin (KI 9) 筑宾 [zhú bīn] A point of Kedney Meridian of Foot-*shaoyin*, the gap-like point of the connecting the medial ankle and tendon sheath. Regional anatomy: Between the gastrocnemius muscle of the long flexor muscle of toe. There is the posterior tibial artery and vein in the deeper. The medial cutaneous muscle of calf and the medial cutaneous nerve of leg are distributed. The tibial nerve is in the deeper. Indications: Mania, epilepsy, spitting saliva, hernial pain, infantile umbilical hernia, pain in the medial side of the leg. Puncture: 3—4. 5 cm perpendicularly. Moxibustion: 3—5 moxa cones or 5—10 minutes with warming moxibustion.

Zhushi 注市 [zhù shì] 1. An extra point, located obliquely below the edge of the breast, in the 3rd intercostal space, or directly below

the axilla, in the 7th and 8th intercostal space. Indications: Chronic summer fever, pains in the chest and hypochondrium, abdominal pain. Puncture: 1—1. 5 cm minutes with warming moxibustion; 2. I. e., Pangting.

Zhuxia 注夏 [zhù xià] An extra point, located at the palmar side, in the midpoint of the radial edge of the 2nd metarcarpal bone opposite to Hegu(LI 4). Indications: Anorexia in summer, indigestion, vomiting, diarrhea. Puncture: 1—1. 5 cm perpendicularly. Moxibustion: 3—7 moxa cones or 5—15 minutes with warming moxibustion.

Zusuikong 足髓孔 [zú suí kǒng] See Shouzusuikong.

Zulianghuaijian 足两踝尖 [zú liǎng huái jiān] A collective term for Waihuaijian and Neihuaijian.

Zudierzhishang 足第二趾上 [zú dì èr zhǐ shàng] An extra point. "Zudierzhishang is used for water disease (edema), which can be treated by administering moxibustion with the number of *zhuang* equaling to the patient's age." It is located 1 cm above the suture between the 2nd and 3rd toes, Neiting (ST 44) and Xiangu (ST 43).

Zuxin 足心 [zú xīn] An extra point, located on the midline of the sole, at the midpoint between the tip of the 2nd toe and the posterior edge of the heel. Indications: Metrorrhagia, headache, vertigo, epilepsy, pain in the sole, shock. Puncture: 1—1. 5 cm perpendicularly or 5—15 minutes of warming moxibustion.

Zudazhicongmao 足大趾丛毛 [zú dà zhǐ cóng máo] Referring to Dadun (LR 1).

Zushanglian 足上廉 [zú shàng lián] I. e., Shangjuxu (ST 37).

Zuwuli (LR 10) 足五里 [zú wǔ lǐ] A point of Liver Meridian of Foot-*jueyin*. Location: On the medial side of the at the midpoint of the superior edge of symphysis publis, 9 cm directly below. Regional anatomy: At the long and short adductor muscles and the superficial branches of the medial femoral circumflex artery and vein. The genital femoral nerve, the anterial femoral branch and the obturator nerve are distributed. Indications: Distension and pain in the bilateral lower abdomen, cervical scrofula, prolapse of uterine. Puncture: 3—6 cm perpendicularly. Moxibustion: 3—5 moxa cones.

Zuyu 浊浴 [zuó yù] An extra point, located 7.5 cm bilateral to Zhongshu (GV 72). Indications: Gallbladder trouble with fright, full chest and weakness, bitter mouth, anorexia, hysteria. Puncture 1—1.5 cm obliquely. Moxibustion: 3—7 moxa cones or 5—15 minutes with warming moxibustion.

Zusanli (ST 36) 足三里 [zú sān lǐ] A point of Stomach Meridian of Foot-*yangming*, the sea-like (earth) point of the meridian, also termed Xialing, Xialingsanli. Location: 3 cm directly below Dubi(ST 35)at the lateral side of the patellar ligament, approx. one transvese fingwidth lateral to the anterior crease of tibia. Or the patient takes a sitting position, partially flex its knee joint, presses the knee with his or her plam. The point is where the end of the middle finger touches, or four transverse fingerwidths. Regional anatomy: In the anterior muscle of tibia, reaching at the long extensor muscle of toe. There are the anterial tibial artery and vein, the branches of lateral cutaneous nerve of the gastrocnimius and the saphenous nerve. The fibular nerve is in the deep. Indications: Stomachache, vomiting, abdominal distension, borborygmus, infantile malnutrition, diarrhea, constipation, dysentery, infantile malnutrition, cough with profuse sputum, breast carbuncle, dizziness, tinnitus, palpitations, short breath, mania, apoplexy, foot *qi*, edema, pains in the knee and legs, nasal trouble, postpartum anemia, fainting. Puncture: 3—4.5 cm perpendicularly, slightly deviated to tibia. Moxibustion: 5—15 moxa cones or 10—30 minutes with warming moxibustion.

Zuxialian 足下廉 [zú xià lián] I. e., Xiajuxu

(ST 34).

Zuqiaoyin (GB 44) 足窍阴 [zú qiào yīn] A point of Gallbladder Meridian of Foot-*shaoyang*, also termed Qiaoyin, Zuqiaoyin. The well-like (metal) point of the meridian. Location: At the lateral side of the 4th toe approx. 0.3 cm lateral to the corner of the root of the toenail. Regional anatomy: There is the dorsal artery and vein, and the arterial and venous network formed by the plantar artery and vein. The dorsal digital nerve is distributed. Indications: Headache, anxiety, tinnitus, deafness, vertigo, insomnia, ocular pain, hypochondriac pain, feverish sensation in the palms and soles, irregular menstruation, febrile diseases, hgypertension, neuroasthenia. Puncture: 0.3—0.6 cm obliquely or prick to cause little bleeding. Moxibustion: 1—3 moxa cones or 3—5 minutes with warming moxibustion.

Zuqiao 足窍 [zú qiào] An alternate term for Yangjiao (GB 35).

Zutonggu (BL 66) 足通谷 [zú tōng gǔ] A point originally called Tonggu, pertaining to Gallbladder Meridian of Foot-*taiyang*, the spring-like (water) point of the meridian. Location: At the edge of the lateral side of foot. In the depression in front of the 5th metatarsal phalangeal joint. Regional anatomy: There is the planter digital artery and vein. The proper planter digital nerve and the dorsal lateral cutaneous nerve of foot are distributed. Indications: Headache, vertigo, stiff nape, mania, epistaxis, indigestion, full chest, asthmatic breath, hernia. Puncture: 1—1.5 cm perpendicularly. Moxibustion: 3—5 moxa cones or 5—10 minutes with warming moxibustion.

zuan 纂 [zuàn] See chuan (纂).

Zuojinjin 左金津 [zuǒ jīn jīn] See Jinjin (EX-HN 12), Yuye (EX-HN 13).

Zulinqi (GB 41) 足临泣 [zú lín qì] A point of Gallbladder Meridian of Foot-*shaoyang*, also called Linqi. The stream-like point (wood) of the meridian. One of the points of the eight meridians, communicated with Girdle Vessel. Location: At the dorsal foot, in the depression in front of the conjunction between the 4th and 5th metatarsal bones, 4.5 cm above Xiaxi (GB 43), at the end of the toe suture. Regional anatomy: At the lateral side of the extensor muscle of the toe, reaching at the dorsal interrosseous muscle. There is the dorsal arterial and venous network, and the dorsal artery and vein of the 4th metatarsal bone. The branch of the central cutaneous nerve of the dorsal foot is distributed. Indications: Headache, pain in the outer canthus, vertigo, pains in the chest and hypochondriac region, scrofula, swelling and pain in the dorsal foot, breast carbuncle, malaria, apoplexy and paraplegia. Puncture: 1—1.5 cm perpendicularly. Moxibustion: 1—3 moxa cones or 5—10 minutes with warming moxibustion.

APPENDIX

1. Table 1: A Brief Chinese Chronology

夏 Xià Dynasty		About 21st—16th centuries B. C.
商 Shāng Dynasty		About 16th—11th centuries B. C.
周 Zhōu Dynasty	西 周 Western Zhōu Dynasty	About 11th century to 771 B. C.
	东 周 Eastern Zhōu Dynasty 春 秋 Spring and Autumn Periods 战 国 Warring States	770—256 B. C 722—481 B. C. 475—221 B. C.
秦 Qín Dynasty		221—206 B. C.
汉 Hàn Dynasty	西 汉 Western Hàn	206 B. C.—24 A. D.
	东 汉 Eastern Hàn	25—220
三 国 Three Kingdoms	魏 Wèi	220—265
	蜀 汉 Shú Hàn	221—263
	吴 Wú	222—280
西 晋 Western Jìn Dynasty		265—316
东 晋 Eastern Jìn Dynasty		317—420
南 北 朝 Northern and Southern Dynasties	南 朝 Southern Dynasties	宋 Sòng	420—479
		齐 Qí	479—502
		梁 Liáng	502—557
		陈 Chén	557—589
	北 朝 Northern Dynasties	北 魏 Northern Wèi	386—534
		东 魏 Eastern Wei	534—550

Continued

	北 齐 Northern Qí	550—577
	西 魏 Western Wèi	535—557
	北 周 Northern Zhōu	557—581
隋 Suí Dynasty		581—618
唐 Táng Dynasty		618—907
五 代 Five Dynasties	后 梁 Later Liáng	907—923
	后 唐 Later Táng	923—936
	后 晋 Later Jìn	936—946
	后 汉 Later Hàn	947—950
	后 周 Later Zhōu	951—960
宋 Sòng Dynasty	北 宋 Northern Sòng Dynasty	960—1127
	南 宋 Southern Sòng Dynasty	1127—1279
辽 Liáo Dynasty		916—1125
金 Jīn Dynasty		1115—1234
元 Yuán Dynasty		1271—1368
明 Míng Dynasty		1368—1644
清 Qīng Dynasty		1644—1911
中 华 民 国 Republic of China		1911—1949
中 华 人 民 共 和 国 People's Republic of China		1949—

2. Table 2: The Heavenly Stems and Earthly Branches

The Heavenly Stems

甲 (jiǎ) the first of the ten Heavenly Stems
乙 (yǐ) the second of the ten Heavenly Stems
丙 (bǐng) the third of the ten Heavenly Stems
丁 (dīng) the fourth of the ten Heavenly Stems
戊 (wù) the fifth of the ten Heavenly Stems
己 (jǐ) the sixth of the ten Heavenly Stems
庚 (gēng) the seventh of the ten Heavenly Stems
辛 (xīn) the eighth of the ten Heavenly Stems
壬 (rén) the ninth of the ten Heavenly Stems
癸 (guǐ) the last of the ten Heavenly Stems

The Earthly Branches

子 (zǐ) the first of the twelve Earthly Branches
丑 (chǒu) the second of the twelve Earthly Branches
寅 (yín) the third of the twelve Earthly Branches
卯 (mǎo) the fourth of the twelve Earthly Branches
辰 (chén) the fifth of the twelve Earthly Branches
巳 (sì) (the sixth of the twelve Earthly Branches
午 (wǔ) the seventh of the twelve Earthly Branches
未 (wèi) the eighth of the twelve Earthly Branches
申 (shēn) the ninth of the twelve Earthly Branches
酉 (yǒu) the tenth of the twelve Earthly Branches
戌 (xū) the eleventh of the twelve Earthly Branches
亥 (hài) the last of the twelve Earthly Branches

3. Table 3: The Twenty-Four Solar Terms

Spring	the Beginning of Spring (1st solar term)	Rain Water (2nd solar term)
	the Waking of Insects (3rd solar term)	the Spring Equinox (4th solar term)
	Pure Brightness (5th solar term)	Grain Rain (6th solar term)
Summer	the Beginning of Summer (7th solar term)	Grain Full (8th solar term)
	Grain in Ear (9th solar term)	the Summer Solstice (10th solar term)
	Slight Heat (11th solar term)	Great Heat (12th solar term)
Autumn	the Beginning of Autumn (13th solar term)	the limit of Heat (14th solar term)
	White Dew (15th solar term)	the Autumnal Eqninox (16th solar term)
	Cold Dew (17th solar term)	Frost's Descent (18th solar term)
Winter	the Beginning of Winter (19th solar term)	Slight snow (20th solar term)
	Great Snow (21st solar term	the Winter Solstice (22nd solar term)
	Slight Cold (23rd solar term	Great Cold (24th solar term)

4. Table 4：Sixty Pairs Of Heavenly-Stem-Earthly-Branch-Match

1	甲子	Jiazi	31	甲午	Jiawu
2	乙丑	Yichou	32	乙未	Yiwei
3	丙寅	Bingyin	33	丙申	Bingshen
4	丁卯	Dingmao	34	丁酉	Dinghai
5	戊辰	Wuchen	35	戊戌	Wuxu
6	己巳	Jisi	36	己亥	Jihai
7	庚午	Gengwu	37	庚子	Gengzi
8	辛未	Xinwei	38	辛丑	Xinchou
9	壬申	Renshen	39	壬寅	Renyin
10	癸酉	Guiyou	40	癸卯	Guimao
11	甲戌	Jiaxu	41	甲辰	Jiachen
12	乙亥	Yihai	42	乙巳	Yisi
13	丙子	Bingzi	43	丙午	Bingwu
14	丁丑	Dingchou	44	丁未	Dingwei
15	戊寅	Wuyin	45	戊申	Wushen
16	己卯	Jimao	46	己酉	Jiyou
17	庚辰	Gengchen	47	庚戌	Gengxu
18	辛巳	Xinsi	48	辛亥	Xinhai
19	壬午	Renwu	49	壬子	Renzi
20	癸未	Guiwei	50	癸丑	Guichou
21	甲申	Jiashen	51	甲寅	Jiayin
22	乙酉	Yiyou	52	乙卯	Yimao
23	丙戌	Bingxu	53	丙辰	Bingchen
24	丁亥	Dinghai	54	丁巳	Dingsi
25	戊子	Wuzi	55	戊午	Wuwu
26	己丑	Jichou	56	己未	Jiwei
27	庚寅	Gengyin	57	庚申	Gengshen
28	辛卯	Xinmao	58	辛酉	Xinyou
29	壬辰	Renchen	59	壬戌	Renxu
30	癸巳	Guisi	60	癸亥	Guihai

5. Table 5: International Standardized Nomenclature of Acupuncture Points

Shǒutàiyin Fèijing	Lung Meridian	LU
Shǒuyángming Dàchangjing	Large Intestine Meridian	LI
Zúyángming Wèijīng	Stomach Meridian	ST
Zútàiyin Píjīng	Spleen Meridian	SP
Shǒushàoyīn Xīniīng	Heart Meridian	HT
Shǒutàiyáng Xiǎochángjīng	Small Intestine Meridian	SI
Zútàiyang Pángguāngjing	Bladder Meridian	BL
Zúshàoyīn Shènjīng	Kidney Meridian	KI
Shǒujuéyīn Xīnbāojing	Pericardium Meridian	PC
Shóushàoyáng Sánjiaojing	Triple Energizer Meridian	TE
Zúshàoyáng Dánjing	Gallbladder Meridian	GB
Zújuéyīn Gānjing	Liver Meridian	LR
Dūmài	Governor Vessel	GV
Rènmài	Conception	CV

Lung Meridian, LU.
shǒutàiyīn fèijīng xué

中府	Zhōngfǔ	LU1	列缺	Lièquě	LU7
云门	Yúnmén	LU2	经渠	Jīngqú	LU8
天府	Tianfǔ	LU3	太渊	Tàiyuǎn	LU9
侠白	Xiábái	LU4	鱼际	Yújì	LU10
尺泽	Chīzé	LU5	少商	Shàoshāng	LU11
孔最	Kǒngzuì	LU6			

Large Intestine Meridian, LI.
shǒuyángmīng dàchángjīng xué

商阳	Shangyáng	LI 1	曲池	Quchi	LI 11
二间	Erjian	LI 2	肘髎	Zhǒuliáo	LI 12
三间	Sanjiān	LI 3	手五里	Shǒuwǔlī	LI 13
合谷	Hégǔ	LI 4	臂臑	Bìnào	LI 14
阳溪	Yángxi	LI 5	肩髃	Jiānyù	LI 15
偏历	Pianlì	LI 6	巨骨	Jùgǔ	LI 16
温溜	Wēnliu	LI 7	天鼎	Tiandīng	LI 17
下廉	Xiàlián	LI 8	扶突	Fútū	LI 18
上廉	Shànglián	LI 9	口禾髎	Kǒuhéliáo	LI 19
手三里	Shǒusanli	LI 10	迎香	Yingxiang	LI 20

Stomach Meridian, ST.
zúyángmīng wèijīng xué

承泣	Chéngqì	ST1	滑肉门	Huáròumén	ST24
四白	Sibái	ST2	天枢	Tianshù	ST25
巨髎	Jùliáo	ST3	外陵	Wàiling	ST26
地仓	Dicang	ST4	大巨	Dàjù	ST27
大迎	Dàyuing	ST5	水道	Shuǐdào	ST28

continued

颊车	Jiáche	ST6	归来	Guilái	ST29
下关	Xiàguan	ST7	气冲	Qìchong	ST30
头维	Tóuwéi	ST8	髀关	Bìguan	ST31
人迎	Rénying	ST9	伏兔	Fútù	ST32
水突	Shuǐtū	ST10	阴市	Yīnshì	ST33
气舍	Qìshe	ST11	梁丘	Liángqiú	ST34
缺盆	Quēpen	ST12	犊鼻	Dúbí	ST35
气户	Qìhù	ST13	足三里	Zúsānlǐ	ST36
库房	Kùfáng	ST14	上巨虚	Shàngjùxū	ST37
屋翳	Wūyì	ST15	条口	Tiáokǒu	ST38
膺窗	Yīngchuáng	ST16	下巨虚	Xiàjùxū	ST39
乳中	Rǔzhōng	ST17	丰隆	Fēnglóng	ST40
乳根	Rǔgēn	ST18	解溪	Jiěxi	ST41
不容	Bùróng	ST19	冲阳	Chōngyáng	ST42
承满	Chéngmǎn	ST20	陷谷	Xiàngǔ	ST43
梁门	Liangmén	ST21	内庭	Nèitíng	ST44
关门	Guānmén	ST22	厉兑	Liduì	ST45
太乙	Tàiyǐ	ST23			

Spleen Meridian，SP.
zútàiyīn píjīng xué

隐白	Yǐnbái	SP1	冲门	Chōngmén	SP12
大都	Dàdū	SP2	府舍	Fūshè	SP13
太白	Tàibái	SP3	腹结	Fùjié	SP14
公孙	Gōngsūn	SP4	大横	Dàhéng	SP15
商丘	Shāngqiū	SP5	腹哀	Fù' āi	SP16
三阴交	Sānyīnjiāo	SP6	食窦	Shídòu	SP17
漏谷	Lòugǔ	SP7	天溪	Tiānxī	SP18
地机	Dìjī	SP8	胸乡	Xiōngxiāng	SP19
阴陵泉	Yīnlíngquán	SP9	周荣	Zhōuróng	SP20
血海	Xuèhái	SP10	大包	Dàbāo	SP21
箕门	Jīmén	SP11			

Heart Meridian，HT.
shǒushàoyīn xīnjīng xué

极泉	Jíquán	HT1	阴郄	Yīnxì	HT6
青灵	Qīnglíng	HT2	神门	Shénmén	HT7
少海	Shàohǎi	HT3	少府	Shàofǔ	HT8
灵道	Língdào	HT4	少冲	Shaochōng	HT9
通里	Tōngli	HT5			

Liver Meridian，LR.
zújué yīn gānjīng xué

大敦	Dàdūn	LR1	曲泉	Qūquán		LR8
行间	Xíngjiān	LR2	阴包	Yīnbao		LR9
太冲	Tàichōng	LR3	足五里	Zúwǔlǐ		LR10
中封	Zhōngfēng	LR4	阴廉	Yīnlián		LR11
蠡沟	Lígōu	LR5	急脉	Jímài		LR12
中都	Zhōngdū	LR6	章门	Zhāngmén		LR13
膝关	Xīguān	LR7	期门	Qīmén		LR14

Governor Vessel，GV.
dūmài xué

长强	Chángqiáng	GV1	哑门	Yàmén	GV15
腰俞	Yāoshū	GV2	风府	Fēngfǔ	GV16
腰阳关	Yāoyángguān	GV3	脑户	Nǎohù	GV17
命门	Mìngmén	GV4	强间	Qiángjiān	GV18
悬枢	Xuánshū	GV5	后顶	Hòudǐng	GV19
脊中	Jǐzhōng	GV6	百会	Bǎihuì	GV20
中枢	Zhōngshū	GV7	前顶	Qiándǐng	GV21
筋缩	Jīnsuō	GV8	囟会	Xìnhuì	GV22
至阳	Zhìyáng	GV9	上星	Shàngxīng	GV23
灵台	Língtái	GV10	神庭	Shéntíng	GV24
神道	Shéndào	GV11	素髎	Sùliáo	GV25
身柱	Shēnzhù	GV12	水沟	Shuǐgōu	GV26
陶道	Táodào	GV13	兑端	Duìduàn	GV27
大椎	Dàzhuī	GV14	龈交	Yínjiāo	GV28

Conception Vessel，CV.
rènmài xué

会阴	Huìyīn	CV1	上脘	Shàngwǎn	CV13
曲骨	Qūgǔ	CV2	巨阙	Jùquè	CV14
中极	Zhōngjí	CV3	鸠尾	Jiūwěi	CV15
关元	Guānyuán	CV4	中庭	Zhōngtíng	CV16
石门	Shímén	CV5	膻中	Dànzhōng	CV17
气海	Qìhǎi	CV6	玉堂	Yùtáng	CV18
阴交	Yīnjiāo	CV7	紫宫	Zǐgōng	CV19
神阙	Shénquè	CV8	华盖	Huágài	CV20
水分	Shuǐfēn	CV9	璇玑	Xuánjī	CV21
下脘	Xiàwǎn	CV10	天突	Tiāntū	CV22
建里	Jiànlǐ	CV11	廉泉	Liánquàn	CV23
中脘	Zhōngwǎn	CV12	承浆	Chéngjiāng	CV24

325

Triple Energizer Meridian, TE.
shǒushàoyáng sānjiāo jīng xué

关冲	Guānchōng	TE1	臑会	Nàohuì	TE13
液门	Yèmén	TE2	肩髎	Jiānliáo	TE14
中渚	Zhōngzhǔ	TE3	天髎	Tiānliáo	TE15
阳池	Yángchí	TE4	天牖	Tiānyǒu	TE16
外关	Wàiguān	TE5	翳风	Yìfēng	TE17
支沟	Zhīgōu	TE6	瘈脉	Chìmài（Qìmài）	TE18
会宗	Huìzōng	TE7	颅息	Lúxī	TE19
三阳络	Sānyángluò	TE8	角孙	jiǎosūn	TE20
四渎	Sìdú	TE9	耳门	ěrmén	TE21
天井	Tiānjǐng	TE10	耳和髎	ěrhéliáo	TE22
清冷渊	Qīnglèngyuān	TE11	丝竹空	Sīzhúkōng	TE23
消泺	Xiāoluò	TE12			

Gallbladder Meridian, GB.
zúshàoyáng dǎnjīng xué

瞳子髎	Tóngzǐliáo	GB1	辄筋	Zhéjīn	GB23
听会	Tīnghuì	GB2	日月	Rìyuè	GB24
上关	Shàngguān	GB3	京门	Jīngmén	GB25
颔厌	Hànyàn	GB4	带脉	Dàimài	GB26
悬颅	Xuánlú	GB5	五枢	Wǔshū	GB27
悬厘	Xuánlí	GB6	维道	Wéidào	GB28
曲鬓	Qūbìn	GB7	居髎	Jūliáo	GB29
率谷	Shuàigū	GB8	环跳	Huántiào	GB30
天冲	Tiānchōng	GB9	风市	Fēngshì	GB31
浮白	Fúbái	GB10	中渎	Zhōngdù	GB32
头窍阴	Tóuqiàoyīn	GB11	膝阳关	Xīyángguān	GB33
完骨	Wángǔ	GB12	阳陵泉	Yánglíngquán	GB34
本神	Běnshén	GB13	阳交	Yángjiāo	GB35
阳白	Yángbái	GB14	外丘	Wàiqiū	GB36
头临泣	Tóulínqì	GB15	光明	Guāngmíng	GB37
目窗	Mùchuāng	GB16	阳辅	Yángfǔ	GB38
正营	Zhèngyíng	GB17	悬钟	Xuánzhōng	GB39
承灵	Chénglíng	GB18	丘墟	Qiūxū	GB40
脑空	Nǎokōng	GB19	足临泣	Zúlínqì	GB41
风池	Fēngchí	GB20	地五会	Dìwǔhuì	GB42
肩井	Jiānjǐng	GB21	侠溪	Xiáxī	GB43
渊腋	Yuānyè	GB22	足窍阴	Zúqiàoyin	GB44

continued

肾俞	Shènshù	BL23	承山	Chéngshān	BL57
气海俞	Qìhǎishū	BL24	飞扬	Fēiyáng	BL58
大肠俞	Dàchángshū	BL25	跗阳	Fūyáng	BL59
关元俞	Guānyuánshú	BL26	昆仑	Kūnlún	BL60
小肠俞	Xiǎochángshū	BL27	仆参	Púcán (Púshēn)	BL61
膀胱俞	Pángguāngshú	BL28	申脉	Shènmài	BL62
中膂俞	Zhōnglūshū	BL29	金门	Jīnmén	BL63
白环俞	Báihuànshú	BL30	京骨	Jīnggǔ	BL64
上髎	Shàngliáo	BL31	束骨	Shùgù	BL65
次髎	Cìliào	BL32	足通谷	Zútōnggǔ	BL66
中髎	Zhōngliào	BL33	至阴	Zhìyīn	BL67
下髎	Xiàliáo	BL34			

Kidney Meridian, KI.
zúshàoyīn shènjīng xué

涌泉	Yōngquán	KI1	中注	Zhōngzhù	KI15
然谷	Rángǔ	KI2	肓俞	Huāngshū	KI16
太溪	Tàixī	KI3	商曲	Shānqǔ	KI17
大钟	Dàzhōng	KI4	石关	Shíguān	KI18
水泉	Shuǐquán	KI5	阴都	Yīndū	KI19
照海	Zhàohǎi	KI6	腹通谷	Fùdōnggǔ	KI20
复溜	Fùliū	KI7	幽门	Yòumén	KI21
交信	Jiáoxin	KI8	步廊	Bùláng	KI22
筑宾	Zhùbīn	KI9	神封	Shénfēng	KI23
阴谷	Yīngù	KI10	灵墟	Língxū	KI24
横骨	Hénggǔ	KI11	神藏	Shéncáng	KI25
大赫	Dàhè	KI12	彧中	Yùzhōng	KI26
气穴	Qìxué	KI13	俞府	Shūfǔ	KI27
四满	Sīmǎn	KI14			

Pericardium Meridian, PC.
shǒujuéyīn xīnbāojīng xué

天池	Tiānchi	PC1	内关	Nèiguān	PC6
天泉	Tiānquán	PC2	大陵	Dàiíng	PC7
曲泽	Qūzé	PC3	劳宫	Láogōng	PC8
郄门	Xìmén	PC4	中冲	Zhōngchōng	PC9
间使	Jiānshǐ	PC5			

Small Intestine Meridian，SI.
shǒutàiyáng xiǎochángjīng xué

少泽	Shàozé	SI1	天宗	·Tiānzōng	SI11
前谷	Qiángú	SI2	秉风	Bǐngféng	SI12
后溪	Hòuxī	SI3	曲垣	Qūyuán	SI13
腕骨	Wàngǔ	SI4	肩外俞	Jiānwàishù	SI14
阳谷	Yánggǔ	SI5	肩中俞	Jiānzhōngshū	SI15
养老	Yánglǎo	SI6	天窗	Tiānchuāng	SI16
支正	Zhīzhèng	SI7	天容	Tiānróng	SI17
小海	Xiǎohǎi	SI8	颧髎	Quánliáo	SI18
肩贞	Jiānzhēn	SI9	听宫	Tīnggōng	SI19
臑俞	Nàoshū	SI10			

Bladder meridian，BL.
zútàiyáng pángguāngjīng xué

睛明	Jīngmíng	BL1	会阳	Huìyáng	BL35
攒竹	Cuánzhū（Zànzhú）	BL2	承扶	Chéngfú	BL36
眉冲	Méichōng	BL3	殷门	Yīnmén	BL37
曲差	Qūchā（Qūchāi）	BL4	浮郄	Fúxì	BL38
五处	Wǔchù	BL5	委阳	Wěiyáng	BL39
承光	Chéngguāng	BL6	委中	Wěizhōng	BL40
通天	Tōngtiān	BL7	附分	Fùfēn	BL41
络却	Luòquè	BL8	魄户	Pòhù	BL42
玉枕	Yùzhěn	BL9	膏肓	Gāohuāng	BL43
天柱.	Tiānzhù	BL10	神堂	Shéntáng	BL44
大柱	Dàzhù	BL11	譩譆	Yìxī	BL45
风门	Fēngmén	BL12	膈关	Géguān	BL46
肺俞	Feishū	BL13	魂门	Húnmén	BL47
厥阴俞	Juèyīnshú	BL14	阳纲	Yánggāng	BL48
心俞	Xīnshú	BL15	意舍	Yìshè	BL49
督俞	Dūshú	BL16	胃仓	Wèicāng	BL50
膈俞	Géshù	BL17	肓门	Huāngmén	BL51
肝俞	Gǎnshú	BL18	志室	Zhìshì	BL52
胆俞	Dǎnshū	BL19	胞肓	Bāohuāng	BL53
脾俞	Píshú	BL20	秩边	Zhìbiān	BL54
胃俞	Wèishù	BL21	合阳	Héyáng	BL55
三焦俞	Sānjiāoshù	BL22	承筋	Chěngjīn	BL56

INDEX FOR
CHINESE PINYIN ENTRIES

H

R

W

Y

INDEX FOR ENGLISH ENTRIES

针灸学辞典(英文版)

主　　编:帅学忠　　程志敏

　　　　※

责任编辑:王一方　陈　刚
出　版　者:湖南科学技术出版社
印　刷　者:湖南省新华印刷二厂
发　行　者:中国国际图书贸易总公司
　　　　　(中国北京车公庄西路 35 号)
北京邮政信箱第 399 号　邮政编码 100044
(英文版)1997 年(大 32 开)第 1 版第 1 次印刷
ISBN 7—5357—2046—3/R · 385
05500
14-E-3166S